ARTIFICIAL INTELLIGENCE, MACHINE LEARNING, AND MENTAL HEALTH IN PANDEMICS

ARTIFICIAL INTELLIGENCE, MACHINE LEARNING, AND MENTAL HEALTH IN PANDEMICS

A COMPUTATIONAL APPROACH

Edited by

SHIKHA JAIN
Assistant Professor, Jaypee Institute of Information Technology Noida, India

KAVITA PANDEY
Assistant Professor, Jaypee Institute of Information Technology Noida, India

PRINCI JAIN
Associate Professor, Atal Bihari Vajpayee Institute of Medical Sciences (ABVIMS), New Delhi, India
Dr. Ram Manohar Lohia Hospital, New Delhi, India

KAH PHOOI SENG
Professor, Xian Jiaotong Liverpool University, Suzhou, China
Adjunct Professor, Queensland University of Technology, Brisbane, Australia

ELSEVIER

ACADEMIC PRESS
An imprint of Elsevier

Academic Press is an imprint of Elsevier
125 London Wall, London EC2Y 5AS, United Kingdom
525 B Street, Suite 1650, San Diego, CA 92101, United States
50 Hampshire Street, 5th Floor, Cambridge, MA 02139, United States
The Boulevard, Langford Lane, Kidlington, Oxford OX5 1GB, United Kingdom

ISBN: 978-0-323-91196-2

For information on all Academic Press publications visit our website at https://www.elsevier.com/books-and-journals

Publisher: Nikki Levy
Acquisitions Editor: Joslyn Chaiprasert-Paguio
Editorial Project Manager: Maria Elaine D. Desamero
Production Project Manager: Selvaraj Raviraj
Cover Designer: Matt Limbert

Typeset by TNQ Technologies

Contents

Contributors

Shriyansh Agrawal
Department of Computer Science & Engineering and Information Technology, Jaypee Institute of Information Technology, Noida, Uttar Pradesh, India

C. Akila
Department of Computer Science and Engineering Anna University Regional Campus, Tirunelveli, Tamilnadu, India

Rashid Ali
Department of Computer Engineering, Aligarh Muslim University, Aligarh, Uttar Pradesh, India

Vandana Bhattacharjee
Department of Computer Science and Engineering, Birla Institute of Technology, Mesra, Ranchi, India

Sankalp Singh Bisht
Department of Computer Science & Engineering and Information Technology, Jaypee Institute of Information Technology, Noida, Uttar Pradesh, India

Priyanka Chawla
Lovely Professional University, Jalandhar, Punjab, India

Meher Chopra
Amity University, Noida, Uttar Pradesh, India

Varun Dutt
Applied Cognitive Science Lab, Indian Institute of Technology Mandi, Mandi, Himachal Pradesh, India

Chirantan Ganguly
Institute of Radio Physics and Electronics, University of Calcutta, Kolkata, West Bengal, India

Arshpreet Singh Guglani
Department of Computer Science & Engineering and Information Technology, Jaypee Institute of Information Technology, Noida, Uttar Pradesh, India

Sarishty Gupta
Department of Computer Science & Engineering and Information Technology, Jaypee Institute of Information Technology, Noida, Uttar Pradesh, India

Anil Kumar Gupta
Centre for Development of Advanced Computing (C-DAC), Pune, Maharashtra, India

Vaibhav Gupta
Department of Computer Science & Engineering and Information Technology, Jaypee Institute of Information Technology, Noida, Uttar Pradesh, India

Roshan Jahan
Computer Science and Engineering, Integral University, Lucknow, Uttar Pradesh, India

Megha jain
JSS Academy of Technical Education, Noida, UP, India

Saurabh Jain
Department of Systemics, School of Computer Science, University of Petroleum and Energy Studies, Dehradun, Uttarakhand, India

Shikha Jain
Department of Computer Science & Engineering and Information Technology, Jaypee Institute of Information Technology, Noida, Uttar Pradesh, India

Veenus Jain
Amity University, Noida, Uttar Pradesh, India

Keshav Kaushik
Department of Systemics, School of Computer Science, University of Petroleum and Energy Studies, Dehradun, Uttarakhand, India

V. Kavitha
Department of Computer Science and Engineering University College of Engineering, Kanchipuram, Tamilnadu, India

Adarsh Kumar
Department of Systemics, School of Computer Science, University of Petroleum and Energy Studies, Dehradun, Uttarakhand, India

Aparajita Nanda
Department of Computer Science & Engineering and Information Technology, Jaypee Institute of Information Technology, Noida, Uttar Pradesh, India

Bharti Nanta
Applied Cognitive Science Lab, Indian Institute of Technology Mandi, Mandi, Himachal Pradesh, India

Sagnik Nayak
Institute of Radio Physics and Electronics, University of Calcutta, Kolkata, West Bengal, India

Dhiraj Pandey
JSS Academy of Technical Education, Noida, UP, India

Kavita Pandey
Department of Computer Science & Engineering and Information Technology, Jaypee Institute of Information Technology, Noida, Uttar Pradesh, India

Akhila Sahiti Racherla
Department of Computer Science and Engineering, Birla Institute of Technology, Mesra, Ranchi, India

Tara Rawat
Department of Computer Science & Engineering and Information Technology, Jaypee Institute of Information Technology, Noida, Uttar Pradesh, India

Raj Sahu
Department of Computer Science and Engineering, Birla Institute of Technology, Mesra, Ranchi, India

Herumb Shandilya
Department of Computer Science & Engineering and Information Technology, Jaypee Institute of Information Technology, Noida, Uttar Pradesh, India

Kewal Krishna Sharma
Sanskriti University, Mathura, UP, India

Neha Sharma
Indian Institute of Information Technology Una, Una, Himachal Pradesh, India

Senu Mary Skariah
Amity University, Noida, Uttar Pradesh, India

Rishik Sood
Department of Computer Science & Engineering and Information Technology, Jaypee Institute of Information Technology, Noida, Uttar Pradesh, India

Degala Sriram
Department of Computer Science & Engineering and Information Technology, Jaypee Institute of Information Technology, Noida, Uttar Pradesh, India

Reno Ardian Syaputra
Department of Computer Engineering, Aligarh Muslim University, Aligarh, Uttar Pradesh, India

Manish Madhav Tripathi
Computer Science and Engineering, Integral University, Lucknow, Uttar Pradesh, India

Sonal Tuteja
Department of Computer Science & Engineering and Information Technology, Jaypee Institute of Information Technology, Noida, Uttar Pradesh, India

Shashank Uttrani
Applied Cognitive Science Lab, Indian Institute of Technology Mandi, Mandi, Himachal Pradesh, India

Hrishav Varma
Department of Computer Science & Engineering and Information Technology, Jaypee Institute of Information Technology, Noida, Uttar Pradesh, India

Author biographies

Shriyansh Agrawal is an undergraduate student of Bachelor's in Technology in Computer Science Engineering at Jaypee Institute of Information Technology, Noida, India. He is trained in the field of web development, data science, and machine learning. He has developed a project to find out which employee is most likely to leave and developed an E-commerce site for an edible oil food company.

C. Akila received her B.E. degree in Computer Science and Engineering in 2004 from MS University and M.E degree in Computer Science and Engineering in 2008 from Anna University Chennai. She received her Ph.D. degree in 2017 in the Faculty of Information and Communication Engineering. Right from 2009, she is in the Department of Computer Science & Engineering under various designations. Presently, she is working as Assistant Professor in the Department of CSE at Anna University Regional Campus-Tirunelveli. She has 15 years of experience in teaching. Currently, four research scholars are pursuing Ph.D. under her guidance. Her research interests are Image Processing, pattern Recognition, and Soft Computing. She has published many papers in Conference, National, and International journal in areas such as Image Processing and Soft Computing. She is a lifetime member of ISTE and IE.

Rashid Ali obtained his B.Tech. and M.Tech. from A.M.U. Aligarh, India, in 1999 and 2001 respectively. He obtained his Ph.D. in Computer Engineering in February 2010 from A.M.U. Aligarh. His Ph.D. work was on performance evaluation of Web Search Engines. He has authored about 125 papers in various International Journals and International conference proceedings. He has presented papers in many International conferences and has also chaired sessions in few International conferences. He has reviewed articles for some of the reputed International Journals and International conference proceedings. He has supervised 20 M.Tech Dissertations and six Ph.D. Thesis. Currently, he is supervising three PhD candidates. His research interests include Web-Searching, Web-Mining, soft computing Techniques (Rough-Set, Artificial Neural Networks, fuzzy logic, etc), Recommender Systems, and Online Social Network Analysis

Vandana Bhattacharjee is working as a Professor and presently Head, in the Department of Computer Science and Engineering, Birla Institute of Technology, Mesra, Ranchi. She completed her B. E. (CSE) in 1989 from

BIT Mesra and her M. Tech and Ph. D in Computer Science from Jawaharlal Nehru University New Delhi in 1991 and 1995, respectively. She has several National and International publications in Journal and Conference Proceedings. She has authored a book on Data Analysis. She is a Life Member of Computer Society of India. Her research areas include Machine Learning and its application to healthcare data, Software Engineering domain, and Image regeneration, to name a few.

Sankalp Singh Bisht is an undergraduate student of Bachelor's in Technology in Computer Science Engineering at Jaypee Institute of Information Technology, Noida, India. He has a keen interest in the field of Data Analytics and creating models that deal with automating mundane tasks with intelligence. He has worked with a Delhi-based startup as a Data Scientist where he has contributed to projects including predictive modelling, machine learning, data management, and data integration. His research interests include data modeling, use of artificial intelligence in social and health-related issues, and cloud migration architecture.

Priyanka Chawla is doctorate from the Thapar University, Patiala, India. She is presently working as Professor in Lovely Professional University, India. Her active research areas include Fog Computing, Cloud computing, Big data analytics, Evolutionary algorithms, and Software engineering. Dr. Chawla is having a rich experience of Industry and Academia of around 19 years. She has more than 50 research publications in reputed Journals and Conferences including ACM, Springer, Elsevier, and several others. She is an editorial member of various reputed International journals. She has delivered Invited Talks in various Conferences, FDPs, and workshops. She is a life member of ISTE and ISCA and is actively involved in various activities of these societies.

Meher Chopra has completed MA History from Amity Institute of Social Sciences, Amity University, Noida, Uttar Pradesh, with Silver Medal. She received her Bachelor's degree in History from Gargi College, University of Delhi as well as one more Bachelor's degree in Education from Amity Institute of Education, Amity University, Noida, Uttar Pradesh, with Bronze Medal. She has been instrumental in organizing and coordinating many events as a student coordinator. Her main research interest lies in Sociocultural History, South East Asian History, and Gender Studies.

Varun Dutt works as an Associate Professor in the School of Computing and Electrical Engineering and School of Humanities and Social Sciences at Indian Institute of Technology Mandi. Dr. Dutt has applied his knowledge and skills in the fields of psychology, public policy, and computer science to explore how humans make decisions on social, managerial, and environmental issues. Dr. Dutt's Ph.D. thesis focused on answering the question: why do we want to defer actions on climate change, and he has investigated the question by applying literature on people's risk-preferences, time-preferences, social-cultural dilemmas, and linear thinking. Dr. Dutt has used lab-based methods involving experiments with human participants and cognitive models to investigate his research questions. Dr. Dutt serves as a senior member of IEEE and as the principal investigator at Applied Cognitive Science (ACS) Lab. He is currently serving as an associate editor of Frontiers in Cognitive Science journal, a review editor of Frontiers in Decision Neuroscience journal, and a member of the editorial board of the International Journal on Cyber Situational Awareness. Dr. Dutt is among the board of governors of RxDataScience Inc., USA and Intiot Services Pvt. Ltd., India. In the recent past, Dr. Dutt served as a special topics editor in Frontiers in Psychology (Cognitive Science) journal for a special issue on "Application of Cognitive Approaches to Cyber Security." He was also a lead author on the IPCC WG III fifth Assessment Report.

Chirantan Ganguly is currently pursuing his Bachelor's in Electronics and Communication Engineering from Institute of Radio Physics and Electronics, University of Calcutta. He was selected as the Head of Code Club of University of Calcutta in the past session for his active involvement. He successfully managed to grow the club by organizing numerous competitions, hackathons, and technical talk shows with industry leaders. Chirantan as a part of the mentors' team of Code Club has tutored his peers on various Machine Learning concepts and helped them execute their projects. He has represented his University in a national robotics competition organized by IIT Bombay and was a finalist there. His research interests include Embedded Systems Design, Biomedical electronics, Robotics, Deep Learning, and 5G technology. He has undertaken a research internship under the guidance of Dr. Anamaria Berea, (George Mason University, USA) and is currently undertaking one under Dr. Anil Gupta at CDAC, Pune.

Anil Kumar Gupta is a Senior Member, IEEE and Senior Member ACM. He has more than 24 years of Industry experience. He received his master's degree from IIT Roorkee, India, which is an Institute of National Importance as declared by the Govt. of India. He also holds a Ph.D. in strategy from west coast University Panama. He has done MBA(HR) from Calorx Teachers University. Dr. Anil is working with CDCAC Pune as Associate Director. His research interests are in HPC, SDN, IOT, 5G, Data Analytics NLP, computer vision, System Software Blockchains, cyber security. He has more than 70 publications and two book chapters in various national/International conferences and journals. He has filed four patents in India, and multiple patents are in various stages of evaluation. He has guided more than 15 Masters' Dissertations. He also has guided 25+ B.Tech students for their projects.

Sarishty Gupta is an Assistant Professor in Department of Computer Science Engineering and Information Technology at Jaypee Institute of Information Technology, Noida. Formerly she worked as Guest Faculty at MNIT, Jaipur, Rajasthan. Her research areas are Software Engineering and Data Science and analysis.

Vaibhav Gupta is an undergraduate student of Bachelor's in Technology in Computer Science Engineering at Jaypee Institute of Information Technology, Noida, India. He has a good amount of experience in Machine Learning and is planning a Minor specialization in the same. His main research interests include Artificial Intelligence and Deep Learning and working on Data-Centric systems, along with the influence of Machine Learning on preexisting methodologies.

Roshan Jahan is an Assistant Professor in Department of Computer Science, Integral University, Lucknow. She is gold medalist in B.Tech and overall topper in master's (M.Tech), she has more than 10 years of Teaching. Mrs. Jahan has Won Best Paper Award for paper presentation in International Conference ACEIT-2016 and ACEIT-2018. Her research area is image processing, machine learning, and expert systems. Three of her projects got selected for DAAD-RISE fellowship program run by Germany. She is currently involved in a project related to implementing sensor networks in forests to save wildlife and also medical imaging to detect tumors and Alzheimer diseases. She has published more than 18 papers in reputed international journals and conferences. She has also attended various seminars organized by professional bodies and industry associations worldwide. Mrs. Roshan, holds professional associations with IEEE, ACM, and ISTE. Mrs. Roshan got invitation from ACM UK chapter to pursue her research in the United Kingdom and supervise undergraduate students in university from September 2019 to September 2020.

Megha Jain is working as Assistant Professor in the Department of Information Technology, of JSS Academy of Technical Education, Noida. She was awarded M.Tech in Computer Science degree in 2012 from MDU, Rohtak. She is a graduate in Information Technology program at the B.M Institute of Technology, MDU, Rohtak, in 2006. She has over 14 years of academic experience and published more than 10 research papers in various national, international conferences, and journals. Articles are published in publications such as Springer, IEEE, IGI global USA, and most of the articles are Scopus indexed. She has contributed as an author in several book chapters in leading international publications.

Saurabh Jain has received a master's degree (M.Tech) in Information Security from MANIT, Bhopal, Madhya Pradesh, India, in 2012. He is pursuing his Ph.D. in CSE from the University of Petroleum and Energy Studies, Dehradun, India. He has worked as an Assistant Professor in the Department of CSE at Oriental College of Technology, Bhopal. In the past, he has worked as HOD, M.Tech Coordinator, and Remote Center Coordinator in the CSE Department at Oriental College of Technology, Bhopal, Madhya Pradesh, India, and currently working as an Assistant Professor in the School of Computer Science at the University of Petroleum and Energy Studies, Dehradun. He has published 30+ International research papers and patents. He has also conducted many International/National Conferences, Workshops, FDPs, and STPs. He was a certified QCSP (Quick Heal Academy Certified Cyber Security Professional) in 2018, and his research interest lies in network security, web security, cryptography, and Blockchain Technology.

Shikha Jain is presently working with Jaypee Institute of Information Technology (JIIT), Noida, India as Assistant Professor. She has more than 18 years of research and academic experience. She has received her Ph.D. in computer science from Jaypee Institute of Information Technology, Noida, India. She has published a number of research papers in the renowned journals and conferences. She was advisory board member of a book entitled "Nature-Inspired Algorithms for Big Data Frameworks," IGI Global. She was a guest editor of a special issue "Advances in Computational Intelligence and its applications" in International Journal of Information Retrieval Research (Publishing phase). She is active reviewer of many International Journals and technical program committee member of various International Conferences. Her research area includes Affective Computing, Emotion Modeling, Cognitive Affective Architectures, Machine Learning, and Soft Computing. She is a senior member of IEEE society.

Veenus Jain is a historian, commenced her career with Galaxy Education System Rajkot, India. She was the Principal, Human Resources Manager and Director (Education), of Global Indian International School, Gandhidham (Gujarat). She joined Amity University as Junior Vice-President and established department of History at Amity University and is currently serving there as Professor of Indian History. She is also serving as an editorial board member of many referred and indexed international and national journals and has authored several books. She has been felicitated with numerous awards and honours such as Gold Medal for her MA Ancient History and M Phil degrees, President Award by the President of India, Outstanding Educator and Scholar Award, and Distinguished Woman Educator and Scholar Award.

Keshav Kaushik is an Assistant Professor in the School of Computer Science at the University of Petroleum and Energy Studies, Dehradun, India. He is pursuing a Ph.D. in Cybersecurity and Forensics. He is an experienced educator with over 7 years of teaching and research experience in Cybersecurity, Digital Forensics, the Internet of Things, and Blockchain Technology. Mr. Kaushik received his B.Tech degree in Computer Science and Engineering from the University Institute of Engineering and Technology, Maharshi Dayanand University, Rohtak. He obtained his M.Tech degree in Information Technology from YMCA University of Science and Technology, Faridabad, Haryana. He has qualified GATE (2012 & 2016). He has published several research papers in International Journals and has presented at reputed International Conferences. He is a Certified Ethical Hacker (CEH) v11, CQI and IRCA Certified ISO/IEC 27,001:2013 Lead Auditor, and Quick Heal Academy certified Cyber Security Professional (QCSP). He acted as a keynote speaker and delivered professional talks on various national and international platforms. He has various international and national patents under his belt.

V. Kavitha obtained her B.E. degree in Computer Science and Engineering in 1996 from MS University and M.E degree in Computer Science and Engineering in 2000 from Madurai Kamaraj University. She is the University Rank Holder in UG and Gold Medallist in PG. She received her Ph.D. degree in Computer Science and Engineering from Anna University, Chennai, in 2009. Right from 1996, she is in the Department of Computer Science & Engineering under various designations. Presently, she is working as Professor in the Department of CSE at University College of Engineering, Kancheepuram, and she has 25 years of overall experience of teaching. Under her guidance, 15 research scholars, full time and part time, have been awarded Ph.D. Currently, four research scholars are pursuing Ph.D. under her guidance. Her research interests are network security, cloud computing, wireless sensor networks, image processing, mobile computing. She has published 100+ papers in national and international journals.

Adarsh Kumar is an Associate Professor in the School of Computer Science with University of Petroleum & Energy Studies, Dehradun, India. He received his master's degree (M. Tech) in Software Engineering from Thapar University, Patiala, Punjab, India, and earned his Ph.D. degree from Jaypee Institute of Information Technology University, Noida, India, followed by Post-Doc from Software Research Institute, Athlone Institute of Technology, Ireland. From 2005 to 2016, he was associated with the Department of Computer Science Engineering & Information Technology, Jaypee Institute of Information Technology, Noida, Uttar Pradesh, India, where he worked as Assistant Professor. His main research interests are cyber security, cryptography, network security, and ad-hoc networks. He has many research papers in reputed journals, conferences, and workshops. He participated in one European Union H2020 sponsored research project, and he is currently executing two research projects sponsored by UPES SEED division and one sponsored by Lancaster University.

Aparajita Nanda received the Ph.D. degree in Computer Science and Engineering from NIT Rourkela, India. She has an experience of 4+ years as an Assistant Professor with the Computer Science Department. She has authored or coauthored in research articles in journals, conferences, reference books, and book chapters. She has worked on a R&D project funded by SERB. Her research focuses on Computer Vision, Data Mining, Machine Learning, and Visual Surveillance.

Bharti Nanta is working as a Project Associate at Indian Institute of Technology Mandi. She has earlier worked as an Assistant Professor in A P Goyal Shimla University, where besides teaching, she has also handled the Unnat Bharat Abhiyan projects. Ms. Nanta has also worked as a Research Assistant at IIT Mandi for a Digital Identity Research Initiative (DIRI)-funded project, which involved Secondary Data Collation, Questionnaire Designing, Primary Data Collection, data Visualisation for Data Analysis using Tableau, and participation in Focus Group Discussions, Conferences.

Sagnik Nayak is currently a student in the third year of B.Tech. in Electronics and Communication Engineering from the Institute of Radio Physics and Electronics, University of Calcutta. In the previous session, he served as a Python Mentor and an Executive Member of CodeClub of the University of Calcutta. He successfully guided the newcomers into understanding Python and applying them in various fields of the industry and played a significant role in the growth of the coding culture in his institution by organizing various competitions and technical talks with the leaders of the industry. Sagnik also tutored his peers into understanding various Machine Learning and Deep Learning concepts and their applications. His research interests include Deep Learning, the Internet of Things, Embedded Systems, Biomedical Electronics, 5G technology, and Robotics. He is currently undertaking a research internship under Dr. Anil Kumar Gupta at CDAC, Pune.

Dhiraj Pandey is currently serving as Associate Professor, Department of Information Technology, JSS Academy of Technical Education, Noida. He has completed B.Tech, M.Tech, and Ph.D. in CSE. He has over 18 years of academic experience and published over 25 research articles in International Journals and Conferences of repute. Articles are published in publications such as Elsevier, Springer, Taylor & Francis, Inderscience, IGI global USA, and most of the articles are SCI/Scopus indexed. He has contributed as an author in several book chapters in leading international publications. He has also been contributing as a reviewer for several international journals of repute and associated with several technical societies of repute such as IEEE (Senior Member), ISTE (Life Member) etc. Currently, he is supervising three candidates for their doctoral research work in the field of natural language processing and deep learning along with handling consultancy with IIT Delhi for election-commission-related prestigious ongoing project as coprincipal investigator.

Kavita Pandey received her B.Tech. in Computer Science and Engineering from M.D. University in 2002 and M.Tech.(CS) from Banasthali Vidyapeeth University in year 2003. She has obtained her Ph.D. (CS) from Jaypee Institute of Information Technology (JIIT), Noida, India, in January, 2017. She is currently working as an Assistant Professor (Senior Grade) in JIIT, Noida. Her research interests include Soft Computing, Machine Learning, Vehicular Ad hoc Networks, Internet of Things, and Optimization Techniques. She has published various papers in International journals and conferences including Wiley, IEEE, Springer, Inderscience, etc. She worked as a guest editor of special issue, "Advances in Computational Intelligence and Applications" in International Journal of Information Retrieval Research (IJIRR), IGI Global, ESCI (Web of Science). She worked as a reviewer in many international journals of renowned publishers including Elsevier, Inderscience, IEEE Access, etc. She is an active TPC member of many conferences such as REDSET, IC3, UPCON, TEAMC, ICTCS, and many more. She is also a senior member of IEEE society.

Tara Rawat is currently pursuing her Ph.D. in the field of Emotion Disorder from Department of Computer Science and Information Technology at Jaypee institute of Information Technology (JIIT), Noida, India. She received her M.E. (Software Systems) from BITS, Pilani. She has more than 10 years of academic experience. She has published research papers in the reputed journals and conferences. Her research interest includes NLP, Affective Computing, Machine Learning, Emotion Mining, and Data Analytics.

Akhila Sahiti Racherla is a postgraduate student at the Department of Computer Science and Engineering in the stream of Information Technology from Birla Institute of Technology, Mesra, Ranchi, Jharkhand. She has been a scholarship holder during her graduation. She has also done various courses and projects related to Machine Learning, Deep Learning. She is an active participant in various online coding sites. Most of her projects are based on exploring deep learning areas and her research interests include Computer Vision, Natural Language Processing, and Machine Learning.

Raj Sahu is an undergraduate student in the Department of Computer Science and Engineering, Birla Institute of Technology, Mesra, Ranchi. He has a passion for coding, and his current area of interest is to explore the emerging areas in machine learning. He is highly interested in various research areas of computer science and would like to pursue higher studies.

Herumb Shandilya is an undergraduate student pursuing Computer Science Engineering from Jaypee Institute of Information Technology, Noida, India. He has done an internship at DRDO in CAIR Labs in 2021 and has been Data Science Intern at CrowdAnalytix in 2021. His domains of interest include Computer Vision, Natural Language Processing, and Robotics.

Kewal Krishna Sharma is currently serving as Associate Professor, Department of Computer Science, Sanskriti University, Mathura. He has completed B.Sc, M.B.A, M.C.A, and Ph.D. in CSE. He has over 30 years of academic and industry experience, two patents, and published over 20 research articles in International Journals and Conferences of repute. He has also been contributing as a reviewer for several international journals of repute and associated with several technical societies of repute such as International Association of Engineers, ISTE (Life Member), etc. Currently, he is supervising six candidates for their doctoral research work and evaluated three Ph.D. theses.

Neha Sharma works as an Assistant Professor in the Department of Computer Science at Indian Institute of Information Technology, Una. She completed her doctorate in the field of computer science under the guidance of Prof. Varun Dutt. Her area of research includes human decision-making, machine learning, and computational modeling of human decisions under risk and uncertain conditions. She was also awarded a TCS research fellowship for her doctoral research.

Arshpreet Singh is an undergraduate student pursuing Computer Science Engineering from Jaypee Institute of Information Technology, Noida, India. He has worked with the Centre for Artificial Intelligence and

Robotics (CAIR) Lab, DRDO, India, as an NLP Research Intern. He's also worked with several other organizations in the domain of Machine Learning and NLP. His research interest includes health-tech and ergonomics and has taken up multiple projects for the same.

Senu Mary Skariah has completed M.A. in History from Amity Institute of Social Sciences, Amity University, Noida, Uttar Pradesh with Gold Medal. She received her Bachelor's degree in History from Jesus Mary College, University of Delhi. She has been instrumental in organizing and coordinating many events as a student coordinator. Her main research interest lies in Sociocultural History, South East Asian History, and Gender Studies.

Rishik Sood is an undergraduate student of Bachelors in Technology in Computer Science Engineering at Jaypee Institute of Information Technology, Noida, India. He is skilled in the field of Data Structures and Algorithms, which can be highlighted by his achievements of becoming Candidate Master and reaching the ICPC Regionals. He is also interested in the field of Machine Learning Problems and has received certifications from Coursera in Machine Learning and Deep Learning.

Degala Sriram is an undergraduate student of Bachelor's in Technology in Computer Science Engineering at Jaypee Institute of Information Technology, Noida, India. He achieved a rank of around 70,000 in JEE mains exam in 2018. He got certified as an intern in Artificial Intelligence (AI) from IBM in 2021. His research interests are in Machine Learning and Artificial Intelligence applications in health care, forensics, security sectors.

Reno Ardian Syaputra obtained his B.Tech. from Universitas Muhammadiyah Magelang, Indonesia, in 2017. He obtained M. Tech in September 2021 from Aligarh Muslim University, India. His M. Tech dissertation was on intelligent techniques for social media data analysis. He has 1 year of work experience as IT support specialist in a private bank Indonesia. His interest includes Web-Mining, Natural Language Processing, and Augmented Reality.

Manish Madhava Tripathi serves as Associate Professor of Computer Science & Engineering at Integral University, Lucknow, Uttar Pradesh. He has two decades of work experience. He functioned briefly as Software Engineer before commencing his stint in Academia. Prior to Integral University, he served at VBS Purvanchal University, Jaunpur. His academic background is Bachelor of Science in 1996 from VBS Purvanchal University with silver medal, Bachelor of Technology in 2001 from U.N.S Institute of Engineering and Technology, Master's in Technology from the former AAI

Deemed University in 2005, Ph.D. in 2018 themed on "Designing a Model to Improve Medical Image Watermarking." He is the senior member of IEEE as well as life member of Computer Society of India. His areas of interest include Digital Image Processing, Pattern Recognition, Machine Learning, etc. He has served as Member, Syllabus Review Committee; Member, Board of Studies as well as member of various other committees. He has published five book chapters, one patent, and more than 35 peer-reviewed journal papers. He has presented myriad conference papers and attended multiple workshops and Quality Improvement Programs. He has himself conducted various workshops and has guided and implement several projects including those on proxy servers and face authentication systems. He is also a Ph.D. research supervisor as well as M.Tech. Dissertation Supervisor.

Sonal Tuteja is an Assistant Professor in Department of Computer Science and Information Technology at Jaypee institute of Information Technology (JIIT), Noida, India. Prior to joining JIIT, she worked as a research fellow at JNU, New Delhi. Her research focuses on Data Mining, Graph Databases, and Graph Applications.

Shashank Uttrani is a research scholar in the School of Computing and Electrical Engineering at Indian Institute of Technology, Mandi. He has worked as a software engineer after graduating as a computer science engineer from Birla Institute of Technology Mesra. Currently, his research focuses on modeling human behaviour using computational and cognitive models to better understand human preference reversals under risky and uncertain situations using instance-based learning theory, quantum decision theory, deep learning, and reinforcement learning.

Hrishav Varma is an undergraduate of Bachelor's in Technology in Computer Science Engineering at Jaypee Institute of Information Technology, Noida, India. He is skilled in statistical data analysis and modeling and experienced in the fields of Computer Vision, Natural Language Processing, and Predictive Modeling using Machine Learning and Deep Learning Techniques with hands-on projects to demonstrate the same.

Editor biographies

Dr. Shikha Jain is presently working with Jaypee Institute of Information Technology (JIIT), NOIDA, INDIA, as Assistant Professor. She has more than 18 years of research and academic experience. She has received her Ph.D. in computer science from Jaypee Institute of Information Technology, Noida, India. She has published a number of research papers in the renowned journals and conferences. She was advisory board member of a book entitled "Nature-Inspired Algorithms for Big Data Frameworks," IGI Global. She was a guest editor of a special issue "Advances in Computational Intelligence and its applications" in International Journal of Information Retrieval Research (Publishing phase). She is active reviewer of many International Journals and technical program committee member of various International Conferences. Her research area includes Affective Computing, Emotion Modelling, Cognitive Affective Architectures, Machine Learning and Soft Computing. She is a senior member of IEEE society.

Dr. Kavita Pandey received her B.Tech in Computer Science and Engineering from M.D. University in 2002, and M.Tech. (CS) from Banasthali Vidyapeeth University in year 2003. She has obtained her Ph.D. (CS) from Jaypee Institute of Information Technology (JIIT), Noida, India, in January, 2017. She is currently working as an Assistant Professor (Senior Grade) in JIIT, Noida. Her research interests include Soft Computing, Machine Learning, Vehicular Ad hoc Networks, Internet of Things, and Optimization Techniques. She has published various papers in International journals and conferences including Wiley, IEEE, Springer, Inderscience, etc. She worked as a guest editor of special issue, "Advances in Computational Intelligence and Applications" in International Journal of Information Retrieval Research (IJIRR), IGI Global, ESCI (Web of Science). She worked as a reviewer in many international journals of renowned publishers including Elsevier, Inderscience, IEEE Access, etc. She is an active TPC member of many conferences such as REDSET, IC3, UPCON, TEAMC, ICTCS, and many more. She is also a senior member of IEEE society.

Dr. Princi Jain is an Associate Professor at Atal Bihari Vajpayee Institute of Medical Sciences (ABVIMS) and Dr. Ram Manohar Lohia Hospital, Delhi, India. She has obtained MD (Internal Medicine) from Vardhman Mahavir Medical College and Safdarjang Hospital, Delhi. She has more than 8 years of academic and research experience. She is an active member of Association of Physicians of India and American College of Physicians. She has published a number of research papers in renowned journals and conferences.

Prof. Kah Phooi Seng is an established senior academic with proven track record of teaching, research, and leadership in Data Science including Machine Learning and Artificial Intelligence (AI), Engineering, Computer Science, and IT disciplines. She has a Ph.D. in AI and Signal Processing from the University of Tasmania, Australia. She has about more than 15 years of substantial academic experience in Australia-based and UK-based universities. Currently, she is the Adjunct Professor in School of Engineering and IT at University of New South Wales (UNSW). Her previous academic experiences include being Professor in Computer Science and Head of Department of Computer Science and Networked Systems at Sunway University (affiliated with Lancaster University, UK). Research-wise, she has a strong record of publications and published over 250 papers in journals and international refereed conferences in the areas of data science/analytics, machine learning, AI and intelligent systems, mobile software development, Big data, IoT and cloud computing, multimodal signal processing, visual information engineering, sensor networks, reconfigurable embedded systems, etc. She has made significant contributions to research in those fields as testified by publications in premier journals such as the IEEE Transactions. More than 50 of her journal papers are Tier One and Two (Q and Q2) papers. Her recent research papers have been published by IEEE Transactions journals with Impact Factors ranging from 2.563 to 7.596. The total count of her citations is about 4500, with h-index of 25 and i10-index of 60 following Google Scholar.

Acknowledgment

First of all, we want to thank the *Almighty*, the *Supreme Power*, whose blessings show us a path and provide strength to proceed ahead. We express our sincere gratitude to all *authors* who contributed their knowledge and time. We would like to thank all the *reviewers* for their valuable comments and time to enrich the content of the book. All this work would not be possible without the consistent support of our *parent organization*, thus sincere thanks go to them as well. We would also like to thank our *family members* for their love, continuous support, and encouragement.

We want to convey our sincere thanks to the *entire production team of Elsevier* without their invaluable support this book would not be possible. Special thanks go to our Editorial Project Manager for providing their time to time guidance and help whenever needed. We would also like to thank our senior acquisitions editor, copyrights coordinator, rights associate, payments information manager, and production manager. At last, we want to thank everyone who contributed in the success of this book with a special quote "Great things can never be achieved by a single person; they are done by a team of people."

Glossary

Artificial Intelligence: There are certain tasks that cannot be performed by machines without providing the human intelligence. To perform these kinds of tasks, machines are provided with an intelligence known as Artificial Intelligence, which is a mimic of human intelligence.

Blockchain: It is a specific kind of database, which takes the information in groups known as blocks. Each block has some storage capacity, when it becomes full; it gets linked with the previous filled blocks of data. Thus, it forms a chain of data, known as blockchain.

Convolution neural network: It is a special kind of feed forward artificial neural network, which is designed to process the structured data such as images. There is a special type of layer known as convolutional layer, which is the power of doing tasks by Convolution Neural Network.

COVID-19: It is a contagious infection spread in humans by the SARS-CoV-2 virus.

Deep Learning: It is a subset of machine learning techniques based on artificial neural networks. Unlike artificial neural networks, it has more number of layers allowing it to analyze massive amount of data.

Depression: It is a major mood disorder in which a person experiences loneliness and sad. This mood disorder affects the daily activities of a human being as well. If it is left untreated for a long time, it becomes a serious medical illness.

GRU: GRU (Gated Recurrent unit) is a type of recurrent neural network in which gates are added to solve the vanishing gradient problem of standard RNN. There are two gates, update and reset gate, which decide what information is to be passed to the output. It is also known as a variant of LSTM.

LSTM: LSTM (Long Short Term Memory networks) is a special type of recurrent neural network, which has the capability to learn the long-term dependencies. It can process the entire sequence of data with the help of three gates input, output, and forget gate.

Machine learning: It is a branch of Artificial Intelligence, which provides the capability to machines to learn from the past data and improve its performance through experience.

Mental health: The term "mental health" reflects the state of human beings that how an individual reacts, thinks, or feels while facing different situations of life. It includes the person emotional and behavioural well-being. The state of mental health affects our social well-being, personal life, and physical health.

Pandemic: When an infectious disease covers a large geographical area and becomes a public health concern, it is defined as a pandemic. Recently, World Health Organization declared COVID-19 as a pandemic as it covers a large population across the continents and took more lives.

Stress: It is an individual body's response while facing any new or unexpected situation. Sometimes, the stress is good, for example, it alerts you to work harder and meet your deadlines. On the other hand, continuous stress makes you feel overwhelmed and sooner it becomes a problem.

Word embedding: Word embedding is a term for word representation used in Natural Language Processing. The syntactic and semantic similarity of the words will be used to represent the words in a numeric vector.

Introduction

Artificial Intelligence (AI) is a field of Computer Science that enables the machine to demonstrate intelligence. It makes the machines smarter and capable to perform tasks, which require human intelligence. Machines leveraged with AI can mimic the human decision-making process.

In 1950, Alan Turing prompted a question "Can machines think?" and offered a test "Turing Test" to distinguish between a computer and a human via conversation. In 1956, John McCarthy formally announced the term "Artificial Intelligence" at a conference at Dartmouth College, in Hanover, New Hampshire. He defined it as "the science and engineering of making intelligent machines."

Over the years, AI has evolved from deductive reasoning to knowledge acquisition to machine learning and deep learning. Deep Learning is a subset of machine learning algorithms. Machine Learning is a powerful tool that allows machines to learn from data while identifying some common patterns. These are the AI-based algorithms that can perform various tasks such as classification, prediction, or clustering and much more. Nowadays, ML and DL algorithms become such a powerful tools that mingled in almost all domains such as networking, psychology, health care, agriculture, security, and many more.

Natural disasters and pandemics have high impact on human toll and economics. However, at the same time, their adverse impact on psychological health of people cannot be denied. Rather, the psychological impact takes longer time to recover and sometimes it becomes worse.

With the increase in number of natural disasters and ongoing pandemic, people are experiencing uncertainty, which leads to fear in their lives. It further raises many psychological health challenges such as stress, anxiety, and many a times, it leads to depression. A mental disorder not only impacts a human but his family also. However, this issue has not been considered seriously in our society and left ignored. Moreover, many countries have very limited resources on mental health services.

The aim of this book is to provide a handy guide to public health authorities, researchers, and health professionals, which details the research findings on psychological health. Moreover, the book discusses AI and ML-based solutions for monitoring, detection, and intervention for mental health at an early stage so that it can be timely cured.

The main challenge faced by the people in today's scenario is the need of one umbrella where they can find all information related to psychological impact of pandemics and natural calamities. This all includes datasets, feature selection, algorithms, and many more. Audience needs to know about the availability of datasets that can be directly or indirectly incorporated in their research.

All the questions such as what are the important features for prediction of useful information about pandemics or what are the new designed algorithms and solutions for a particular kind of scenario will be answered through this handbook. One side of the coin is that year 2020 threatened the whole world but the other side of the coin says this year teaches everyone one way or the other. So, this book provides a platform where researchers, medical practitioners have marked their findings, and the people can refer their experiences.

The proposed book can be of great use as:

1. Innovative healthcare solutions and research can be used as a stepping stone for the advancement of existing healthcare.
2. Machine Learning solutions can help in determining the precautionary measures and in-depth insight into psychological health problems.
3. Data-driven healthcare solutions can easily help in finding the unanswerable questions and help the medical experts to make better decision.
4. Innovative AI solutions and bistatistics computations can strengthen day-to-day medical procedures and decision-making.
5. AI in medicine can decide on effective treatment options of mental health patients depending on various genetic features.

This book is a collection of fourteen chapters; each chapter is summarized as follows.

Chapter 1

Chapter 1 provides a systematic review of the current literatures investigating the COVID-19 pandemic's impact on mental well-being of the general population, these studies explore machine learning and deep learning techniques to detect and treat mental illnesses when traditional therapies are inaccessible for the general populace due to lockdowns and social distancing norms imposed. Machine learning is a vital data-driven approach allowing the virtual analysis of various kinds of textual, audio, visual, and health data collected from a myriad of sources for performing sentiment analysis and understanding the mental health of people utilizing numerous critical parameters in this situation.

The different machine learning algorithms approaches utilized in these studies are thoroughly analyzed and discussed in this chapter. Detailed explanation of the data sources used and a review of the types of features investigated in mental disorder identification are included as well. The obstacles of employing machine learning techniques in biomedical applications are reviewed, and possibilities to enhance and progress the discipline in future are explored. This chapter provides a broad yet detailed overview of the key literatures among many published during the pandemic and therefore provides directions to the future researchers about the problems they can address and the ideas they can explore.

Chapter 2

Chapter 2 proposes a model for recognizing the depressed client through an online media review by identifying highlights of the client's conduct and the client's online schedule (messages). Depression is a mood disorder, such as feelings of sadness, loss, or anger. It interferes with a person's daily activities. People express their frustration in various ways. Some people react on social media, while few people react in their personal lives. People use social media to share information with friends, chatting with friends. It creates huge amount of data each day. This data can be gathered in the form of images, videos, or text. These data reflect the mental status of the person. However, people are working hard to use such computational models on user-generated content to automatically learn patterns. Although many previous works have conducted small-scale research to a large extent by assuming that the unimodality of the data may not bring us truthful results.

Author used a certifiable information index for depressed and disheartened customers and applied it to the model. Author has proposed a mixed model that is represented by presenting an interplay between the BiGRU and CNN models. Authors designate the multimodality property that addresses the customer's conduct in BiGRU and the customer calendar presents to CNN on removing semantic highlights. Proposed model demonstrates that the preparation of this Metis network enhances order fulfillment and distinguishes depressed customers from other sound techniques. Moreover, the use of another as the end of the famous word representation procedures offered otherwise called preprepared language templates. While there will be difficulties when utilizing such preprepared language models can present due to the limitation that they force on the arrangement length; by the by, contemplating these models on this undertaking assists with uncovering their upsides and downsides. At the end, the future work expects to identify other psychological instability associated with melancholy to catch the complex mental problems that have plagued a person's life.

Chapter 3

Chapter 3 proposes a Graph Convolutional Networks(GCNs)-based framework to solve the problem of classifying people based on their mental stress condition. With the current pandemic scenario where people are being faced with strange situations, unforeseen and never thought of before, it is all the more pertinent that mental health be given special importance. With the advent of social networking platforms, people very often tend to vent out their feelings in the form of tweets, posts, etc. In this work, the authors aim to utilize these tweets/posts as attributes to build the classification framework. Although, the use of machine learning techniques to healthcare data has been in vogue for quite some time now, however, for some application domains, graphs are a very useful representation and are increasingly grabbing the attention of researchers. One can think of people as points and their interrelationships as lines joining these points.

In the present work, graph structure with people as nodes is created. GCNs are used for generating node embeddings, and these node embeddings are used for labeling the nodes (people) as "Mentally stressed" or "Normal." As node features, attributes such as age, gender, occupation, history of chronic ailment, and the tweet words used by the user in a certain time frame have been considered. A GCN-based model for learning the node features is presented, which would be used for node classification. The authors have taken up a study of the graph of persons as nodes, labeled as "Stressed" or "Normal," and use GCN to label the unlabeled nodes. The goal is to build up a Machine Learning model that helps in predicting stress or other problems on various sets of people. The methodology of the research is as follows: A graph structure with people as nodes is created and links between two nodes depend upon the similarity of the nodes.

The node features are aggregated using GCNs, and final node embeddings are obtained. These node embeddings are used for labeling the nodes (people) as "Stressed" or "Normal." Experiments on three datasets show training accuracy of 95.0% and testing accuracy of 93.75%.

Chapter 4

Chapter 4 depicts that the pandemic increased the stress in all sectors of work for both men and women. But, working women faced more stress as they were expected to look after the children and do other daily chores compared to the men. Women in all the spectrum of work go through innumerable issues such as gender bias, unequal pay, lack of maternity leaves, etc., the arrival of pandemics created havoc and increased the problems of women. Healthcare workers are the backbone of society as they are serving people with biological illnesses. They are the most vulnerable part of society, as there is no work-from-home option available to them during lockdown.

This study investigated the issues faced by women working as nurses, doctors, etc., during the pandemic COVID-19. The main focus lies on issues and challenges faced by these women during the pandemic, which include the number of increased working hours, quarantine issues, issues they faced while working, challenge of stealing time to be spent with family, and the nightmare of coping with the truth that the virus might be transmitted to their children and other family members. The problems of fear of working in coronavirus ward, the issues faced in wearing the double mask and personal protective equipment have also been dealt with. Healthcare workers being in the frontline to handle the pandemic faced major issues while working, being quarantined, and managing it during the lockdown. It not only drained them physically but also emotionally. As there was no definite cure or medicine, the healthcare workers went through psychological and physical stress due to their work environment. Even though the new vaccination brought some relief, the fear of catching the virus has always been there. The research showed that the emotional, mental, and physical stress of women healthcare workers increased during the pandemics.

Chapter 5

Chapter 5 deals with the problems faced by women educators during COVID-19. Educational institutions all over the world adopted the "remote learning" strategy so that there are no interruptions in education during the pandemics. During this pandemic when the workload of almost all other sectors decreased significantly, education sector worked full time. With immense pressure from the institute and an increase in working hours, teachers juggled between their professional and personal life resulting in the problem of a time crunch in their personal lives. This paper discusses the issues faced by teachers during the pandemic time. This study investigated issues faced by women educators having newborn babies, school-going children, and college-going children during pandemics. They have been facing different issues such as technical issues, time management, increase in work load, lack of security of job, managing household chores, and looking after the academics of their children. They were also responsible to keep a check on student's mental health. Managing these issues led to an imbalance between their personal and professional lives. Teachers in this pandemic have been pushed in an unfamiliar zone with constant observation from school authorities and parents, which has laid serious effects on their mental health. Further, it even led to teachers being cyber-attacked by students, which increased their emotional stress. The COVID-19 outbreak and the economic crisis risk increased gender inequality in the education sector in all its forms: pay and pension gaps, horizontal and vertical gender segregation. This research clearly highlighted that educators were affected emotionally, physically, and mentally and called for a need to revolutionize the education system. The institutions need to have empathy toward the problem of educators and should put forth more realistic demands. Further, family should also understand the situation and put more effort to help these educators create a balance.

Chapter 6

Chapter 6 focuses on deep learning predictive analysis of mental health for Higher Education students where online mode of Education was an alternative to impart knowledge to student's community during the pandemic of COVID-19 to till date. This chapter has made a detailed study and predictive analysis of offline vs online mode of education by collecting synthetic data from both staff and students via social media platforms. The statistical analysis on the performance of online mode of teaching is presented, and detailed information regarding the parameters that affect the mental health of the faculty and students to impart knowledge via online mode is discussed.

A detailed explanation regarding the implementation of deep learning algorithm (CNN) to extract the best features and to learn the input data and to predict the objective is concentrated in this chapter. The live data collected was subjected to CNN algorithm to extract the highly relevant features to analysis of the reachability of knowledge to the students, use of technology to impart education in pandemic period, analysis of mental health issues of students and faculty during online mode of teaching, and recommendations to the Government to suggest blended mode of Education to Higher Education with guidelines that does not affect the physical and mental health of students and staff involved in Education Sector.

Chapter 7

Chapter 7 focuses on the radical change in education system from traditional to online during COVID-19 pandemic and its affect in Indian student's mental health. This chapter proposes a modular framework for analyzing and predicting the students' mental health based on a set of benchmark questions. These questions are employed to assess and analyze the parameters associated with mental health among college students and surveyed on students from Indian universities. The responses are preprocessed and collected into a dataset. Further, categorization is done on the responses as high mental stress and low mental stress using k-means clustering algorithm. The labels obtained from k-means are validated by the students. Then, different machine learning classification models such as Naive Bayes, Logistic regression, Support Vector Machine, and Random Forest are applied to predict the mental stress level of students. Additionally, student's responses are analyzed to understand the parameters that are of more concern for the Indian students.

This chapter also presents brief descriptions of different methodologies on machine learning based mental health analysis and COVID-19 analysis based on Machine Learning. The proposed Framework is conveyed in detail. The responses of students to each of the benchmark questionnaire and the statistics are analyzed and described through graphs. The modular framework is validated through experimentation on the collected student's responses. Experimentation and results detail the clustering techniques and analysis with respect to set of surveyed questions. The proposed framework with various classification models and its performance are also presented and followed by a discussion. The concluding remarks and the future scope are drawn at the end of the chapter.

Chapter 8

Chapter 8 investigates the impact of COVID-19 pandemic and socioeconomic factors on global mobility and its effect on human mental health by modeling the phenomenon using linear regression. The COVID-19 pandemic has created a global physical and mental health crisis that has had a huge impact on the way we see and perceive our world and our everyday lives. Also, the pandemic has made public health governance all over the world seem insufficient. Although there has been discussion regarding the impact of COVID-19 on people's lifestyle, changed work environment, and economic decline, however, little is known about how the COVID-19 pandemic and socioeconomic factors influence global mobility and, in turn, impact our mental health. Also, little is known about how computational models would predict global mobility under the influence of COVID-19 and socioeconomic variables.

The primary objectives of this chapter are to investigate the influence of the COVID-19 pandemic and socioeconomic factors on people's mobility worldwide and to develop a regression model to predict the future impact on mobility due to the COVID-19 lockdown. The two datasets used for this study are the mobility and the COVID-19 dataset. The data taken into consideration was for 14 months, i.e., from April 1, 2020 May 31, 2021. The mobility dataset contained retail and recreation, grocery and pharmacy, parks, transit stations, workplaces, and residential areas. In contrast, the COVID-19 and socioeconomic dataset contained total confirmed cases, total deaths, total tests, population density, human development index, and other variables. Multiple regression models were built to predict the pandemic's impact on different mobility variables around the world. Variables such as the total number of cases and total deaths per million were negatively correlated with people's mobility at retail and recreation centers, indicating fear and uncertainty. There was a significant negative correlation between reported cases of domestic violence and mobility to the workplace. This indicates the increased stress and anxiety level among individuals due to imposed lockdown during the pandemic.

Chapter 9

Chapter 9 explores the prospects of social media in online personas and presents a review of the various approaches for understanding and working with depression, covering questionnaire, psychological, machine learning, and microexpression-based approaches. The outcome of each approach draws a robust and structured formulation of concepts to understand mental health in a clear way. Additionally, the challenges and research directions are also discussed in order to develop an efficient and evidence-based depression detection system. In terms of clinical relevance, this study highlights the need for automatic early-stage depression detection and use of psychological aspects for strong clinical insights.

Chapter 10

Chapter 10 proposes to use word embedding-based clustering for tweets classification. The proposed models classify the tweets into two classes, tweets-related to mental health and tweets-not related to mental health. In this work, context-aware pretrained models are used to convert tweets into word vectors before clustering. In this work, we intend to analyze social media data related to mental health using intelligent techniques. Early detection of mental health tweets, which are published on Twitter, can be crucial in preventing the spread of mental health tweets, particularly among adults in pandemic COVID-19. The majority of previous research has ignored the importance of context while analyzing the tweets. In order to understand the intended meaning from a tweet that has been posted by a user, we need to have some background information (e.g., context). Latest text classification research showed that tweets can be classified accurately by using word embedding combined with the K-means algorithm. Word embedding is a way for representing words into numbers, so that the word representation can be further fed into the clustering algorithm. However, given the number of choices of word embedding models (Word2Vec, ELMo, and BERT), it raises the question of which type of word embedding has the best performance for text classification tasks. Many kinds of thoughts are spread through Twitter especially, which are related to anxiety during the pandemic.

This study aims to determine the most accurate web embedding methods in classifying tweets related to COVID-19 pandemic anxiety into a more specific cluster. Each cluster is evaluated whether it has relation to the feeling of loneliness. To analyze the performance of the classification, each model is judged for their quality in which the representation method gets the best quality of clusters. Lastly, three word embedding methods are compared in terms of performance using confusion matrix (precision, recall, F1, and accuracy).

Chapter 11

Chapter 11 presents the techniques to detect whether a person is experiencing a feeling of solitude or loneliness. According to psychology, there are two contexts in which loneliness can be defined, positive and negative. The positive sense of loneliness, i.e., solitude is defined as the situation where the person wants to spend time with himself for feeling good or introspection. On the other hand, sometimes a person experiences loneliness due to circumstances and if it goes undetected can lead to depression. Due to pandemics, these kinds of feelings among people get increased as all people got affected one way or the other. A large number of businesses get shut down and in most of the sectors, people are working from home. Due to adaption of mechanical lifestyle and not meeting with family and friends, people are moving toward various psychological disorders. Among these disorders, depression due to loneliness becomes a big challenge for society, which requires immediate attention.

Due to prevalent use of social media among people, they proactively share their feelings on it. Using the web text shared by individuals on the social media, one can dig out the feelings and expressions wrapped in the text. This chapter presents the techniques to recognize the state of loneliness of an individual using the web text (tweets). Firstly, a sequence of preprocessing steps is applied to clean the raw tweets. Subsequently, word embeddings such as GloVe and Word2Vec are applied to obtain the word vectors. These word vectors are further used by classifiers BiLSTM, GRU, Random Forest, XGBoost to detect whether an individual is actually feeling lonely or is talking about only solitude or other positive emotions. Interesting results are obtained, which show that BiLSTM and GRU with GloVe embedding demonstrate the best accuracy and F1 score. Also, high recall for loneliness class is obtained using BiLSTM with Glove model. The proposed application can help an individual, his relatives, or medical professionals to detect depression at an early stage and provide timely support.

Chapter 12

Chapter 12 proposes the deep-learning-based model to diagnose the level of depression. Depression is a fact that is very hard to accept for any individual and is always a multistep process. The initial stage of Depression is Loneliness, and thus the information about these emotions can be leveraged and can help in the early detection of Depression, which in turn leads to suicidal thoughts. Also, tweet data analysis is one of the most popular ways to determine the presence of depression and suicidal thoughts, through the concepts of Machine Learning.

In this chapter, authors have predicted level of depression as loneliness, depression, and suicidal thoughts from a user's specific tweet. These tweets are analyzed to check the level of depression as moderate or severe when people start thinking of suicide. The simulation is carried out using four different models for one level of classification, and eight models are used at the second level of classification. It is observed that GRU with BERT outperformed all the models and showed the accuracy of 99% and 97%. However, for class-1 recall with XLNet gave the best result with class-1 recall being 0.99. This application can help the individual in early detection of depression without any human intervention and seek medical help. Moreover, it also provides an insight about the feelings of the individual to the medical practitioners, which, in turn, can help them provide better decision-making.

Chapter 13

Chapter 13 surveyed the recent developments in COVID-19 vaccine distribution, challenges, and optimization approaches. Here, those solutions are discussed that give importance to technologies for handling COVID-19 vaccine preservation and distribution system. Further, those architectures are emphasized that consider minimizing the healthcare costs and optimizing the system performance for efficiently handling different subsystems.

Chapter 14

EHR using blockchain technology provides data security, integrity, and management challenges. We provide a new approach, methodology, and system for calculating dyslexia symptoms in this research with machine learning algorithm and secure dyslexia data storage using blockchain technology. Dyslexia not only causes major difficulties for students, it also results in severe consequences for their parents (mothers, in particular). Guardians of children having dyslexia are seen to have greater levels of stress and anxiety. Because of the enormous and widespread health threat posed by the coronavirus (COVID-19) pandemic, several governments throughout the world have imposed home-based quarantines as a means of limiting COVID-19's spread. Schools and universities all around the world were forced to close campuses and libraries, reduce face-to-face interactions, and transition to virtual instruction in a short period of time as a result of the epidemic.

This chapter provides a concise overview of the approaches that can be used to detect dyslexia. Fuzzy rule-based learning was used for collecting data, and the model's accuracy demonstrates that this model is quite effective at recognising dyslexic children. The execution incorporate data obtaining, prehandling of the data, applying rule-based for figuring out how to name the information and afterward utilizing this checked data to prepare appropriate AI model. After the model is prepared, the information is stored in EHR structure. The principle thought behind utilizing blockchain is to fundamentally make the current EHR framework to be more exact and precise. We concentrated on strengthening the security of health-records data, and using blockchain technique, a framework has been created to secure, decentralized, and distributed platform for medical records. This method aids in the monitoring of medical practitioner's lack of transparency by limiting access to the EHR system to only the genuine number of users.

CHAPTER ONE

Mental health impact of COVID-19 and machine learning applications in combating mental disorders: a review

Chirantan Ganguly[1], Sagnik Nayak[1] and Anil Kumar Gupta[2]
[1]Institute of Radio Physics and Electronics, University of Calcutta, Kolkata, West Bengal, India
[2]Centre for Development of Advanced Computing (C-DAC), Pune, Maharashtra, India

1. Introduction

As the COVID-19 virus continues to spread throughout the world, the general populace is filled with dread, anxiety, and concern. The pandemic's mental health repercussions are so severe and widespread that a new fear epidemic (which has led to the coining of the term "fearodemic" on social media) has swept across society. People are worried about their health and what the future beholds for them; they fear losing their loved ones, being alone, and losing their source of income. The rise in stress, anxiety, and a myriad of other mental illnesses has given the continuing health crisis a new dimension.

Despite recent increases in mental health literacy in Western countries, attitudes toward people suffering from mental illnesses have remained relatively unchanged [1]. Discrimination, stigma, and human rights violations continue to plague people with mental illnesses all across the world. According to a study by Tesfaye et al., [2] there is widespread stigma against individuals suffering from mental disorders in Ethiopia, with the majority of people preferring not to interact with people with mental disorders. A work by Bagchi et al., [3] on the knowledge, practice, and attitude toward mental health illnesses in an urban community in West Bengal, India, shows that 54.5% will go to a general practitioner in case of any mental illness though only 2.5% thought individuals can totally recover from serious mental illnesses. These studies show the extensive prejudice and challenge that the individuals with mental health disorders face and the pervasive societal misunderstanding about mental health care.

Artificial Intelligence, Machine Learning, and Mental Health in Pandemics
ISBN: 978-0-323-91196-2
https://doi.org/10.1016/B978-0-323-91196-2.00016-8

Despite the fact that mental health is undervalued and misunderstood, it is critical to global growth. Many mental health issues may be treated effectively for a low cost, but owing to existing stigma and prejudice, access to therapy remains severely limited.

The COVID19 pandemic has significantly aggravated the long-standing issue of indifference and prejudice against persons with mental disorders and has also made the general population more prone to mental illness. Not only has the massive loss of life and hopelessness traumatized many, disrupting their mental well-being, but the imposed lockdowns have also made accessing care for those who have already been affected exceedingly difficult.

Thus, at this time of crisis, we must explore utilizing existing technologies while also working to build better ones for detecting and treating mental illness.

In this digital world, social media, cell phones, wearables, and neuroimaging have enabled mental health researchers and practitioners to collect a massive quantity of data at a quick pace [4]. When these data are analyzed for trends, we can learn a lot about the individuals' mental health. Not only can mental diseases be discovered easily, but more accurate diagnostic tools can be devised [5]. The ability to learn and construct systems from existing data makes Machine Learning (ML) and Deep Learning (DL) methodologies an exceptionally effective tool in health domains such as bioinformatics.

This review aims to provide a systematic, clear, and replicable strategy for locating, analyzing, and evaluating the existing corpus of recorded documents [6] in the domain of ML applications in mental health research, with the following goals in mind:

(i) Investigating the implications of the COVID-19 pandemic and other large-scale natural catastrophes on the mental well-being of specific and larger populations.

(ii) Examine how artificial intelligence (AI) and ML can be used to detect, diagnose, and cure mental disorders.

(iii) Emphasize the challenges of implementing ML techniques to study mental health.

(iv) Inform practitioners and researchers about the possibility for additional study in this field.

2. Methods

A systematic quantitative review was conducted of literature published up until 2021, using the methods outlined by Pickering and Byrne [7].

The questions that we want to address through this study are as follows:

1. What effect did COVID-19 have on our mental health?
2. What effect does COVID19 have on persons of different ages, professions, and medical histories, and who are the most seriously affected?
3. Which mental illnesses are experiencing the greatest increase in prevalence?
4. How can we use ML techniques to diagnose these mental diseases remotely?

2.1 Search strategy

The search for relevant literature was conducted on the electronic databases using the following main keywords:

"COVID-19," "Pandemic," "Mental Health," "Machine Learning," and "Deep Learning."

The articles that cite the initial set of included papers were also looked into for finding relevant works. This can be categorized as our secondary search algorithm for finding more relevant literature apart from searching with keywords in electronic databases.

The search of literature was undertaken in both Health and Information Technology (IT) databases since ML application in the research of how pandemics influenced people's mental health spans interdisciplinary domains. IT databases IEEE Xplore and the ACM Digital Library were searched. We included literature from health-related research databases, such as PsycInfo, PLOS Medicine, The Lancet, JAMA Network, The American Journal for Public Health and PubMed. Databases such as ScienceDirect (Elsevier), Springer, Sage, Science (AAAS), and Nature were used to search for relevant literature in both domains. The search did not have a set date range.

2.2 Study selection

Papers were considered for reviewing if they fulfilled the following criteria:

1. The paper was written in English.
2. The paper emphasized the dangers that the COVID-19 pandemic or other natural disasters have had to the general public's mental health.
3. The study explored the use of ML techniques to diagnose and treat mental health disorders; throughout the chapter, we utilize the World Health Organization's (WHO) definition of mental health to conceptualize it [8].
4. The work was accepted for publication in a peer-reviewed journal.

The following exclusion criteria were used to filter out papers not relevant to this study:

1. The article was not written in English.
2. The paper did not focus on mental health applications.
3. The article did not address any specific mental health disorder and outlined mental illness as one broad category.
4. The article used data from sophisticated clinical equipment to train the ML model.
5. The paper's complete text was not published (e.g., conference abstracts).
6. The paper was a tutorial or a course material.

This selection criterion is in compliance to PRISMA guidelines [124] and in accordance with the mental health literature and prior systematic reviews on affective mental health. Fig. 1.1 illustrates the flowchart of our search procedure.

In the findings section, the finalized corpus is summarized narratively. This method was chosen to illustrate the range and complexity of the trends and issues that had been documented, as well as to aid in the identification of any gaps in the existing literature.

3. Findings

3.1 Overview of article characteristics

Upon searching the databases, a total of 439 studies were identified using either one or more of the following keywords: "COVID-19," "Pandemic," "Mental Health," "Machine Learning," and "Deep Learning." Following that upon screening and study eligibility review, we ended up with a corpus of a total of 111 papers. The study corpus includes studies reviewed the impact of COVID-19 and other analogous worldwide natural catastrophes (with significant mortality rates), epidemics, and economic failures in the past, which have had an influence on the mental health of both specific and larger populations (51 studies). These papers highlighted the severe risk the COVID-19 pandemic can pose on the mental well-being of people. However, as COVID-19 is a unique combination of a global epidemic, which is causing widespread deaths and also has caused a severe economic downturn, the study of the events from the past cannot appropriately demonstrate the severe threat to mental health that COVID-19 poses, as none of the previous events had this nature. A detailed discussion of the same is given in Section 3.2.

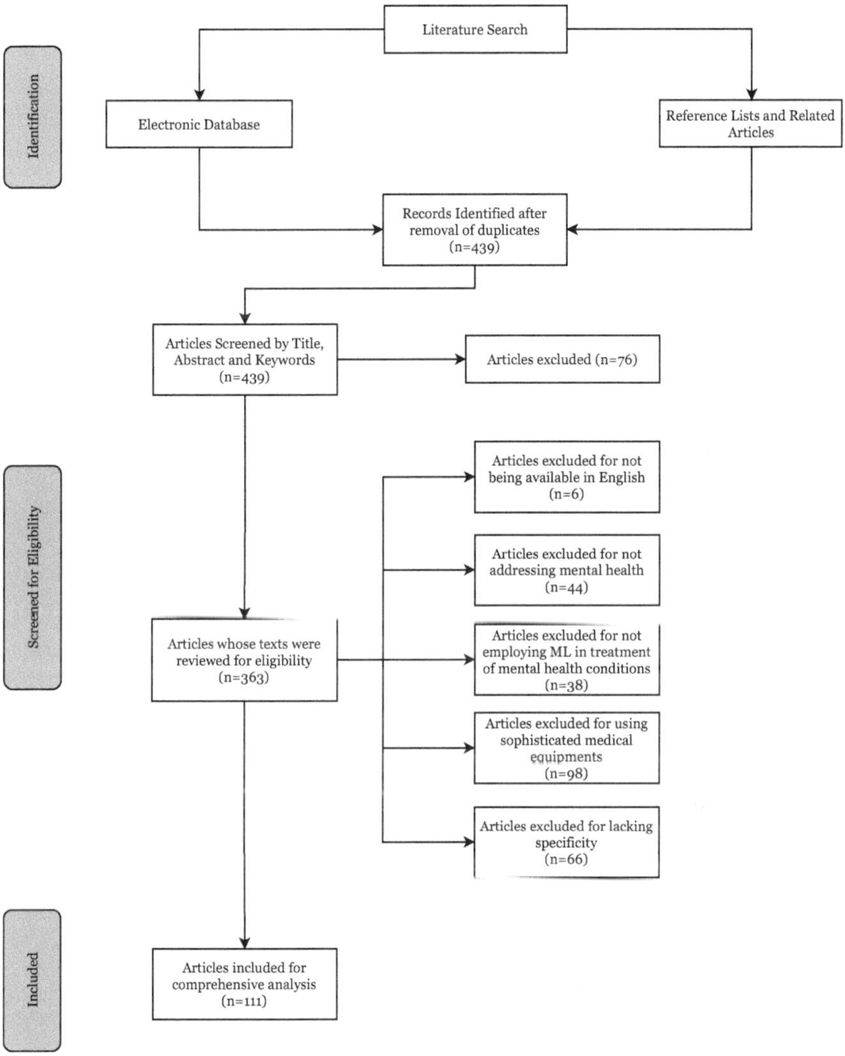

Figure 1.1 Procedural flowchart of literature search following PRISMA guidelines.

This study of threats posed by the COVID-19 pandemic is followed by a study of ML-based methods for detection and treatment of mental health disorders in a remote manner during the pandemic (60 papers). These studies explain and argue for the use of ML techniques to mitigate and address the pandemic's severe mental health impacts. The number of papers examining the use of ML techniques to treat mental health disorders has increased dramatically in recent years, almost two-thirds of all research were published

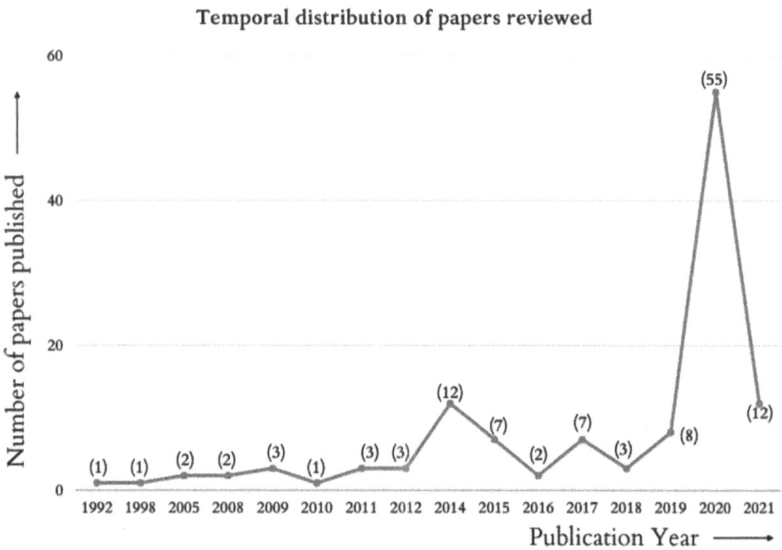

Figure 1.2 Graph depicting the increase in the number of ML mental health publications over time.

in the previous 3 years (2019, 2020, 2021) (Fig. 1.2). A detailed overview of these papers is presented in Section 3.3 of this study.

The works related to studying the mental health impacts of COVID-19 have been categorized based on the section of population those studies are addressed to, and those related to development and deployment of ML algorithms in detecting and treating mental disorders are categorized on the basis of the mental health condition the study targets. Fig. 1.3B depicts the distribution of papers into the major categories discussed.

3.2 An assessment of the pandemic's impacts on mental health

In order to assess the impact of the COVID-19 pandemic, we must study public mental health, which includes assessing the mental health of both specific and broader populations and developing risk models to improve health system delivery. Social media data, electronic health records, and online surveys were commonly employed as data sources in studies relevant to public health applications.

The COVID-19 pandemic's devastation has resulted in a widespread deterioration in mental health [11,12,30], but people from specific backgrounds have been disproportionately affected. As a result, we stratified

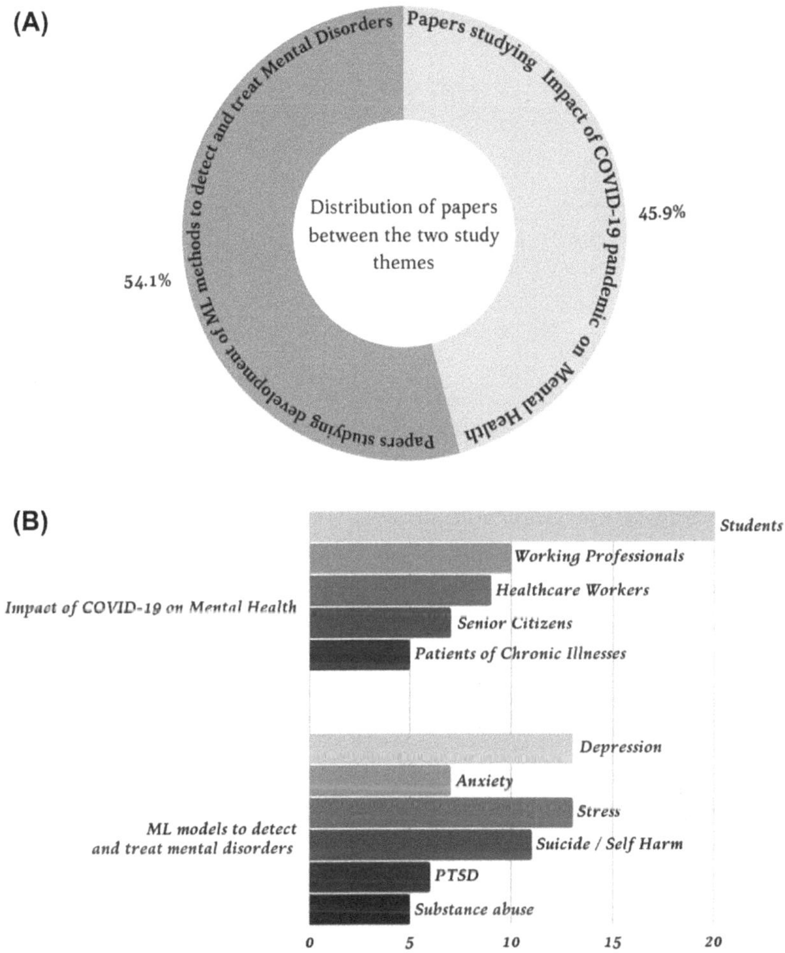

Figure 1.3 (A) Distribution of papers between the two study themes. (B) Frequency distribution of the papers reviewed in different categories as discussed.

the articles depending on the background (age, profession, and health) of the participants involved in the studies in order to gain a more comprehensive understanding of the issue (Fig. 1.4).

The population has been stratified according to the age and profession of the participants involved in the following categories:

(i) Students (school (age group up to 18) and college (age group 18–29))
(ii) Working Professionals (due of the disproportionate impact of COVID-19 on healthcare personnel' mental health, they are classified as a distinct group) (age group 25–60)
(iii) Retired individuals/senior citizens (age group 60+)

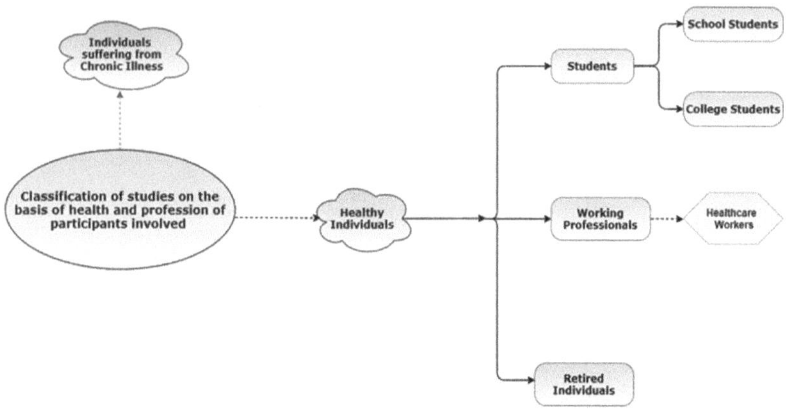

Figure 1.4 Stratification of articles on the basis of age, profession, and health.

Chronic illness patients have been given a distinct category since they are one of society's most vulnerable groups, with heightened vulnerability to both the virus and the pandemic's psychological impacts (Distribution of the studies is demonstrated in Fig. 1.5).

The following section is a detailed analysis of the pandemic's impact on mental health in the several categories we devised to make the information more presentable:

3.2.1 Students

3.2.1.1 School students

People of all ages have had their everyday routines disturbed as a result of the COVID-19 outbreak and the social distancing measures put in place by

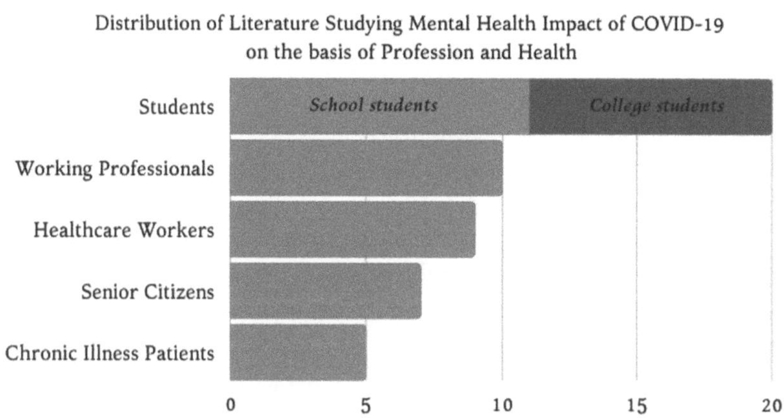

Figure 1.5 Number of papers in each stratified class of literature.

various nations to stop it from spreading further. According to UNESCO [9], about half of the world's students are still affected by partial or complete school closures as of March 2021. "The global scale and speed of the current educational disruption is unparalleled," UNESCO Director-General Audrey Azoulay said. This perturbation is not only causing significant learning loss among school pupils, but it is also impacting them during their formative years, potentially damaging their mental health in the long run.

Aside from regular checkups and immunizations, children and adolescents are generally healthy and do not require much medical attention. When it comes to mental health, children and teenagers, on the other hand, require specific attention. Since the majority of mental disorders begin in childhood [13], it is essential to recognize and handle mental health concerns early on in a child's development.

Due to the unusual mix of public health catastrophe, social isolation, and economic distress, the COVID-19 pandemic has the potential to worsen preexisting mental health problems in patients and also lead to an increase in cases among children and adolescents. Economic downturns are connected to adult unemployment, adult mental health, and child maltreatment, all of which can contribute to a rise in mental health difficulties among the younger population [14,41]. A lot of research has supported this idea by analyzing and deriving conclusions from pertinent data demonstrating the deterioration of school pupils' mental health.

A few relevant studies highlighting the same are as follows:

1. Following the outbreak of COVID-19, Qi et al., [10] performed an online survey to investigate the mental health of Chinese teenagers and discovered a greater frequency of depression and anxiety symptoms in adolescents, with more severe symptoms in those exposed to COVID-19 (diagnosed with COVID-19 or had a history of close contact with COVID-19 infected person). A statistically significant difference in the incidence of sadness and anxiety symptoms between female and male students was also observed.
2. Students and healthcare workers, according to Rehman et al., [11] experience substantially more stress, anxiety, and depression than the overall population.
3. Another study by Liang et al. [15] found that in comparison to the 21–35-year-old group, the 14–20-year-old group had the higher probability to acquire psychiatric difficulties as a result of COVID-19 limitations.

4. A study by Khattar et al., [16] on the mental health of young Indian students showed that more than 69.3% (32.4% somewhat and 36.9% very much) have adapted well to the stay-at-home restrictions and are hopeful that life will soon return to normal; however, these results are somewhat skewed toward students from financially secure residences. Students however have faced enormous disruptions in teaching and learning, and their primary worries right now are the uncertain schedule of upcoming examinations and admittance to the next higher level courses, which has resulted in heightened worry.
5. According to a study conducted by Kapasia et al., [19] students in West Bengal, India, have been experiencing depression, anxiety, poor network connectivity, and an unpleasant study environment at home. During this pandemic, students from rural places and marginalized groups face the greatest hurdles in their studies.
6. A study by Jha et al., [29] shows an increase in the conditional probability of anxiety arising from canceled, or postponed school 7%, and studying from home >7%.
7. In the United Kingdom, a survey of 2111 people [age = 25 years] with a history of mental health problems was conducted [17]; results from the survey show that the current pandemic and lockdown worsened their condition. About 26% of them have been unable to obtain mental health care after the end of "face-to-face" therapy. Some young people considered tele or online services to be inadequate.

Though the pandemic's overall impact on school students' mental health has been overwhelmingly negative, some studies point to a pattern of increased self-care among students as they diversify their minds toward skilled learning, self-exploration, self-care, spiritual connection, and enhancing creative and critical thinking processes, among other things [18].

3.2.1.2 College students

The COVID-19 epidemic has had a particularly negative impact on college students.

A lot of work has been published quantifying the same, a few prominent articles and their findings are as follows:

1. As a result of the COVID-19 epidemic, 71% of students in the United States of America reported heightened stress and anxiety, [20]. A multitude of causes have been blamed for the increased levels of stress among students.

2. According to a purposive sampling Internet survey of university students in Bangladesh revealed that the perception of "e-Learning crack-up" has a significant influence on students' mental distress, and the fear of losing an academic year is one of the primary causes of psychological anguish during COVID-19 confinement [24].
3. A study by Wang et al., [25] shows that Chinese college students have higher anxiety in new semesters of online learning during COVID-19.
4. According to Herbert et al., [26] the average anxiety scores of university students in Egypt and Germany were considerably higher than the threshold values that differentiate between high and low anxious individuals, and 51.82% of students experienced symptoms of depression. In comparison to before the epidemic, there were significant concerns about mental and physical health, as well as reported difficulties in comprehending feelings and obstacles in learning behavior.
5. Study conducted by Akour et al. [27] shows that implementing remote learning systems as educational aids during the COVID-19 pandemic might greatly enhance teaching and learning. However, because of the emotions that university students experience, such as dread of low grades, stress from family situations, and grief from the loss of friends, the usefulness of such systems may be diminished.
6. According to a study done by Khattar et al. [16] on Indian college students, those graduating in 2020 are the most concerned about their future prospects of all college students, as they will be starting careers at the onset of a major global recession.
7. According to research by George et al., [28] due to the pandemic and the lockdown, most students are suffering from anxiety, stress, depression, fear of infection, and uncertainty. The students, on the other hand, participate in a variety of activities that assist them cope with the circumstance.

It is also worth mentioning that the COVID-19 outbreak has had a positive influence on the well-being of some university students [21,22]. There is even evidence that student exam performance may have improved under lockdown, showing the pandemic's heterogeneous effects on student experience [23].

3.2.2 Working professionals

During previous instances of war, natural calamities, and epidemics in the world, a stark increase in the suicide rate among working professionals is not uncommon [34–36]; thus similar trend is also expected due to the COVID-19 pandemic, and we must make every effort possible to prevent mental health deterioration and the rise of suicidal inclinations by giving the essential social assistance to individuals who are particularly sensitive to self-harm.

The worldwide workforce has faced considerable problems as a result of the COVID-19 pandemic, with instances of job losses and wage cutbacks progressively becoming more frequent across industries [31,42]. The economic recession brought about by COVID-19, as well as the lockdowns imposed to control its spread, is taking a toll on people's mental health around the world [32]. Suicide rates have traditionally risen in response to widespread economic recession/depression [37–40], with males experiencing a higher rate of self-harm than females.

A similar trend is already being noticed in the case of COVID-19 where the fear of poverty due to loss of income is spiking up the suicide rates (especially in developing countries) [33]. There have also been reports of an increase in domestic violence and substance misuse during the COVID-19 lockdown period, according to studies.

We may also witness a rise in the number of mental illnesses such as anxiety and posttraumatic stress disorder (PTSD) among working adults after the COVID-19 issue is resolved.

3.2.3 Healthcare professionals

Healthcare workers, such as nurses, nursing technicians, and medical doctors, who come into close contact with patients and their bodily fluids, are the ones most prone to infection. Because of the exponential increase in demand for healthcare, they are required to work long shifts with limited resources and poor infrastructure [43]. There also exists the fear of becoming infected, as well as the risk of spreading the infection to their relatives, friends, or colleagues [44,45]. This might cause them to become estranged from their family, alter their routine, and reduce their social support network [46]. Healthcare professionals who have been infected with COVID-19 and have survived it have experienced harassment, stigmatization, and, in some cases, physical assault. In Mexico, for example, physicians and nurses were discovered riding bicycles after being refused access to public transportation and subjected to physical attacks. Similarly, healthcare professionals in Malawi have been denied access to public transportation, ridiculed on the street, and evicted from rented residences. According to media accounts in India, physicians and medical personnel who worked with COVID-19 patients were subjected to severe social exclusion, were ordered to quit their leased houses, and were even assaulted while performing their responsibilities [47].

All of these variables contribute to increased mental stress, which may lead to feelings of helplessness and isolation, as well as negative emotional states such as tension, irritability, and physical and mental weariness [46].

Work overload and stress symptoms render health workers more sensitive to psychological distress, increasing their risk of acquiring mental illnesses [44,45,48,49]. Studies have also shown that health personnel who provide treatment during epidemics might have significant levels of stress, depression, anxiety, and PTSD after the emergency has passed [50,51].

Healthcare employees' mental health has been the most severely impacted of all professions. Because they are the ones who have witnessed the virus's carnage up close and are taking care of those who are in need among all of the other obstacles.

3.2.4 Retired individuals/senior citizen

Certain groups of people, such as the elderly, are as sensitive to the infection as they are to the pandemic's psychological impact and the containment measures put in place to halt the disease's spread. The fear and uncertainty of a pandemic can have a greater impact on the minds of the elderly, who are more aware of their susceptibility [52].

Because of their increased risk of cardiovascular, autoimmune, neurocognitive, and mental health conditions, studies have shown that isolation among older individuals during the pandemic is a "major public health concern" [53,55]. A study by Santini et al. [54] demonstrates that older individuals who are socially isolated are prone to suffer from depression and anxiety.

Older adults, who exclusively engage with others outside of their family, such as at daycare facilities, recreation centers, and places of worship, will be disproportionately affected by self-isolation. Those who do not have close family or friends and rely on volunteer services or social services for help, as well as those who are already lonely, secluded, or introverted, may be put at greater danger [56].

Similar results have been observed in earlier epidemics when social distance limitations were enforced on the elderly [57,58], suggesting that immediate intervention is required to reduce the mental and physical health consequences for the aged.

3.2.5 Individuals suffering from chronic illness

Chronically sick individuals feel threatened due to the outbreak of the pandemic as they believe they are at more danger of infection and in greater need of health care in this circumstance. Physicians have realized this early on that chronic patients' primary concern throughout the quarantine time was availability of alternate support when needed. In a study conducted by Ciacci et al., [59] patients stated that they were afraid about COVID-19. Fear of mortality, fear of being more susceptible to COVID-19 than the general population, fear of being alone due to the social isolation caused by the quarantine, fear of medicine shortages, and the fear that physicians and caregivers would be unable to provide adequate treatment for them due to the current stress on the health infrastructure were the primary worries expressed.

Anxiety and sadness have been linked to 50% of uncontrolled asthma patients in another study [60], indicating a possible psychological influence on asthma patients.

In a study of the mental health of patients with type 1 and type 2 diabetes [61], 43% of patients showed signs of substantial psychological distress, with type 2 diabetes patients having a much higher propensity. Diabetes-related mental discomfort was identified in 29.2% of patients, while eating disorders were detected in 75.8%, and moderate/severe sleeping problems were found in 77.5%.

Another study [62] looked into mental health concerns in cancer patients during the COVID-19 pandemic and found that 23.4% of 6213 cancer patients had depression, 17.7% had anxiety, 9.3% had PTSD, and 13.5% had hostility; however, only 1.6% of them sought psychological help during COVID-19.

Another study by Jha et al. [29] found that cancer patients have a greater conditional probability of experiencing less than one anxiety-ridden day per week than the broader population. This finding might be due to lower work-related stress or more time spent with family members at home during lockdown.

The findings of the studies revealed that COVID-19 causes significant discomfort in patients with chronic diseases, indicating that particular psychological treatments for this susceptible group should be devised.

3.3 ML application domains in mental health

We can see just how death, fear of losing loved ones, rising unemployment, economic downturn, stress, uncertainty about the future, and social isolation caused by the COVID-19 pandemic and subsequent lockdown have affected everyone's mental well-being in some way or another from the study of the impact of the COVID-19 pandemic on mental health provided in the previous section.

As the social distancing norms continue to restrict the transmission of the virus, accessing mental health counseling from qualified experts and committed organizations has become increasingly difficult for those who are in desperate need of it. In this situation, ML and AI techniques have shown to be critical in managing the mental health crisis caused by COVID-19 at its different phases.

In this section, we systematically analyze the available literature using ML techniques in dealing with mental health disorders.

Though ML and AI may be used to study a wide variety of mental health disorders, we will concentrate on those that have seen a substantial increase in the general population as a result of COVID-19 and the lockdown measures that went along with it (discussed in the previous section). This section focuses on the studies dealing with the use of ML to identify mental illnesses such as anxiety, depression, stress, PTSD, substance abuse, suicide thoughts, and self-harm.

Fig. 1.6 depicts the distribution of articles reviewed in this area, which are categorized according to mental health problems.

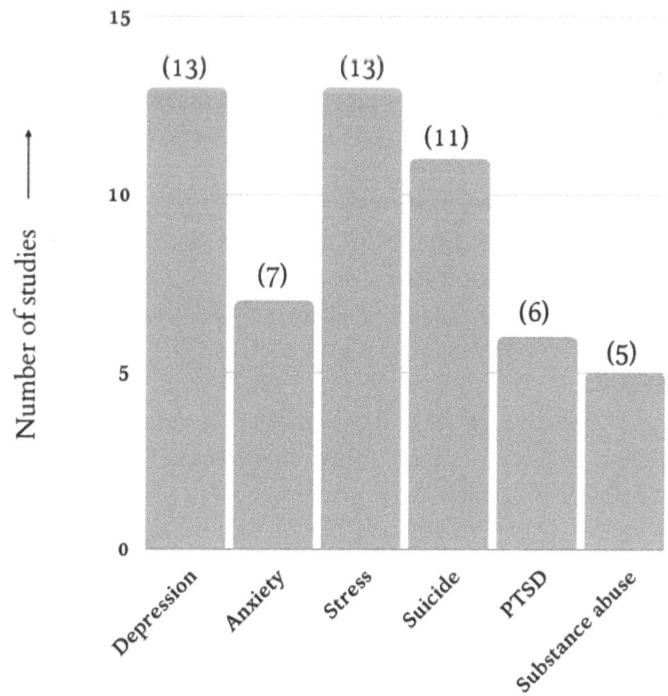

Figure 1.6 Frequency distribution of the mental health focus of the papers in the review corpus.

We concentrated on studies that employed the data categories that can be easily accessed in a remote fashion and systematically analyzed to effectively diagnose predict long-term outcomes of a patient mental illness in people using machine learning:

(i) Audio/Video—Audio, video, and speech-related studies are promising as since such data may be obtained from target individuals easily in a remote fashion through recorded telephonic or online-video interviews, as well as a variety of other methods. Due to the ease with which high-quality visual and speech data can be accessed remotely in recent times, efficient diagnosis of various mental health disorders may be done using the same.

(ii) Smartphones/Smart Wearables—As of June 2021, nearly half of the world's population owns a smartphone or other smart gadget (such as a smart watch). These smart devices collect a range of data, which if accessed and analyzed ethically, can provide us with a valuable tool for investigating the onset and progression of mental disorders in individuals in an unobtrusive, passive manner if desired by using effective machine learning algorithms.

(iii) Questionnaires/Surveys—Online surveys and questionnaires may be readily conducted by creating dedicated websites or utilizing tools such as Google Forms. People can fill out these surveys and questionnaires from the comfort of their own homes, in a remote manner. When the data obtained through these surveys regarding emotional state and socioeconomic status are analyzed using ML algorithms, we can gain valuable insight about the mental health status of the individuals participating in the survey.

(iv) Electronic Health Records—Over the last decade, the use of electronic health records (EHRs) in healthcare systems around the world has increased rapidly. Comprehensive, longitudinal data captured in EHRs provide a constantly expanding library of clinical and phenotypic data. These data may be used to develop and train ML algorithms for detecting and tracking mental health issues. A study of prospective patients' EHRs using such ML models can provide valuable insight into the possibility of mental health problems developing in the patients as well as forecast illness progression.

(v) Social Media Data—Individuals' mental health has become a significant component of research using social media platforms. Through the creation of virtual networks and communities, social media has allowed the exchange of ideas, opinions, and information in the form of texts and other types of multimedia. Using various ML techniques, we may get insight into the emotional and mental condition of the individual expressing these thoughts and ideas on such social sites and digital channels.

We try to avoid literature that advocates the use of advanced medical equipment combined with ML to detect mental health issues, even though they may provide more accurate results, because we propose techniques that must be accessible to people during times of crisis, such as the COVID-19 pandemic. This constraint is introduced intentionally since some of these instruments are unavailable to the public at large, and many of these devices require specialized settings and skilled personnel to operate, which is not possible, especially when movement is limited due to lockdowns (Fig. 1.7).

A large proportion of the papers discussed here describes the application of ML to assist in the detection or diagnosis of mental health symptoms or conditions (n = 47), the remaining studies seek to anticipate a patient's long-term prognosis as due to mental health conditions, and some seek the development of ML solutions to optimize the procedure of therapeutic interventions for people with mental disorders (n = 3).

For each selected article studying use of ML methods to detect and treat mental disorders, we extracted data regarding the following:

(i) Area of mental health focus;
(ii) The aim/purpose of research;
(iii) Type of data used and how it was collected;
(iv) ML methods and algorithms used;
(v) Results;
(vi) Participant demographics of the study (if any).

All the information is presented in a tabular format in Table 1.1.

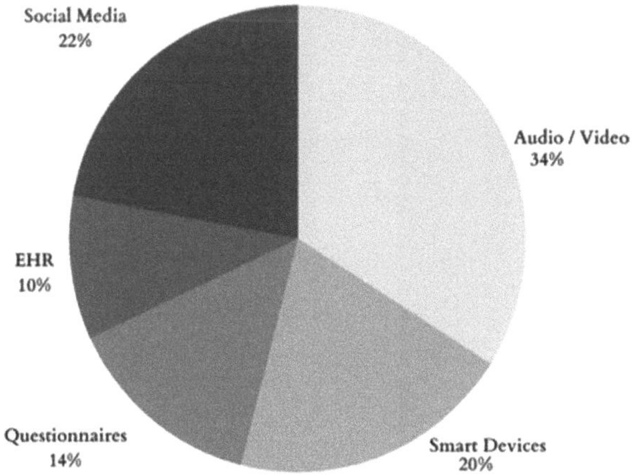

Figure 1.7 Distribution of studies on the basis of data types employed to develop ML models.

Table 1.1 A summary of papers in review corpus that use machine learning to diagnose and treat mental health disorders.

Reference	Mental health target	Purpose	Data domain and description	ML algorithms	Results
Literatures focusing on the usage of audio/Video data (n = 17)					
Zhao et al., [63]	Depression	Developing a multimodal fusion algorithm for the diagnosis of depression, a multimodal fusion algorithm based on voice signal and face picture sequence	Audio/Video The National Institute of Mental Health's experimental voice databases, as well as YouTube recordings of 30 self-described depressed persons, were utilized to create a 600-speech database of independent speakers.	Neural networks	The depression detection algorithm of fusion speech and facial emotions achieved an accuracy rate of 81.14%, compared to the present accuracy rate of doctors at 47.3%.
Chang et al., [64]	Depression	To assist in the early detection and long-term monitoring of mental disease symptoms in ordinary speech discussion.	Audio A total of 62 voice recordings of 25 subjects (21 males and 4 females) all diagnosed with major depressive disorder were collected in a period of 4 months. In addition, there were a total of four health practitioners who participated in the study.	Using supervised learning to develop classification of speech utterances.	The findings reveal that depressed people have low emotional expressiveness, a bad cadence, and a lot of pauses in their speaking.
Bedi et al., [65]	Substance use	Abused drugs can have a dramatic effect on one's mental state. These impacts are traditionally measured using self-report, which is prone to biases. Speech analysis when inebriated may provide a more direct and objective assessment.	Audio Participants of the study were healthy volunteers (18–38 years old) reporting ecstasy use more than twice. The data was gathered by recording a 10-minute chat between participants and a research assistant about a significant person in their lives.	Support vector machine (SVM)	With an accuracy of 88%, the classifiers were able to distinguish between drug users and placebos.

Baggott et al., [66]	Substance use	To examine how MDMA affects the content of speech, which might indicate how it affects social interactions.	Audio A double-blind trial was conducted which included 35 healthy volunteers with past MDMA experience who were given 1.5 mg/kg oral MDMA and a placebo. Participants took part in a 5-min standardized talking activity in which they explained their close personal relationship with a research assistant. The conversations were recorded and analyzed for selected content categories.	Random forest	Results show that MDMA boosted the use of social terms and phrases associated with both positive and negative emotions.
Pestian et al., [67]	Suicide/Self-harm	Teenagers' words and gestures are used by mental health experts to get insight into their emotional condition and to provide the best treatment. This prescription is frequently inconsistent across caregivers, resulting in a wide range of results. As a result, an automated variation is attempted to be developed, in order to reduce variation by using machine learning as a clinical decision support tool.	Audio 30 suicidal adolescents and 30 matched controls (aged 13–17) completed the suicidal ideation questionnaire and the ubiquitous questionnaire. Participants were then asked a follow-up to these questions the conversation which occurred were audio-recorded and then transcribed.	Natural language processing (NLP); support vector machine (SVM)	96.67% of the subjects are accurately classified

(Continued)

Table 1.1 A summary of papers in review corpus that use machine learning to diagnose and treat mental health disorders.—cont'd

Reference	Mental health target	Purpose	Data domain and description	ML algorithms	Results
Venek et al., [68]	Suicide/Self-harm	To investigate differences between suicidal versus nonsuicidal adolescents and suicidal repeaters' behaviors in comparison to suicidal nonrepeaters	Audio A dataset of 60 audio-recorded interviews of 30 suicidal (13 repeaters and 17 nonrepeaters) and 30 nonsuicidal adolescents interviewed by a social worker was used.	AdaBoost algorithm, statistical analysis	An accuracy of 90% is achieved for the suicidal versus nonsuicidal distinction while the suicidal repeaters versus suicidal nonrepeaters layer classification deliver an accuracy of 60%
Mitra et al., [70]	Depression	A diverse set of features based on spoken audio is explored to understand which features correlate with self-reported depression scores according to the Beck depression rating scale.	Audio The AVEC-2014 challenge dataset of audio-visual depression corpus [69], which comprises 150 videos of people undertaking a human—computer interaction task while being captured by a camera and a microphone. Each recording consists of only one person. The duration of all clips sums to 240 h.	Decision tree, Gaussian processes, regression	The individual system ranges from 9.18 to 11.87 in root mean squared error (RMSE), and from 7.68 to 9.99 in mean absolute error (MAE).
McGinnis et al., [71]	Anxiety and depression	Investigating a new approach for identifying young children with internalizing disorders using a 3-minute speech task.	Audio Participants in the study were 71 children (3—8 years old) and their primary caregivers, child voice was recorded during a 3-minute speech task during a home visit by research assistants, the participants were instructed to prepare and give a 3-min speech and are told that they will be judged based on how interesting it is.	Logistic regression, support vector machine (SVM), random forest	This tool outperforms clinical thresholds on parent-reported child symptoms, which identify children with an internalizing disorder with lower accuracy (67%—77% vs. 80%), and similar specificity (85%—100% vs. 93%), and sensitivity (0%—58% vs. 54%) in this sample.

Sun et al., [73]	Depression	A random forest method with a selected-text feature is proposed to analyze the transcripts of interviews of individuals in different depressive levels.	Audio The publicly available multimodal depression data set, AVEC-2017 [72] was used	Random forest	The model's root mean square error (RMSE) reaches 4.7, and the mean absolute error (MAE) reaches 3.9, which is better than the baseline result, i.e., 7.05/5.66.
Xu et al., [74]	Posttraumatic stress disorder (PTSD)	To make PTSD diagnosis cheaper and more easily and remotely accessible	Audio The TPM system is accessible via the public switched telephone network (PSTN) or the internet. The obtained voice data is subsequently transferred to a secure server, which invokes the PTSD scoring Engine (PTSD-SE), which computes a PTSD mental health score.	Neural networks, support vector machine, Gaussian mixture models	The Tele-PTSD Monitor (TPM) system was supported using a limited dataset with an average detection accuracy of up to 95.88%.
Schultebraucks et al., [75]	Posttraumatic stress disorder (PTSD), major depressive Disorder (MDD)	To examine if machine learning-based computer vision (CV), semantic, and acoustic analysis can capture clinical aspects from free speech replies to a brief interview 1-month posttrauma that accurately categorize major depressive disorder (MDD) and posttraumatic stress disorder (PTSD).	Audio/Video 1 month after admission, 81 patients admitted to a Level-1 trauma Unit's emergency department (ED) after a life-threatening traumatic event engaged in an open-ended qualitative interview with a professional about their experience.	Computer Vision (OpenCV)	The accuracy of discriminatory classification was improved by using both video and audio-based markers. The algorithm has an AUC of 0.90 for discriminating PTSD status 1 month after ED admission and an AUC of 0.86 for discriminating depression status 1 month after ED admission.

(*Continued*)

Table 1.1 A summary of papers in review corpus that use machine learning to diagnose and treat mental health disorders.—cont'd

Reference	Mental health target	Purpose	Data domain and description	ML algorithms	Results
Tomba et al., [79]	Stress detection	To develop a model to detect stress in candidates during automated HR interviews	Audio/Video Three different datasets were used, the Berlin emotional database (EmoDB) [76], the Keio University Japanese emotional speech database (KeioESD) [77] and the Ryerson audio-visual database of emotional speech and song (RAVDESS) [78]	Artificial neural networks (ANNs), hidden Markov model (HMM), Gaussian mixture model (GMM), support vector machines (SVMs) and even nearest neighbors (kNN)	Best accuracy scores obtained KeioESD dataset with SVM (95.83%) and ANN (83.33%).
Madhavi et al., [81]	Stress detection	To detect work-related stress in highly automated digital environments, such as smart factories and cyber-physical ecosystems where verbal communication is not only constrained but also impaired by background noise and other disturbances common to factory settings using a deep learning approach.	Audio The distress assessment interview corpus (DAIC-WOZ) dataset [80], released as part of the 2016 audio/Visual emotional challenge and workshop (AVEC 2016) was used as a benchmark dataset to evaluate the effectiveness and accuracy of the proposed deep learning approach.	Convolutional neural network (CNN), growing self-organizing map (GSOM) algorithms	The accuracy and effectiveness of the proposed approach are demonstrated using a benchmark dataset (DAIC-WOZ) [80]. We report F1 scores of 82% and 64% for normal and distressed classes respectively, which outperform the state-of-the-art models.
Lefter et al., [83]	Stress detection	To design a system for selecting the calls that appear to be urgent, based on emotion detection.	Audio South-African database which contains genuine recordings from call centers was used. The data was labeled according to two classes: Emotional and neutral. The dataset contains 215.02 min of speech. Based on the call identities, 1200 speakers were estimated to have been recorded.	Gaussian mixture models (GMM), support vector machine (SVM)	An improvement in the equal error rate (EER) from 19.0% on average for four individual detectors to 4.2% when fused using linear logistic regression was observed

Dhole et al., [85]	Stress detection	To develop stress identification and classification algorithms with the aid of machine learning (ML) and artificial intelligence (AI) together with MFCC feature extraction methods	Audio Two speech datasets were used for this study: (i) The Berlin Database [76] is in German language consisting of sentences audio wave files of both genders under seven stressed sentiment classes (ii) Toronto emotional speech set [84] is a collection of 200 words spoken by two actresses are from Toronto speaking English language with musical preparation. (iii) audacity software is used in recording female as well as male in languages such as Hindi, Marathi, and English.	Neural network	Results show that the proposed classifiers possess an accuracy of 97.52% in stress identification.
Zhang et al., [82]	Stress detection	To leverage contact-free video cameras for stress detection, by developing a two-leveled stress detection network (TSDNet) by using a deep learning strategy to avoid the labor-intensive hand-crafted feature engineering approach	Video 122 volunteers (58 males and 64 females, aged 18–26) participated in the study. The participants were college students from China. Infrared cameras were used to record the affective reactions of the participants when they watched three different types of 2-min video clips about 1. scenery or food making 2. highlights of variety show 3. science programs with rich knowledge, followed by a question-answering test, questions were designed the questions in such a way that it was very hard to answer. To stimulate the cognitive stress, before the test, the participants were told that they could get some extra rewards they scored >50% in the test as an incentive.	Computer vision, unsupervised learning	TSDNet outperformed the hand-crafted feature engineering approaches with a detection accuracy of 85.42% and F1-Score 85.28%. Considering both facial expressions and action motions could improve detection accuracy and F1-Score of that considering only face or action method by over 7%

(Continued)

Table 1.1 A summary of papers in review corpus that use machine learning to diagnose and treat mental health disorders.—cont'd

Reference	Mental health target	Purpose	Data domain and description	ML algorithms	Results
Sharma et al., [87]	Stress detection	To understand the use of nonintrusive means (i.e., not using medical equipment in medical setup) for stress recognition by reducing restrictions to natural human behavior.	Video The *ANUStressDB* database [86] was used, it contains videos of 35 subjects (22 males, 13 females, aged 23–39) watching *stressed* and *not-stressed* film clips, recorded in visual and thermal spectrum.	Support vector machine (SVM); genetic algorithm	Results show that the system has a recognition rate of around 73% when only visual spectrum videos are used and a recognition rate of around 88% when both visual and thermal spectrum videos are used.
Literatures focusing on the usage of data collected from smartphones/Smart wearables (n = 10)					
Gjoreski et al., [90]	Stress detection	To detect perceived stress in students using data collected with smartphones	Smartphones Data used in this study is freely available on the web [88]; it was collected as part of a larger study (StudentLife) [89]. Several data such as: accelerometers, audio recorder, Wi-Fi, GPS, call log and light sensor were used.	Support vector machine (SVM), random forest	Accuracy of 60% is achieved
Sağbaş et al., [92]	Stress detection	To detect stress in individuals by using accelerometer and gyroscope sensor data of the writing behavior on a smartphone touchscreen panel.	Smartphones Sample data were collected from 46 individuals using motion sensors (accelerometer and gyroscope) and touchscreen panel of a smartphone to determine the stressful or non-stressful situation.	Decision trees, Bayesian networks, k-nearest neighbor (kNN)	Result of the experiments showed, 74.26%, 67.86%, and 87.56% accuracy classification results for decision tree, Bayesian networks and K-nearest neighbors respectively.

Canzian et al., [91]	Depression	To evaluate personalized and general machine learning models to predict the patient health questionnaire (PHQ) score changes from mobility metrics variations.	Smartphones Data used in this study was collected as part of the study (StudentLife) [90]. Only mobility patterns from GPS traces were used in the study.	Support vector machine (SVM)	General model achieves sensitivity and specificity values of 0.74 and 0.78. The average sensitivity and specificity values of the personalized models are 0.71 and 0.87.
Phan et al., [93]	Substance use	Using a smartphone sensing dataset representing nightlife and drinking habits, the study explores the phenomena of heavy drinking at night (4+ drinks for women and 5+ drinks for males in a single evening).	Smartphones A mobile application was developed, which asked the participants (240 individuals) about the number of drinks consumed in the day through a questionnaire, it also asked the participants to take a picture that clearly captured a container with liquid (with or without alcohol) for visual affirmation. The sensor logger of the application also collected a variety of sensor and log data, including GPS coordinates, accelerometer, activity, using a background running process without any user interaction.	Random forest (RF), support vector machines (SVM)	The results demonstrate that a fully automated technique using phone sensors achieves a 71% accuracy rate. Manual input of context of drinking events, on the other hand, yields 70% accuracy, while visual characteristics of manually supplied photos yield 72% accuracy. This indicates that automated sensing is a viable option.

(*Continued*)

Table 1.1 A summary of papers in review corpus that use machine learning to diagnose and treat mental health disorders.—cont'd

Reference	Mental health target	Purpose	Data domain and description	ML algorithms	Results
Phan et al., [94]	Substance use	Two contemporary ways to quantify alcohol consumption in everyday life are to use mobile crowdsensing and social media analytics.	Smartphones/Social media Two data sources are used: (a) Alcohol-related posts from Instagram: Initial corpus of 1.7 million Instagram posts consisting of pictures, hashtags, and metadata collected between November 1, 2010 and March 31, 2016 within the swiss borders, (b) crowdsensing study - an android-based application to collect data related to nightlife activities for Friday and Saturday nights for a period of 3 months. This data also included mobile sensor data like accelerometer, wifi, etc. as well as app logs.	Random forest (RF), support vector machines (SVM)	Models give an accuracy of 82.3% on alcohol category classification (against a baseline of 48.5%) and 90% on alcohol/nonalcohol classification (against a baseline of 65.9%) using a fusion of image features and contextual cues in this task.
Fukazawa et al., [95]	Anxiety/Stress	To predict the change of stress levels using real-world and online behavioral features extracted from smartphone log information.	Smartphones 20 healthy individuals (with no history of mental illness) (15 males and five females; age 20 to 24) participated in the study. A log collection application, which runs in background, was developed and was installed in the smartphones of the participants. The application stores sensor logs (illuminance, acceleration, rotation and execution	Random forest	With an F-score of 74.2%, the results show that anxiety-related stress levels can be predicted using a combination of features derived from smartphone log data.

			status) and stores the daily STAI (state Trait anxiety Inventory) responses by the participants. By pressing the "send" button, the daily smartphone logs and STAI results are sent.		
Zakaria et al., [102]	Depression/Stress	To help detect individuals' stress and depression early.	Smartphones/Laptop StressMon, a scalable detection solution is developed to automatically and non-intrusively identify individuals exhibiting signs of severe stress or depression in a work setting; it uses the location information, directly sensed from the WiFi infrastructure. 3 studies were conducted for validation of the application: (i) 76 students (aged 19 −25) studied for 81 days (ii) 13 students (aged 20−24) studied for 36 days (iii) 51 students (aged 19 −26) studied for 81 days	Support vector machine; random forest; logistic regression	Evaluation demonstrated StressMon detecting severely stressed students with a 96.01% true positive rate (TPR), an 80.76% true negative rate (TNR), and a 0.97 AUC score using a 6-day prediction window. In addition, StressMon was able to detect depression at 91.21% TPR, 66.71% TNR, and 0.88 AUC using a 15-day window.
Gjoreski et al., [96]	Stress detection	To design and develop a stress detection technology that can accurately, continuously, and inconspicuously monitor psychological stress in real life.	Smartweables 21 individuals (mean age: 28) participated in the study. The data is collected solely using the Empatica wrist band device, and the following health data were extracted for the experiment: Blood Volume Pulse (BVP), Heart rate (HR), Inter-beat Interval (IBI), electrodermal activity (EDA), skin Temperature (ST), and Acceleration.	Decision tree, k-nearest neighbor, Naïve Bayes, Boosting, support vector machine, random forest	Results showed that the method detects (recalls) 70% of the stress events with a precision of 95%.

(*Continued*)

Table 1.1 A summary of papers in review corpus that use machine learning to diagnose and treat mental health disorders.—cont'd

Reference	Mental health target	Purpose	Data domain and description	ML algorithms	Results
Jacobson et al., [121]	Anxiety (*Prognosis*)	To demonstrate the capacity of digital biomarkers collected from passive sensing from smart wearables to predict long-term prognosis.	Smart wearable The data for this research came from a long-term study called Midlife in the United States (MIDUS), the participants completed a phone-based interview that assessed generalized anxiety disorder and panic disorder symptoms at enrollment, followed up by a participation in a 1-week actigraphy study 9–14 years later where data was collected using wearable sensors and completed a long-term follow-up, phone-based interview to quantify generalized anxiety disorder and panic disorder symptoms 17–18 years from initial enrollment.	Deep learning	Results suggest that wearable movement data may substantially predict which patients will have symptom worsening, verified by out-of-sample cross-validation (AUC = 0.696).
Gargot et al., [123]	Posttraumatic stress disorder (*Prognosis*)	Design and creation of a smartphone app for collecting longitudinal data in order to forecast and track the	Smartphone When users initially use the app, they must fill in their information; after that, the software assigns one of three treatments aimed at preventing the	Arranging hackathons for a successful development and deployment of the	The results are currently unavailable, but the application development and deployment in the mass can assist production of large

		progression of PTSS toward PTSD is proposed.	development of PTSS to PTSD. Following that, supplementary surveys and sleep data are collected to track the course of PTSS. The app will advise the participant to seek professional mental health treatment if significant indications or symptoms are identified. A 1-month follow-up will be conducted to determine if they have developed persistent PTSD.	application described is proposed	datasets that might give insights about the best methods to treat PTSS, and cause critical interventions when needed to stop worsening of mental health condition.
Literatures focusing on the usage of data collected from surveys and questionnaires (n = 7)					
Ahuja et al., [97]	Stress detection	To calculate students' mental stress 1 week before the exam and while they are using the internet.	Questionnaire Data was taken from the 206 students of Jaypee Institute of information Technology Noida, they were asked 14 basic PSS (perceived stress scale) test questions about their feelings in situations that they might have encountered in the last month and their reactions to it. Their responses are weighted, and the weights are used to generate a score that may be used to assess an individual's stress level.	Linear regression, random forest, Naïve Bayes, and support vector machine (SVM)	Results showed that the highest accuracy recorded was by support Vector machine (85.71%).

(*Continued*)

Table 1.1 A summary of papers in review corpus that use machine learning to diagnose and treat mental health disorders.—cont'd

Reference	Mental health target	Purpose	Data domain and description	ML algorithms	Results
Karstoft et al., [98]	Posttraumatic stress disorder (PTSD)	To evaluate the potential of machine learning (ML) technologies for pre- and early postdeployment prediction of resilience or posttraumatic stress disorder development in soldiers.	Questionnaire 561 Danish soldiers who deployed to Afghanistan participated in the study. Of the study sample, 95% were male, and the mean age was 26.2 years. Participants were assessed at six time points: 5–6 weeks before deployment, during deployment, 1–3 weeks after return, 3 months after deployment, 7 months after deployment, and 2.5 years after return by a survey.	Support vector machine	The model accurately predicted long-term posttraumatic stress responses (predeployment: AUC = 0.84 (95% CI = 0.81–0.87), post-deployment: AUC = 0.88 (95% CI = 0.85–0.91)).
Andrews et al., [99]	Depression	To demonstrate the potential of survey based data to predict future depression status in older adults.	Questionnaire The data used in this study was initially collected for the validation of the NANA system [100]. Data used included mood scores self-reported by 40+ adults, comprising ratings each day of how 'happy', 'sad', 'tired', 'alert', 'relaxed' and 'hungry' each participant was on a scale of 0–10. Participants completed this self-report daily over three individual weeks.	Logistic regression	The cross-validated area under the ROC curve for this model was 0.88 (CI: 0.69–0.97).

Dipnall et al., [101]	Depression	To design and develop a flexible, modular risk index for depression based on structural equation models of major factors.	Questionnaire Community-based data from the 2009–10 National health and Nutrition examination survey (NHANES) (2009–10) were used for this cross-sectional study ($N = 5546$, age range 18–80years). To improve the precision and reliability of population estimates, data were collected from 15 locations throughout 50 US states, with oversampling of subsets of the population of specific public health importance.	Logistic regression	The AUCs for the individual demographics, diet and biomarker determinants were below 0.7. The AUCs were above 0.7 for somatic symptoms ($AUC = 0.741$) and lifestyle-environs ($AUC = 0.780$).
Tate et al., [104]	Multiple (depression/Anxiety/Hyperactivity) study of medical risk factors	To design and develop a model that can detect mental health issues in mid-adolescents.	Questionnaire The study looked into 7638 twins from Sweden's child and adolescent Twin study. The data from parental reports and registers yielded 474 predictors. The strengths and difficulties questionnaire determined the result.	Random forest, support vector machines, neural network, XGBoost	The random forest model resulted in $AUC = 0.739$, followed closely by support vector machines $AUC = 0.735$
Shen et al., [117]	Suicide/Self-harm	To design a machine learning model that can reliably predict the likelihood of attempting suicide in medical college students in China.	Questionnaire The study included 4882 medical students, the majority of whom were female. Self-reported socio-demographic and clinical variables were gathered online via a website or the popular social media app, WeChat.	Random forest	Results show that the random forest model performed well [(AUC) = 0.9255] in predicting suicide attempts with an accuracy of 90.1%.

(*Continued*)

Table 1.1 A summary of papers in review corpus that use machine learning to diagnose and treat mental health disorders.—cont'd

Reference	Mental health target	Purpose	Data domain and description	ML algorithms	Results
Nobles et al., [122]	Suicide/Self-harm (*Prognosis*)	To design a prospective ML model to predict periods of suicidality versus depression using data from textual communications. The model is built utilizing retrospective data from suicide ideators, by recreating the chronology to a period before they had suicidal thoughts.	Questionnaire/Smartphone Undergraduate students of department of Psychology of university of Virginia were screened using online surveys for detecting students who have had suicidal thoughts in the past but had no current suicide plan or intent and were ready to share their previous SMS data for the study. After the screening processes 26 students were qualified and their past SMS data was accessed and analyzed for the study.	LIWC, SVM, deep neural network	The results demonstrate that the model achieved an accuracy of 70%.
Literatures focusing on the usage of data from electronic health records (EHRs) (n = 5)					
Burke et al., [105]	Suicide/Self-harm	To apply machine learning approaches to create algorithms that categorize youth with recent and lifetime suicide attempts based on their overall behavioral health symptom profile.	Questionnaire/Electronic health records The study included 13,325 emergency department and primary care patients between the ages of 14 and 24. The behavioral health screen (BHS) was performed electronically by the participants. The study relied on the data from the questionnaire and participants' electronic medical records.	Decision trees, random forests	Across methods, key behavioral health symptom for suicide classification were identified as follows: a history of active and passive suicidal ideation, suicide planning, and nonsuicidal self-injury emerged as important in classifying suicide attempt history. The performance was similar across ridge and random forests.

Schultebraucks et al., [103]	Posttraumatic stress disorder	To develop and test of a machine learning algorithm for predicting posttraumatic stress disorder.	Electronic health records For the development and validation of the algorithm, electronic health records were obtained from two separate cohorts of ED patients hospitalized following trauma (n = 377 from Grady Memorial hospital in atlanta; n = 377 from Bellevue hospital center in New York City).	Logistic regression	Results show that the algorithm achieved extremely high discriminating accuracy on the development dataset (AUC = 0.96), and reasonably good performance (AUC = 0.78) on the independent external validation set.
Zheng et al., [106]	Suicide/Self-harm	To develop an early-warning system for high-risk suicide attempt patients through the establishment of a population-based risk stratification surveillance system	Electronic health records The studied dataset was obtained from the EHR of all patients who visited any of the three Berkshire health system hospital between.January 1, 2015 and December 31, 2017	Deep neural network, multivariate logistic regression	The area under the curve (AUC ROC) of the 1-year suicide attempt risk model was 0.792 and 0.769 in the retrospective and prospective cohorts, respectively
Su et al., [108]	Suicide/Self-harm	To develop machine learning models for predicting suicidal behavior in children and adolescents based on long-term clinical data, as well as identifying long- and short term risk factors.	Electronic health records The researchers utilized electronic health records from the Connecticut Children's medical center from October 1, 2011, to September 30, 2016. The study includes clinical information from 41,721 young patients (10−18 years old).	Logistic regression	Suicidal behavior was predicted by the proposed predictive models across all prediction windows, with AUCs ranging from 0.81 to 0.86.
Wu et al., [107]	Depression	To extract symptom profiles and cognitive impairment from electronic health records using text mining.	Electronic health records The National Taiwan University Hospital's Integrated Medical Database (NTUH-iMD) from January 1, 2006 to September 30, 2016 was used. The study included a total of 4836 discharge notes from a psychiatric facility with a primary mental diagnosis.	Natural language processing	The text mining technique performs well in recognizing depressed symptoms; however, the recall for functional impairment is lower, resulting in F-scores of 0.774−0.753.

(Continued)

Table 1.1 A summary of papers in review corpus that use machine learning to diagnose and treat mental health disorders.—cont'd

Reference	Mental health target	Purpose	Data domain and description	ML algorithms	Results
Literatures focusing on the usage of data collected from social media platforms (n = 11)					
Ophir et al., [109]	Suicide/Self-harm	To forecast the risk of suicide among social media users based on their everyday language.	Social media The dataset includes 83,292 postings from 1002 verified Facebook users, as well as accurate psychosocial data about the participants.	Artificial neural network	The model produced improved prediction accuracy of $0.697 \leq AUC \leq 0.746$. The findings also showed that predictions were based on a variety of text characteristics rather than obvious suicide-related themes.
Fauziah et al., [110]	Anxiety	To demonstrate the use of text mining and machine learning technologies to identify anxiety during the pandemic.	Social media The study examined a sample of 4862 YouTube comments, comprising 3211 negative comments and 1651 favorable remarks.	Random forest, XGBOOST	The random forest and XGBOOST techniques were shown to be 83% and 73% accurate, respectively.
Praveen et al., [111]	Anxiety/Stress	To get a better understanding of Indian citizens' attitudes on COVID-19-related anxiety, stress, and trauma, as well as the primary causes of it.	Social media 840,000 tweets by Indian Citizens were used as the data for this study.	Natural language processing	Even while describing the stress, worry, and trauma produced by COVID-19, the majority of tweets were in neutral feelings. The two most prominent components of the COVID-19 that generated tension, anxiety, and trauma among Indian civilians were death and lockdown.

Chang et al., [112]	Anxiety	To help identify social anxiety disorder patients for early intervention	Questionnaire/Social media For the study, 200 online social network users were recruited, and they completed standard anxiety disorder scale questionnaires. The participants' facebook data was also used in the study for training and testing machine learning models.	Support vector machine (SVM)	One-class SVM obtains a 0.794 F1-score, according to the results.
Kamal et al., [113]	Posttraumatic stress disorder	To develop a novel ML methodology to classify the patient's mental illness on the basis of their posts (along with their relevant comments) shared on "Reddit."	Social media Data from the social media platform "Reddit" is used in this study, posts from four clinical subreddits were collected: r/Schizophrenia, r/Autism, r/OCD and r/PTSD.	XGBoost	Results show that the model created detects PTSD (with F-score 0.63), effectively and can be used for the diagnosis of mental illnesses.
Verma et al., [114]	Depression	To develop a machine learning model for investigating depression that is both effective and scalable.	Social media The data used in this study are tweets extracted from the user. Two datasets are used as inputs to the model. The tweets of depressed and nondepressed users are used. Tweepy, a Python library, was used to access the Twitter API.	Support vector machine, random forest, K-neural network, Naïve Bayes	The overall accuracy achieved using Naïve Bayes, SVM, KNN and random forest were 58%, 69%, 70% and 78% respectively
Reece et al., [115]	Depression	To use machine learning methods including color analysis, metadata components, and face identification to successfully identify depression signals from Instagram pictures.	Social media A total of 43,950 photographs from 166 Instagram users were collected for the study, 71 of whom had a history of depression.	Logistic regression	The models that resulted exceeded the average unassisted diagnostic success rate for depression among general practitioners. These findings held true even when the study was limited to posts published before depressed people were identified.

(Continued)

Table 1.1 A summary of papers in review corpus that use machine learning to diagnose and treat mental health disorders.—cont'd

Reference	Mental health target	Purpose	Data domain and description	ML algorithms	Results
Gupta et al., [116]	Suicide/Self-harm	To discover social media users who are on the brink of inflicting self-harm or commit suicide due to fragile mental health conditions.	Social media Reddit posts were used as data points in this study to identify users with higher relative risk of inflicting self-harm	Naïve Bayes	The Naïve Bayes classifier stably categorized Reddit users at greater risk of self-harm with a precision value of 71.40%, according to the findings.
Roy et al., [118]	Suicide/Self-harm	To design the algorithm termed "Suicide artificial intelligence prediction Heuristic (SAIPH)," which analyses publicly accessible Twitter data to forecast future risk of suicide ideation.	Social media A total of 512,526 tweets from 283 suicidal individuals and 3,518,494 tweets from 2655 controls were used to train the algorithm.	Random forest, neural network	With an AUC of 0.88, the model predicted $N = 830$ suicide ideation events generated from a separate sample of 277 suicide ideators compared to $N = 3159$ control events in all control subjects.
Tadesse et al., [119]	Suicide/Self-harm	Using deep learning and machine learning-based categorization techniques applied to Reddit social media, for early identification of suicidal thoughts.	Social media The study's dataset includes 3549 suicide-indicative posts and 3652 non-suicidal posts from reasonably big subreddits dedicated to helping possibly at-risk people.	Natural language processing, convolutional neural network, SVM, Naive Bayes, random forest, gradient boosting	The results reveal that long short-term memory—CNN outperforms other algorithms, with an accuracy of 93.8% and an F1 score of 92.8%.

Sarker et al., [120]	Substance use	To obtain real-time temporal and geographical data on opioid usage from social media data using natural language processing.	Social media The study examined publicly available tweets that were geolocated in Pennsylvania and dated from January 1, 2012, to October 31, 2015. Prescription and illegal opioid names, including street names and misspellings, were used to extract tweets mentioning opioids. The tweets (n = 9006) were manually classified into four categories, and different machine learning methods were trained and evaluated.	Natural language processing, Naïve Bayes, decision tree, support vector machine, random forest, CNN, k-nearest neighbor	Supervised machine learning algorithms accomplished automatic 4-class categorization of opioid-related social media discourse with a highest F1 score of 0.726.

4. Challenges of using machine learning in studying mental health

Though the use of ML techniques in mental health applications can be beneficial, both as a primary technique for assessing a person's mental well-being when clinical therapy is not available and as a secondary mechanism to assist health professionals and specialists in diagnosing and treating individuals with mental health issues, there are some challenges and risks to be considered, addressed, and eventually solved.

4.1 Unavailability of large and diverse datasets

The quality of data currently available to train and test ML algorithms inevitably limits the same. Researchers require larger and more diverse datasets to create better machine learning models, which may need increased collaboration and cooperation between researchers and clinicians in order to exchange and harmonize data [107,119,120]. Currently, almost no datasets are being created with the purpose of being utilized in the development of ML models; therefore, new comprehensive datasets targeted toward training and testing various ML algorithms in the mental health context must be produced.

4.2 Real-life implementation of ML models to study mental health

A model that may look very promising in the laboratory setting, upon implementation in real-world scenarios, is likely to create additional problems due to multifaceted reasons. The majority of the models studied have been on a population scale rather than an individual level; however in real life, ML algorithms are anticipated to identify mental health in an individual context when the patients opt for diagnosis by healthcare professionals. Most existing research has only utilized retrospective data to train and test models; such models are unaware of current global events, such as natural disasters and related incidents, which may have a stark influence on public mental health, and therefore the model's dynamic efficacy is reduced. Moreover, some studies only provide limited evidence to make causal claims to be used in real-life clinical scenarios [89,90]. Further study is therefore needed to assess the therapeutic usefulness of ML models in a real-world environment. Furthermore, because mental health status can change dramatically over time, future models should be capable of identifying weak signals as well as continually evolving mental health detection situations.

Moreover, because ML is being used more than ever in studying and understanding people's mental health, special care must be taken to develop models that can not only effectively detect people at true risk of various mental disorders but also have a reduced rate of false positives. Mental health, unlike physical health, is still misunderstood by the general public, a false positive report can have far-reaching consequences for the person falsely diagnosed, affecting their self-esteem, reputation, and even employment in some cases, due to widespread ignorance and stigma.

4.3 Lack of specificity

There is a general lack in specificity in the studies that have been done; researchers have outlined mental health problems as a general problem rather than concentrating on a specific form of mental illness. Except for a few studies, most prior studies did not include and consider the multiple categories of mental health disorders, and thus were not included in this review in accordance to the previously mentioned exclusion criteria. To make the results more relevant in real-world settings, the challenge of extracting various characteristics in order to increase the study's specificity must be accepted.

4.4 Nonutilization of data that are not in English

Most of the studies done till date have been using only the datasets (EHRs, questionnaire answers, social media posts) that are in English, thus in future, the fascinating challenge to utilize datasets in other languages and those that are multilingual should take up.

4.5 Lack of data security and unambiguous ethical code

Researchers should also focus on developing ways for increasing the security in storing health and behavioral data acquired from smart devices in order to create ML models, sometimes in an unobtrusive manner with the informed permission of patients.

Furthermore, a complete and unambiguous ethical framework should be created so that (i) patients' privacy is effectively protected and (ii) researchers have a clear understanding of how they may utilize the data obtained responsibly.

5. Limitations

The corpus covered in this study is far from exhaustive, and new research is continually being published in this domain, now more than ever. We realize that the significance of our research is somewhat constrained by our paper selection criteria, since we were only able to evaluate works published in peer-reviewed publications and were written in English for this study. Furthermore, our study excluded studies that outlined mental health issues as a general problem rather than concentrating on discovering specific illnesses from the available data. Since, in this study we try to explore plausible ways to handle mental health degradation during the COVID-19 pandemic and illustrate how data-driven, ML-based methods can serve a critical purpose in doing the same, we made a deliberate decision to exclude studies that used data from advanced medical instruments to train the ML algorithms, as those kind of instruments are not accessible during the pandemic; however, the studies involving the use of data from clinical instruments can help to build ML models that have better accuracy than the ones that use remotely accessible data.

The analysis we provide includes more detailed descriptions of the specific studies we reviewed, restricting our ability to investigate the nature and pattern of the research activity more broadly. Nonetheless, this chapter provides an overview of the present obstacles in utilizing ML to research mental health (in Section 4), as well as a discussion of potential future directions (in Section 6).

To decrease the potential of bias in the collection of data, three researchers systematically assessed and identified potential article, with disagreements addressed by full-text examination and discussion. Important information was carefully retrieved from each article, and a standard data extraction sheet was utilized to store the same in a systematic and structured manner. All members of the study analyzed and reevaluated reports and interpretations on a regular basis to ensure that descriptions of various approaches and findings were balanced.

6. Conclusion and future directions

In conclusion, the study that we present here can be divided into two broad themes: first, we try to understand the impact of the COVID-19 outbreak on our mental health, and second, we try to find feasible solutions to this mental health problem, largely utilizing a data-driven, ML approach. We here conduct a systematic analysis of the current corpus of articles to gain more insight about the said topics.

We discovered upon reviewing articles illustrating the impact of the COVID-19 pandemic and previous comparable natural calamities on the mental well-being of the population in general and some groups in particular that the COVID-19 pandemic has resulted in a pervasive decline in the mental health of the population at large.

It has sparked fears of losing loved ones, of not being able to access healthcare services (especially among the elderly and people suffering from chronic illnesses) when they are needed owing to the present overcrowding, and due to the economic uncertainty brought about by the lockdown has caused many to be concerned about salary cuts and job losses (especially among the working professionals), this has led to the development of mental stress and potentially long-term mental health issues such as anxiety and depression.

A study of the population's mental health status following prior global/regional scale natural and economic crises suggests that we may witness a sharp increase in suicide rates and drug misuse (especially among college students and working professionals). According to a study of the mental health of healthcare professionals who treated people during previous epidemics, they are more prone to suffer from serious cases of PTSD because they are the ones combating the virus with inadequate facilities and witnessing its devastation up close.

These severe mental health implications of the first part of the chapter, motivated our exploration of papers discussing data-driven methods to detect and treat mental health issues (in a remote manner) using ML and AI. We comprehensively analyzed the relevant literature dealing with the development of such ML algorithms. For each reviewed paper, we provide discussion about five main aspects of it—the mental health condition the paper addresses, the purpose of the research, the type of data used and how it was collected, ML algorithms and methods used, and the results the corresponding study yielded.

While conducting the study we only included those studies that used data types that are remotely accessible, such as recorded audio/video data, data collected from smart wearables, questionnaires, which can be hosted online, electronic medical records, and social media data. We refrain from including the studies that included the involvement of clinical machinery such as the studies suggesting the use of brain imaging using fMRI, etc., since such machinery is not remotely accessible to the general population, especially during a period when movement is severely restricted.

Most of the papers that we review have used audio/video data, social media data, and data collected from smart wearables for developing and validating the ML models. Moreover, audio/video data, social media data, and data from smart wearables are the ones that can be most readily accessed during the pandemic situation. The currently available electronic medical records in most parts of the world are severely ill-maintained and flawed; studies that employ online surveys and questionnaires solely to study mental well-being also suffer from severe biases and thus cannot be implemented effectively in real-life scenarios.

The current challenges in using ML techniques for studying and treating mental health conditions have also been outlined in Section 4, and should be addressed in future studies on mental health using ML. Furthermore, the majority of present research focuses solely on detecting mental health concerns; little work has been done to dynamically investigate the course of mental health illnesses and build ML approaches for therapeutic treatment of patients.

Future researchers and enthusiasts might try to capitalize the data-driven mental health assessment techniques by developing products such as a smartphone applications to continually study multimodal data collected from the patient's smartphone with their informed consent and develop ML algorithms, which will not only help in detection of mental health disorders but also track the progression of such disorders. A well-integrated application should not only make use of critical data collected from the sensors of the smartphone, but add additional features such as daily questionnaires to assess the perception of the patient. The application might also be used to provide critical interventions if suicidal tendencies starts to develop by daily affirmations or by building support groups for people who are lonely. With collaboration of doctors and data scientists, such an application can be developed to provide all-round help to the people who need assistance during the COVID-19 pandemic in a remote manner. If such an application can be developed, and promoted for use in a large and diverse population, a well-maintained structured dataset can also be developed, following ethical guidelines and protecting privacy of the users, which is currently not present. Production of such a dataset would be unimaginably helpful in promoting further research in this domain.

Future researchers can also study the effect the pandemic has had on mental health by segregating the studies on the basis of race, economic standing, and social status and thereby highlight the difference that exists (if any). This method can bring forth if people of some race or social status are being disproportionately affected, and we can study and theorize the reasons why.

Finally, we must say that increased investment is needed to perform research on all fronts in mental health to promote understanding of it on a medical and social level and publish those results to spread awareness and thereby decrease the prevalent stigma against mental health patients. Efforts must be made to promote accessibility to quality mental health care and effective therapies even during periods of global crisis; research must also be done to find novel treatments and improve existing treatments for all mental diseases, and data-driven methods using ML analysis will have a key role to play in achieving these objectives.

References

[1] M.C. Angermeyer, A. Holzinger, H. Matschinger, Mental health literacy and attitude towards people with mental illness: a trend analysis based on population surveys in the eastern part of Germany, Eur. Psychiat. 24 (4) (2009) 225–232, https://doi.org/10.1016/j.eurpsy.2008.06.010.

[2] Y. Tesfaye, L. Agenagnew, G. Terefe Tucho, S. Anand, Z. Birhanu, G. Ahmed, M. Getenet, K. Yitbarek, Attitude and help-seeking behavior of the community towards mental health problems, PLoS One 15 (11) (2020) e0242160, https://doi.org/10.1371/journal.pone.0242160.

[3] A. Bagchi, P. Sarkar, R. Basu, Knowledge, attitude and practice towards mental health illnesses in an urban community in West Bengal: a community based study, Int J Commun. Med. Publ. Heal. 7 (3) (2020) 1078–1083, https://doi.org/10.18203/2394-6040.ijcmph20200970.

[4] M. Chen, S. Mao, Y. Liu, Big data: a survey, Mobile Netw. Appl. 19 (2) (2014) 171–209, https://doi.org/10.1007/s11036-013-0489-0.

[5] M.I. Jordan, T.M. Mitchell, Machine learning: trends, perspectives, and prospects, Science 349 (6245) (2015) 255–260, https://doi.org/10.1126/science.aaa8415.

[6] A. Fink, Conducting Literature Research Reviews: From Paper to the Internet, Sage Publications, Inc, Thousand Oaks, CA, 1998.

[7] C. Pickering, J. Byrne, The benefits of publishing systematic quantitative literature reviews for PhD candidates and other early-career researchers, High Educ. Res. Dev. 33 (3) (2014) 534–548, https://doi.org/10.1080/07294360.2013.841651.

[8] Mental Health: Strengthening Our Response, World Health Organization, August 2014. Retrieved 4 May 2014.

[9] UNESCO's data on school closures worldwide. https://en.unesco.org/covid19/educationresponse.

[10] M. Qi, S.J. Zhou, Z.C. Guo, L.G. Zhang, H.J. Min, X.M. Li, J.X. Chen, The effect of social support on mental health in Chinese adolescents during the outbreak of COVID-19, J. Adolesc. Health 67 (4) (2020) 514–518, https://doi.org/10.1016/j.jadohealth.2020.07.001.

[11] U. Rehman, M.G. Shahnawaz, N.H. Khan, K.D. Kharshiing, M. Khursheed, K. Gupta, D. Kashyap, R. Uniyal, Depression, anxiety and stress among Indians in times of Covid-19 lockdown, Commun. Mental Health J. 57 (1) (2021) 42–48, https://doi.org/10.1007/s10597-020-00664-x.

[12] M. Alkwiese, S.H. Alsaqri, M. Aldalaykeh, M. Hamzi, M. Mahdi, Z. Shafie, Anxiety among the general population during coronavirus-19 disease in Saudi Arabia:

implications for a mental support program, medRxiv (2020), https://doi.org/10.1101/2020.05.07.20090225.
[13] Centers for Disease Control and Prevention. Data and statistics on children's mental health. Accessed March 27, 2020. https://www.cdc.gov/childrensmentalhealth/data.html.
[14] E. Golberstein, G. Gonzales, E. Meara, How do economic downturns affect the mental health of children? Evidence from the National Health Interview Survey, Health Econ. 28 (8) (2019) 955–970, https://doi.org/10.1002/hec.3885.
[15] L. Liang, H. Ren, R. Cao, Y. Hu, Z. Qin, C. Li, S. Mei, The effect of COVID-19 on youth mental health, Psychiatr. Q. 91 (3) (2020) 841–852, https://doi.org/10.1007/s11126-020- 09744-3.
[16] A. Khattar, P.R. Jain, S.M.K. Quadri, Effects of the disastrous pandemic COVID 19 on learning styles, activities and mental health of young Indian students-a machine learning approach, in: 2020 4th International Conference on Intelligent Computing and Control Systems (ICICCS), IEEE, May 2020, pp. 1190–1195, https://doi.org/10.1109/ICICCS48265.2020.9120955.
[17] Coronavirus: Impact on Young People with Mental Health Needs, 2020. Survey, https://youngminds.org.uk/about-us/reports/coronavirus-impact-on-young-people-with-mental-health-needs/.
[18] A. Kakunje, R. Mithur, M. Kishor, Emotional well-being, mental health awareness, and prevention of suicide: Covid-19 pandemic and digital psychiatry, Archiv. Med. Health Sci. 8 (1) (2020) 147, https://doi.org/10.4103/amhs.amhs_98_20.
[19] N. Kapasia, P. Paul, A. Roy, J. Saha, A. Zaveri, R. Mallick, B. Barman, P. Das, P. Chouhan, Impact of lockdown on learning status of undergraduate and postgraduate students during COVID-19 pandemic in West Bengal, India, Child. Youth Serv. Rev. 116 (2020) 105194, https://doi.org/10.1016/j.childyouth.2020.105194.
[20] C. Son, S. Hegde, A. Smith, X. Wang, F. Sasangohar, Effects of COVID-19 on college students' mental health in the United States: interview survey study, J. Med. Internet Res. 22 (9) (2020) e21279. https://www.jmir.org/2020/9/e21279.
[21] Z. Lyons, H. Wilcox, L. Leung, O. Dearsley, COVID-19 and the mental well-being of Australian medical students: impact, concerns and coping strategies used, Australas. Psychiat. 28 (6) (2020) 649–652, https://doi.org/10.1177/1039856220947945.
[22] Y. Zhang, H. Zhang, X. Ma, Q. Di, Mental health problems during the COVID-19 pandemics and the mitigation effects of exercise: a longitudinal study of college students in China, Int. J. Environ. Res. Publ. Health 17 (10) (2020) 3722, https://doi.org/10.3390/ijerph17103722.
[23] T. Gonzalez, M.A. De La Rubia, K.P. Hincz, M. Comas-Lopez, L. Subirats, S. Fort, G.M. Sacha, Influence of COVID-19 confinement on students' performance in higher education, PLoS One 15 (10) (2020) e0239490, https://doi.org/10.1371/journal.pone.0239490.
[24] N. Hasan, Y. Bao, Impact of "e-Learning crack-up" perception on psychological distress among college students during COVID-19 pandemic: a mediating role of "fear of academic year loss", Child. Youth Serv. Rev. 118 (2020) 105355, https://doi.org/10.1016/j.childyouth.2020.105355.
[25] C. Wang, H. Zhao, H. Zhang, Chinese college students have higher anxiety in new semester of online learning during COVID-19: a machine learning approach, Front. Psychol. 11 (2020) 3465, https://doi.org/10.3389/fpsyg.2020.587413.
[26] C. Herbert, A. El Bolock, S. Abdennadher, How do you feel during the COVID-19 pandemic? A survey using psychological and linguistic self-report measures, and machine learning to investigate mental health, subjective experience, personality, and behaviour during the COVID-19 pandemic among university students, BMC Psychol. 9 (1) (2021) 1–23, https://doi.org/10.1186/s40359-021-00574-x.

[27] I. Akour, M. Alshurideh, B. Al Kurdi, A. Al Ali, S. Salloum, Using machine learning algorithms to predict people's intention to use mobile learning platforms during the COVID-19 pandemic: machine learning approach, JMIR Med. Educ. 7 (1) (2021) e24032, https://doi.org/10.2196/24032.
[28] G. George, M.R. Thomas, Quarantined effects and strategies of college students—COVID-19, Asian Educ. Dev. Stud. (2020), https://doi.org/10.1108/AEDS-04-2020-0054.
[29] I.P. Jha, R. Awasthi, A. Kumar, V. Kumar, T. Sethi, Learning the mental health impact of COVID-19 in the United States with explainable artificial intelligence: observational study, JMIR Mental Health 8 (4) (2021) e25097, https://doi.org/10.2196/25097.
[30] J. Xue, J. Chen, R. Hu, C. Chen, C. Zheng, Y. Su, T. Zhu, Twitter discussions and emotions about the COVID-19 pandemic: machine learning approach, J. Med. Internet Res. 22 (11) (2020) e20550, https://doi.org/10.2196/20550.
[31] A. Chakraborty, A.K. Kar, How did COVID-19 impact working professionals — a typology of impacts focused on education sector, Int. J. Inform. Learn. Technol. 38 (3) (2021) 273—282, https://doi.org/10.1108/IJILT-06-2020-0125.
[32] D. Posel, A. Oyenubi, U. Kollamparambil, Job loss and mental health during the COVID-19 lockdown: evidence from South Africa, PLoS One 16 (3) (2021) e0249352, https://doi.org/10.1371/journal.pone.0249352.
[33] M.A. Mamun, I. Ullah, COVID-19 suicides in Pakistan, dying off not COVID-19 fear but poverty?—The forthcoming economic challenges for a developing country, Brain Behav. Immun. 87 (2020) 163, https://doi.org/10.1016/2Fj.bbi.2020.05.028.
[34] R.C. Kessler, S. Galea, M.J. Gruber, N.A. Sampson, R.J. Ursano, S. Wessely, Trends in mental illness and suicidality after Hurricane Katrina, Mol. Psychiatr. 13 (4) (2008) 374—384, https://doi.org/10.1038/sj.mp.4002119.
[35] Preliminary Statistics of Cases of Suicide in Puerto Rico, 2017 (in Spanish), http://www.salud.gov.pr.
[36] I.M. Wasserman, The impact of epidemic, war, prohibition and media on suicide: United States, 1910—1920, Suicide Life-Threatening Behav. 22 (2) (1992) 240—254, https://doi.org/10.1111/j.1943-278X.1992.tb00231.x.
[37] F. Luo, C.S. Florence, M. Quispe-Agnoli, L. Ouyang, A.E. Crosby, Impact of business cycles on US suicide rates, 1928—2007, Am. J. Publ. Health 101 (6) (2011) 1139—1146. https://ajph.aphapublications.org/doi/abs/10.2105/AJPH.2010.300010.
[38] S.S. Chang, D. Gunnell, J.A. Sterne, T.H. Lu, A.T. Cheng, Was the economic crisis 1997—1998 responsible for rising suicide rates in East/Southeast Asia? A time—trend analysis for Japan, Hong Kong, South Korea, Taiwan, Singapore and Thailand, Social Sci. Med. 68 (7) (2009) 1322—1331, https://doi.org/10.1016/j.socscimed.2009.01.010.
[39] P. Corcoran, E. Griffin, E. Arensman, A.P. Fitzgerald, I.J. Perry, Impact of the economic recession and subsequent austerity on suicide and self-harm in Ireland: an interrupted time series analysis, Int. J. Epidemiol. 44 (3) (2015) 969—977, https://doi.org/10.1093/ije/dyv058.
[40] D. Stuckler, S. Basu, M. Suhrcke, A. Coutts, M. McKee, The public health effect of economic crises and alternative policy responses in Europe: an empirical analysis, Lancet 374 (9686) (2009) 315—323, https://doi.org/10.1016/S0140-6736(09)61124-7.
[41] E.K. Fry-Bowers, Children are at risk from COVID-19, J. Pediatr. Nurs. 53 (2020) A10, https://doi.org/10.1016/2Fj.pedn.2020.04.026.

[42] M.P. Crayne, The traumatic impact of job loss and job search in the aftermath of COVID-19, Psychol. Trau. Theory Res. Prac. Policy 12 (S1) (2020) S180. https://psycnet.apa.org/doi/10.1037/tra0000852.

[43] J. Shigemura, R.J. Ursano, J.C. Morganstein, M. Kurosawa, D.M. Benedek, Public responses to the new coronavirus 2019 (2019-nCoV) in Japan: consequences for mental health and target populations, Psychiat. Clin. Neurosci. 74 (4) (2020) 281–282, https://doi.org/10.1111/pcn.12988.

[44] L. Kang, Y. Li, S. Hu, M. Chen, C. Yang, B.X. Yang, Y. Wang, J. Hu, J. Lai, X. Ma, J. Chen, The mental health of medical workers in Wuhan, China dealing with the 2019 novel coronavirus, Lancet Psychiat. (2020). https://psycnet.apa.org/doi/10.1016/S2215-0366(20)30047-X.

[45] S. Liu, L. Yang, C. Zhang, Y.T. Xiang, Z. Liu, S. Hu, B. Zhang, Online mental health services in China during the COVID-19 outbreak, Lancet Psychiat. 7 (4) (2020) e17–e18, https://doi.org/10.1016/S2215-0366(20)30077-8.

[46] J.Z. Huang, M.F. Han, T.D. Luo, A.K. Ren, X.P. Zhou, Mental health survey of 230 medical staff in a tertiary infectious disease hospital for COVID-19, Zhonghua lao dong wei sheng zhi ye bing za zhi= Zhonghua laodong weisheng zhiyebing zazhi= Chin. J. Indus. Hyg. Occup. Dis. 38 (2020), https://doi.org/10.3760/cma.j.cn121094-20200219-00063. E001-E001.

[47] S. Bagcchi, Stigma during the COVID-19 pandemic, Lancet Infect. Dis. 20 (7) (2020) 782, https://doi.org/10.1016/S1473-3099(20)30498-9.

[48] Y.T. Xiang, Y. Yang, W. Li, L. Zhang, Q. Zhang, T. Cheung, C.H. Ng, Timely mental health care for the 2019 novel coronavirus outbreak is urgently needed, Lancet Psychiat. 7 (3) (2020) 228–229, https://doi.org/10.1016/S2215-0366(20)30046-8.

[49] M. Malta, A.W. Rimoin, S.A. Strathdee, The coronavirus 2019-nCoV epidemic: is hindsight 20/20? EClinicalMedicine 20 (2020) https://doi.org/10.1016/j.eclinm.2020.100289.

[50] Z. Li, J. Ge, M. Yang, J. Feng, M. Qiao, R. Jiang, J. Bi, G. Zhan, X. Xu, L. Wang, Q. Zhou, Vicarious traumatization in the general public, members, and non-members of medical teams aiding in COVID-19 control, Brain Behav. Immun. 88 (2020) 916–919, https://doi.org/10.1016/j.bbi.2020.03.007.

[51] F. Ornell, J.B. Schuch, A.O. Sordi, F.H.P. Kessler, "Pandemic fear" and COVID-19: mental health burden and strategies, Braz. J. Psychiat. 42 (3) (2020) 232–235, https://doi.org/10.1590/1516-4446-2020-0008.

[52] D. Banerjee, 'Age and ageism in COVID-19': elderly mental health-care vulnerabilities and needs, Asian J. Psychiat. 51 (2020) 102154, https://doi.org/10.1016/2Fj.ajp.2020.102154.

[53] K. Gerst-Emerson, J. Jayawardhana, Loneliness as a public health issue: the impact of loneliness on health care utilization among older adults, Am. J. Publ. Health 105 (5) (2015) 1013–1019. https://ajph.aphapublications.org/doi/abs/10.2105/AJPH.2014.302427.

[54] Z.I. Santini, P.E. Jose, E.Y. Cornwell, A. Koyanagi, L. Nielsen, C. Hinrichsen, C. Meilstrup, K.R. Madsen, V. Koushede, Social disconnectedness, perceived isolation, and symptoms of depression and anxiety among older Americans (NSHAP): a longitudinal mediation analysis, Lancet Pub. Health 5 (1) (2020) e62–e70, https://doi.org/10.1016/S2468-2667(19)30230-0.

[55] R. Aylaz, Ü. Aktürk, B. Erci, H. Öztürk, H. Aslan, Relationship between depression and loneliness in elderly and examination of influential factors, Arch. Gerontol. Geriatr. 55 (3) (2012) 548–554, https://doi.org/10.1016/j.archger.2012.03.006.

[56] R. Armitage, L.B. Nellums, COVID-19 and the consequences of isolating the elderly, Lancet Pub. Health 5 (5) (2020) e256, https://doi.org/10.1016/S2468-2667(20)30061-X.

[57] P.S. Yip, Y.T. Cheung, P.H. Chau, Y.W. Law, The impact of epidemic outbreak, Crisis (2010), https://doi.org/10.1027/0227-5910/a000015.

[58] Y.T. Cheung, P.H. Chau, P.S. Yip, A revisit on older adults suicides and Severe Acute Respiratory Syndrome (SARS) epidemic in Hong Kong, Int. J. Geriatr. Psychiat. J Psychiat. Late Life All. Sci. 23 (12) (2008) 1231–1238, https://doi.org/10.1002/gps.2056.

[59] C. Ciacci, M. Siniscalchi, Tips from the battlefront: psychological support of patients with a chronic illness during the COVID-19 lockdown in four steps, Uni. Eur. Gastroenterol. J. 8 (6) (2020) 741–742, https://doi.org/10.1177/2F2050640620927564.

[60] D.S. Sheha, A.S. Abdel-Rehim, O.M. Abdel-Latif, M.A. Abdelkader, R.H. Raafat, S.A. Sallam, N.S. Mostafa, Level of asthma control and mental health of asthma patients during lockdown for COVID-19: a cross-sectional survey, Egyp. J. Bronchol. 15 (1) (2021) 1–10, https://doi.org/10.1186/s43168-021-00058-x.

[61] J. Alessi, G.B. De Oliveira, D.W. Franco, B.B. Do Amaral, A.S. Becker, C.P. Knijnik, G.L. Kobe, T.R. De Carvalho, G.H. Telo, B.D. Schaan, G.H. Telo, Mental health in the era of COVID-19: prevalence of psychiatric disorders in a cohort of patients with type 1 and type 2 diabetes during the social distancing, Diabetol. Metab. Syndr. 12 (1) (2020) 1–10, https://doi.org/10.1186/s13098-020-00584-6.

[62] Y. Wang, Z. Duan, Z. Ma, Y. Mao, X. Li, A. Wilson, H. Qin, J. Ou, K. Peng, F. Zhou, C. Li, Epidemiology of mental health problems among patients with cancer during COVID-19 pandemic, Transl. Psychiat. 10 (1) (2020) 1–10, https://doi.org/10.1038/s41398-020-00950-y.

[63] J. Zhao, W. Su, J. Jia, C. Zhang, T. Lu, Research on depression detection algorithm combine acoustic rhythm with sparse face recognition, Cluster Comput. 22 (4) (2019) 7873–7884, https://doi.org/10.1007/s10586-017-1469-0.

[64] K.H. Chang, M.K. Chan, J. Canny, AnalyzeThis: unobtrusive mental health monitoring by voice, in: CHI'11 Extended Abstracts on Human Factors in Computing Systems, 2011, pp. 1951–1956, https://doi.org/10.1145/1979742.1979859.

[65] G. Bedi, G.A. Cecchi, D.F. Slezak, F. Carrillo, M. Sigman, H. De Wit, A window into the intoxicated mind? Speech as an index of psychoactive drug effects, Neuropsychopharmacology 39 (10) (2014) 2340 2348, https://doi.org/10.1038/npp.2014.80.

[66] M.J. Baggott, M.G. Kirkpatrick, G. Bedi, H. de Wit, Intimate insight: MDMA changes how people talk about significant others, J. Psychopharmacol. 29 (6) (2015) 669–677, https://doi.org/10.1177/2F0269881115581962.

[67] J.P. Pestian, J. Grupp-Phelan, K. Bretonnel Cohen, G. Meyers, L.A. Richey, P. Matykiewicz, M.T. Sorter, A controlled trial using natural language processing to examine the language of suicidal adolescents in the emergency department, Suicide Life-Threatening Behav. 46 (2) (2016) 154–159, https://doi.org/10.1111/sltb.12180.

[68] V. Venek, S. Scherer, L.P. Morency, A. Rizzo, J. Pestian, Adolescent suicidal risk assessment in clinician-patient interaction: a study of verbal and acoustic behaviors, in: 2014 IEEE Spoken Language Technology Workshop (SLT), IEEE, December 2014, pp. 277–282, https://doi.org/10.1109/SLT.2014.7078587.

[69] M. Valstar, B. Schuller, K. Smith, T. Almaev, F. Eyben, J. Krajewski, R. Cowie, M. Pantic, Avec 2014: 3d dimensional affect and depression recognition challenge, in: Proceedings of the 4th International Workshop on Audio/visual Emotion Challenge, November 2014, pp. 3–10, https://doi.org/10.1145/2661806.2661807.

[70] V. Mitra, E. Shriberg, M. McLaren, A. Kathol, C. Richey, D. Vergyri, M. Graciarena, The SRI AVEC-2014 evaluation system, in: Proceedings of the 4th International Workshop on Audio/Visual Emotion Challenge, November 2014, pp. 93–101, https://doi.org/10.1145/2661806.2661818.

[71] E.W. McGinnis, S.P. Anderau, J. Hruschak, R.D. Gurchiek, N.L. Lopez-Duran, K. Fitzgerald, K.L. Rosenblum, M. Muzik, R.S. McGinnis, Giving voice to

vulnerable children: machine learning analysis of speech detects anxiety and depression in early childhood, IEEE J. Biomed. Health Inform. 23 (6) (2019) 2294–2301, https://doi.org/10.1109/JBHI.2019.2913590.
[72] F. Ringeval, B. Schuller, M. Valstar, J. Gratch, R. Cowie, S. Scherer, S. Mozgai, N. Cummins, M. Schmitt, M. Pantic, Avec 2017: real-life depression, and affect recognition workshop and challenge, in: Proceedings of the 7th Annual Workshop on Audio/Visual Emotion Challenge, October 2017, pp. 3–9, https://doi.org/10.1145/3133944.3133953.
[73] B. Sun, Y. Zhang, J. He, L. Yu, Q. Xu, D. Li, Z. Wang, A random forest regression method with selected-text feature for depression assessment, in: Proceedings of the 7th Annual Workshop on Audio/Visual Emotion Challenge, October 2017, pp. 61–68, https://doi.org/10.1145/3133944.3133951.
[74] R. Xu, G. Mei, G. Zhang, P. Gao, T. Judkins, M. Cannizzaro, J. Li, A voice-based automated system for PTSD screening and monitoring, in: Medicine Meets Virtual Reality vol. 19, IOS Press, 2012, pp. 552–558, https://doi.org/10.3233/978-1-61499-022-2-552.
[75] K. Schultebraucks, V. Yadav, A.Y. Shalev, G.A. Bonanno, I.R. Galatzer-Levy, Deep learning-based classification of posttraumatic stress disorder and depression following trauma utilizing visual and auditory markers of arousal and mood, Psychol. Med. (2020) 1–11, https://doi.org/10.1017/S0033291720002718.
[76] F. Burkhardt, A. Paeschke, M. Rolfes, W.F. Sendlmeier, B. Weiss, A database of German emotional speech, in: Ninth European Conference on Speech Communication and Technology, 2005.
[77] Keio university Japanese emotional speech database (keioesd).http://research.nii.ac.jp/src/en/Keio-ESD.html. Accessed: 2018-03-29.
[78] S.R. Livingstone, F.A. Russo, The Ryerson audio-visual database of emotional speech and song (RAVDESS): a dynamic, multimodal set of facial and vocal expressions in north American English, PLoS One 13 (5) (2018) e0196391, https://doi.org/10.1371/journal.pone.0196391.
[79] K. Tomba, D. Joel, M. Elena, A.K. Omar, H. Salah, Stress detection through speech analysis, ICETE (1) (2018) 560–564.
[80] J. Gratch, R. Artstein, G.M. Lucas, G. Stratou, S. Scherer, A. Nazarian, R. Wood, J. Boberg, D. DeVault, S. Marsella, D.R. Traum, The distress analysis interview corpus of human and computer interviews, in: LREC, May 2014, pp. 3123–3128.
[81] I. Madhavi, S. Chamishka, R. Nawaratne, V. Nanayakkara, D. Alahakoon, D. De Silva, September. A deep learning approach for work related stress detection from audio streams in cyber physical environments, in: 2020 25th IEEE International Conference on Emerging Technologies and Factory Automation (ETFA), vol. 1, IEEE, 2020, pp. 929–936, https://doi.org/10.1109/ETFA46521.2020.9212098.
[82] H. Zhang, L. Feng, N. Li, Z. Jin, L. Cao, Video-based stress detection through deep learning, Sensors 20 (19) (2020) 5552.
[83] I. Lefter, L.J.M. Rothkrantz, D.A.V. Leeuwen, P. Wiggers, Automatic stress detection in emergency (telephone) calls, Int. J. Intell. Def. Supp. Syst. 4 (2) (2011) 148, https://doi.org/10.1504/ijidss.2011.039547.
[84] Toronto Emotional Speech Set. Database available on http://tspace.library.utoronto.com.
[85] N.P. Dhole, S.N. Kale, Stress Detection in Speech Signal Using Machine Learning and AI. Machine Learning and Information Processing, Springer, Singapore, 2020, pp. 11–26.
[86] R. Irani, K. Nasrollahi, A. Dhall, T.B. Moeslund, T. Gedeon, December. Thermal super-pixels for bimodal stress recognition, in: 2016 Sixth International Conference

on Image Processing Theory, Tools and Applications (IPTA), IEEE, 2016, pp. 1–6, https://doi.org/10.1109/IPTA.2016.7821002.

[87] N. Sharma, A. Dhall, T. Gedeon, R. Goecke, Thermal spatio-temporal data for stress recognition, EURASIP J. Image Video Process. 2014 (1) (2014) 1–12, https://doi.org/10.1186/1687-5281-2014-28.

[88] StudentLife Study information is available at: https://studentlife.cs.dartmouth.edu/.

[89] R. Wang, F. Chen, Z. Chen, T. Li, G. Harari, S. Tignor, X. Zhou, D. Ben-Zeev, A.T. Campbell, September. StudentLife: assessing mental health, academic performance and behavioral trends of college students using smartphones, in: Proceedings of the 2014 ACM International Joint Conference on Pervasive and Ubiquitous Computing, 2014, pp. 3–14, https://doi.org/10.1145/2632048.2632054.

[90] M. Gjoreski, H. Gjoreski, M. Lutrek, M. Gams, Automatic detection of perceived stress in campus students using smartphones, in: 2015 International Conference on Intelligent Environments, IEEE, July 2015, pp. 132–135, https://doi.org/10.1109/IE.2015.27.

[91] L. Canzian, M. Musolesi, Trajectories of depression: unobtrusive monitoring of depressive states by means of smartphone mobility traces analysis, in: Proceedings of the 2015 ACM International Joint Conference on Pervasive and Ubiquitous Computing, September 2015, pp. 1293–1304, https://doi.org/10.1145/2750858.2805845.

[92] E.A. Sağbaş, S. Korukoglu, S. Balli, Stress detection via keyboard typing behaviors by using smartphone sensors and machine learning techniques, J. Med. Syst. 44 (4) (2020) 1–12, https://doi.org/10.1007/s10916-020-1530-z.

[93] T.T. Phan, F. Labhart, S. Muralidhar, D. Gatica-Perez, Understanding heavy drinking at night through smartphone sensing and active human engagement, in: Proceedings of the 14th EAI International Conference on Pervasive Computing Technologies for Healthcare, May 2020, pp. 211–222, https://doi.org/10.1145/3421937.3421992.

[94] T.T. Phan, S. Muralidhar, D. Gatica-Perez, Drinks & crowds: characterizing alcohol consumption through crowdsensing and social media, Proc. ACM Inter. Mobile Wearable Ubiquitous Technol. 3 (2) (2019) 1–30, https://doi.org/10.1145/3328930.

[95] Y. Fukazawa, T. Ito, T. Okimura, Y. Yamashita, T. Maeda, J. Ota, Predicting anxiety state using smartphone-based passive sensing, J. Biomed. Inf. 93 (2019) 103151, https://doi.org/10.1016/j.jbi.2019.103151.

[96] M. Gjoreski, M. Luštrek, G. Matjaž, G. Hristijan, Monitoring stress with a wrist device using context, J. Biomed. Inf. 73 (10.1016) (2017), https://doi.org/10.1016/j.jbi.2017.08.006.

[97] R. Ahuja, A. Banga, Mental stress detection in university students using machine learning algorithms, Proced. Comput. Sci. 152 (2019) 349–353, https://doi.org/10.1016/j.procs.2019.05.007.

[98] K.I. Karstoft, A. Statnikov, S.B. Andersen, T. Madsen, I.R. Galatzer-Levy, Early identification of posttraumatic stress following military deployment: application of machine learning methods to a prospective study of Danish soldiers, J. Affect. Disord. 184 (2015) 170–175, https://doi.org/10.1016/j.jad.2015.05.057.

[99] J.A. Andrews, R.F. Harrison, L.J.E. Brown, L.M. MacLean, F. Hwang, T. Smith, E.A. Williams, C. Timon, T. Adlam, H. Khadra, A.J. Astell, Using the NANA toolkit at home to predict older adults' future depression, J. Affect. Disord. 213 (2017) 187–190, https://doi.org/10.1016/j.jad.2017.02.019.

[100] A.J. Astell, F. Hwang, L.J. Brown, C. Timon, L.M. Maclean, T. Smith, T. Adlam, H. Khadra, E.A. Williams, Validation of the NANA (Novel Assessment of Nutrition

and Ageing) touch screen system for use at home by older adults, Exp. Gerontol. 60 (2014) 100−107, https://doi.org/10.1016/j.exger.2014.10.008.
[101] J.F. Dipnall, J.A. Pasco, M. Berk, L.J. Williams, S. Dodd, F.N. Jacka, D. Meyer, Getting RID of the blues: formulating a Risk Index for Depression (RID) using structural equation modeling, Aust. N. Z. J. Psychiat. 51 (11) (2017) 1121−1133, https://doi.org/10.1177/2F0004867417726860.
[102] C. Zakaria, R. Balan, Y. Lee, StressMon: scalable detection of perceived stress and depression using passive sensing of changes in work routines and group interactions, Proc. ACM Human-Comput. Inter. 3 (CSCW) (2019) 1−29, https://doi.org/10.1145/3359139.
[103] K. Schultebraucks, A.Y. Shalev, V. Michopoulos, C.R. Grudzen, S.M. Shin, J.S. Stevens, J.L. Maples-Keller, T. Jovanovic, G.A. Bonanno, B.O. Rothbaum, C.R. Marmar, A validated predictive algorithm of post-traumatic stress course following emergency department admission after a traumatic stressor, Nat. Med. 26 (7) (2020) 1084−1088, https://doi.org/10.1038/s41591-020-0951-z.
[104] A.E. Tate, R.C. McCabe, H. Larsson, S. Lundström, P. Lichtenstein, R. Kuja-Halkola, Predicting mental health problems in adolescence using machine learning techniques, PLoS One 15 (4) (2020) e0230389, https://doi.org/10.1371/journal.pone.0230389.
[105] T.A. Burke, R. Jacobucci, B.A. Ammerman, L.B. Alloy, G. Diamond, Using machine learning to classify suicide attempt history among youth in medical care settings, J. Affect. Disord. 268 (2020) 206−214, https://doi.org/10.1016/j.jad.2020.02.048.
[106] L. Zheng, O. Wang, S. Hao, C. Ye, M. Liu, M. Xia, A.N. Sabo, L. Markovic, F. Stearns, L. Kanov, K.G. Sylvester, Development of an early-warning system for high-risk patients for suicide attempt using deep learning and electronic health records, Transl. Psychiat. 10 (1) (2020) 1−10, https://doi.org/10.1038/s41398-020-0684-2.
[107] C.S. Wu, C.J. Kuo, C.H. Su, S.H. Wang, H.J. Dai, Using text mining to extract depressive symptoms and to validate the diagnosis of major depressive disorder from electronic health records, J. Affect. Disord. 260 (2020) 617−623, https://doi.org/10.1016/j.jad.2019.09.044.
[108] C. Su, R. Aseltine, R. Doshi, K. Chen, S.C. Rogers, F. Wang, Machine learning for suicide risk prediction in children and adolescents with electronic health records, Transl. Psychiat. 10 (1) (2020) 1−10, https://doi.org/10.1038/s41398-020-01100-0.
[109] Y. Ophir, R. Tikochinski, C.S. Asterhan, I. Sisso, R. Reichart, Deep neural networks detect suicide risk from textual facebook posts, Sci. Rep. 10 (1) (2020) 1−10, https://doi.org/10.1038/s41598-020-73917-0.
[110] Y. Fauziah, S. Saifullah, A.S. Aribowo, Design text mining for anxiety detection using machine learning based-on social media data during COVID-19 pandemic, in: Proceeding of LPPM UPN "Veteran" Yogyakarta Conference Series 2020−Engineering and Science Series, vol. 1, October 2020, pp. 253−261, https://doi.org/10.31098/ess.v1i1.117. No. 1.
[111] S.V. Praveen, R. Ittamalla, G. Deepak, Analyzing Indian general public's perspective on anxiety, stress and trauma during Covid-19-a machine learning study of 840,000 tweets, Diab. Metab. Syndr. Clin. Res. Rev. 15 (3) (2021) 667−671, https://doi.org/10.1016/j.dsx.2021.03.016.
[112] M.Y. Chang, C.Y. Tseng, June. Detecting social anxiety with online social network data, in: 2020 21st IEEE International Conference on Mobile Data Management (MDM), IEEE, 2020, pp. 333−336, https://doi.org/10.1109/MDM48529.2020.00073.

[113] Nasir, A., Aslam, K., Tariq, S. and Ullah, M.F., Predicting Mental Illness using Social Media Posts and Comments. https://doi.org/10.14569/IJACSA.2020.0111271.
[114] P. Verma, K. Sharma, G.S. Walia, Depression detection among social media users using machine learning, in: International Conference on Innovative Computing and Communications, Springer, Singapore, 2021, pp. 865–874, https://doi.org/10.1007/978-981-15-5113-0_72.
[115] A.G. Reece, C.M. Danforth, Instagram photos reveal predictive markers of depression, EPJ Data Sci. 6 (2017) 1–12, https://doi.org/10.1140/epjds/s13688-017-0110-z.
[116] S. Gupta, D. Das, M. Chatterjee, S. Naskar, Machine learning-based social media analysis for suicide risk assessment, in: Emerging Technologies in Data Mining and Information Security, Springer, Singapore, 2021, pp. 385–393, https://doi.org/10.1007/978-981-33-4367-2_37.
[117] Y. Shen, W. Zhang, B.S.M. Chan, Y. Zhang, F. Meng, E.A. Kennon, H.E. Wu, X. Luo, X. Zhang, Detecting risk of suicide attempts among Chinese medical college students using a machine learning algorithm, J. Affect. Disord. 273 (2020) 18–23, https://doi.org/10.1016/j.jad.2020.04.057.
[118] A. Roy, K. Nikolitch, R. McGinn, S. Jinah, W. Klement, Z.A. Kaminsky, A machine learning approach predicts future risk to suicidal ideation from social media data, NPJ Dig. Med. 3 (1) (2020) 1–12, https://doi.org/10.1038/s41746-020-0287-6.
[119] M.M. Tadesse, H. Lin, B. Xu, L. Yang, Detection of suicide ideation in social media forums using deep learning, Algorithms 13 (1) (2020) 7, https://doi.org/10.3390/a13010007.
[120] A. Sarker, G. Gonzalez-Hernandez, Y. Ruan, J. Perrone, Machine learning and natural language processing for geolocation-centric monitoring and characterization of opioid-related social media chatter, JAMA Netw. Open 2 (11) (2019) e1914672-e1914672.
[121] N.C. Jacobson, D. Lekkas, R. Huang, N. Thomas, Deep learning paired with wearable passive sensing data predicts deterioration in anxiety disorder symptoms across 17–18 years, J. Affect. Disord. 282 (2021) 104–111, https://doi.org/10.1016/j.jad.2020.12.086.
[122] A.L. Nobles, J.J. Glenn, K. Kowsari, B.A. Teachman, L.E. Barnes, Identification of imminent suicide risk among young adults using text messages, in: Proceedings of the 2018 CHI Conference on Human Factors in Computing Systems, April 2018, pp. 1–11, https://doi.org/10.1145/3173574.3173987.
[123] T. Gargot, H. Kisand, A. Miguel, S. Tanyeri, T.R. Soron, B. Serene, G. Feron, N. Žaja, M.J. Valdés-Florido, Ó. Soto-Angona, I. Frankova, Preventing Post Traumatic Stress Disorder in the general population induced by trauma during the COVID pandemic: a simple brief intervention based on cognitive science that could be delivered digitally, Eur. J. Trau. Dissoc. 5 (2) (2021) 100193, https://doi.org/10.1016/j.ejtd.2020.100193.
[124] D. Moher, A. Liberati, J. Tetzlaff, D.G. Altman, Prisma Group, Preferred reporting items for systematic reviews and meta-analyses: the PRISMA statement, PLoS Med. 6 (7) (2009) e1000097, https://doi.org/10.1371/journal.pmed.1000097.

Further reading

[1] B. Schuller, S. Steidl, A. Batliner, F. Burkhardt, L. Devillers, C. Müller, S.S. Narayanan, The INTERSPEECH 2010 paralinguistic challenge, in: Eleventh Annual Conference of the International Speech Communication Association, 2010.

CHAPTER TWO

Multimodal depression detection using machine learning

Roshan Jahan and Manish Madhav Tripathi
Computer Science and Engineering, Integral University, Lucknow, Uttar Pradesh, India

1. Introduction

Dysfunctional behavior is a difficult issue for many people globally. In a study [1], a huge percentage of the adult population is influenced by various mental problems. The risk for dying by suicide among those who are depressed is several times greater than for other causalities. Recognition of misery is normally a painful task because it requires a careful and precise mental examination by therapists who are experienced in the initial phases [2]. Also, it is common individuals for experiencing sorrow not to visit centers, to request help from specialists in the beginning phases of the problem [3]. Frequently, people who experience the ill effects of psychological problems regularly "certainly" (and may even "expressly") express their sentiments and daily struggles with emotional well-being issues via online media as a method of seeking help [4,5]. Subsequently, online media are a useful asset for finding individuals who are despondent.

It would require a great deal of work investment to filter through the online media profiles on individuals who are discouraged, but programmed adaptable computational techniques could give suggested and mass locations of depressed individuals, which could later forestall significant fatalities and help people who need it at the right time.

The daily exercises of clients through online media could be a gold mine for excavating information, because this information provides rich experiences about client-created content. It give them another platform for examining client conduct and assists with an examination of information that probably would not be possible elsewhere. Client standards of personal conduct for therapists and researchers could be explored by inspecting their online exercise posts in many informal communities [6,7]. It could focus on the perfect people in a timely fashion and provide important and urgent attention [8]. Businesses such as Neotas1, with workplaces in London and

Artificial Intelligence, Machine Learning, and Mental Health in Pandemics
ISBN: 978-0-323-91196-2
https://doi.org/10.1016/B978-0-323-91196-2.00005-3

elsewhere, openly mine accessible client information via online media to assist different organizations with historical verification, including understanding the psychological conditions of potential representatives. This shows that considering the emotional well-being states of a client's Web base using robots helps government or well-being associations and has a colossal business scope. The conduct and social qualities hidden in online media data attracts numerous analysts from various areas, including social researchers, showcasing specialists, information mining specialists, and others to break down Web-based media data as a source for inspecting human temperament, feelings, and practices. The determination of sadness could be difficult to accomplish on an enormous scope because most conventional methods depend on interviews, surveys, self-reporting, or statements by companions and family members. In addition to sharing their temperament and activities, the late reviews show that many individuals, via Web media, will generally share or provide advice on data related to well-being [9—12]. These sources offer a pathway for finding psychological well-being information for requirements such as conclusions, drugs, and claims.

Although some approaches have attempted to become familiar with a model on a limited scale, the format of these techniques is flawed. For example, in Deshpande and Rao [13], the authors examined Slithering tweets that contained complaints related to discouragement as a background truth of Twitter. However, the researchers were able to collect only few relevant information.

Accordingly, their model was considered quantitatively inadmissible because of lack of testing. De Choudhury et al. [14] confronted a comparable issue in which they used few information tests to prepare their classifier. Accordingly, their examination experienced the issue of a temperamental model preparing employing inadequate information, prompting poor quantitative execution. Kumar et al. [15] offered a model to distinguish the restless sadness of customers. They proposed a grouping order model that joined the results of three famous models.

A typical problem viewed by specialists in recognizing misery through online media is the variety of client practices through Web-based media, which makes it difficult to characterize dark highlights related to adapting to issues of emotional well-being. It was confirmed that Web media might help us with a social event. Sufficient information and some social media cooperation is required to design the model. Fatima et al. [16] and Wang et al. [17] showed that one could acquire a only few essential points to distinguish individuals with dietary problems. In Simms et al. [18], the authors also experienced the problem of a lack of highlights, including measurement of a significant informational index leading to powerless outcomes. Unlike previous work, we propose a template prepared on a huge exhibitor dataset. When the technique is scaled up, it creates better and more reliable quantitative performance on known and solid strategies available nearby.

Depressed clients act differently when they interact through Web media, creating rich social information that is regularly used to separate various highlights. They are certainly not all identified by qualities of discouragement. Many existing reviews either ignored significant highlights or chose less relevant highlights, which is a popular topic. A few surveys dealt with a range of client behaviors. For example, Shen et al. [19] collected a large set of data with solid basic truth names. At this stage, they identified various highlights related to customer conduct in online media and grouped them into a few terms and conditions.

The use of a deep understanding of how to acquire knowledgeable and meaningful information from mind-boggling and heterogeneous information has become the standard in artificial intelligence (AI) applications for medical services. For instance, the preparation of a clinical presentation and conclusion obtained incredible results. The advantage of deep learning is its remarkable capacity to iterate learning and the computerized improvement of dormant representations of the multifaceted structure of the network [20]. This convinces us to use the learning ability of the dominant neural organization with the rich and heterogeneous standards of personal behavior of online media customers.

This chapter presents a hybrid model to identify depressed users. The models are described in further sections.

2. Literature survey

Information in online media is usually data that customers share for use in public [15]. Two steps separate information available on social media. The first step is to collect information created by clients about systems administration, and the next is to dissect information collected using a computer or physical model. In any literature survey, highlighting the main extracts is more important it will help to understand the proposed model easily.

An understanding of depression on informal online organizations could be complemented using two related methodologies: are posts and user-level behavioral analysis.

2.1 Post-level analysis

Techniques that use this type of investigation focus primarily on the literary highlights of the customer's position, disembodied as measurable information [16,18]. De Choudhury et al. [14] proposed a method for identifying depression in customers using their social media posts. Work by Hu et al. [22], also considers phonetics and highlights information acquired from Web-based media.

To investigate whether the post identifies symptoms of depression, authors used key words in the content [21,23]. Some analysts have explored anticipated mental health problems by breaking down tweets on Twitter to discover terms related to a slowdown. One author developed [24] a model revealing useful and significant inactive constructs in a tweet. In addition, Shen et al. [19] observed various manifestations of poverty mentioned in a client's tweet. Other work [25] investigated customer behavior on Twitter and Weibo. The authors studied customer messages using semantic highlights. They used a mental investigation framework in Chinese called Text Mind during the concluding examination.

Intriguing behavior hypothesized for after the level was completed on Twitter uncovered depressing, important, and stimulating words, and dark indications. Anorexia was recognized through a post-level analysis [26].

2.2 User-level behaviors

There are various post by customers in online media as it reflects in general conduct. It also distinguishes the client's social engagement on Twitter from their tweets and retweets. In most cases, the etymologic style of posts could be considered to remove highlights [27]. Shen et al. [19] segregated six groups of pain components for a comprehensive representation of each client's collected information. The authors used the number of posts on Twitter and other social forums as highlights of person-to-person organization. In terms of client profile highlights, they used personal information shared by the client in an interpersonal organization. Analyzing the customer's behavior seems useful for identifying the food problem. Wang et al. [17] identified customer engagement and exercise highlights via the Web media. They disembodied client etymologic highlights for psychometric properties similar to those represented in Shen et al. [25]. The authors identified 70 areas of strength from two separate informal communities (Twitter and Weibo).

2.3 Depression detection using deep learning

Various literatures has described deep learning to recognize depression across the Internet, ranging from tweets to conventional recording and the client considers it. Whereas some of this works might fall into one of the classes previously discussed, we independently introduce these discoveries using deep learning strategies.

Work proposed by Lin et al. [28] is similar to the model presented in this chapter. Authors has proposed a deep-learning model based on convolutional neural networks (CNNs) to aggregate depressed Twitter customers using multimodular strength. There are two sections of that proposed system. They used bidirectional encoder representations from transformers (BERT) and convolutional neural network (CNN) for visual representation [29]. The two main points are then consolidated in the same way as in this template, for joint learning. There is then an online melancholy discovery step that examines clients' posts on Twitter along with images. A visual representation of depressive users on Instagram presented in an article [30]. The pattern of Instagram also uses multimodalities in the information. Although the model of Lin et al. [28] showed promising results, there are some hurdles. For example, BERT vectors for veiled tokens require computational acquisition in any event during the tuning phase. Another limitation of their work is that they acquire depictions of BERT's penalty. For example, BERT imposes a symbolic limitation of 512 lengths in which longer arrangements are simply shortened, causing a certain amount of data of depressed users.

Multimodular highlights of content, sound, and images were also used in Zheng et al. [31], who based a model on a built-in diagram considering multimodular information to recognize misery. Although they used CNN's global model, overall engineering surveyed data with limited coverage. For instance, their dataset contains 189 meetings with clients, for 7 to 33 min duration (average 16 min). Although they did not test the technique with short and tumultuous Web-based media information, it remains unclear how the strategy extends to such enormous assortments.

Xezonaki et al. [32] suggested a consideration-based model to distinguish the misery of interpreted clinical meetings from online interpersonal organizations. Their policy decision was that people who were committed to grieving use language full of feelings to a greater extent than do people who are not depressed.

Wolohan [33] investigated the mentality of people during COVID-19. The author used a fastText and LSTM model [34]. Shrestha et al. [35] proposed a model based on recurring neural network (RNN) to analyze chat databases.

Trotzek et al. presented a survey on depression detection in the early stage [36] using posts and messages on social media. They formed different words inserted into the dataset to acquire explicit embedding.

2.4 Selection of words detecting depression

The simplest purpose of word embedding is to identify words useful for representing word entrenchments [37,38].

In addition, it has been applied to psychological well-being problems such as misery. Bahgat et al. [39] focused on Reddit (also used in articles [40]) a couple of networks that contain conversations about the psychological well-being of battles like pain and self-defeating thoughts.

Farruque et al. [41] explored integrating words into situations in which information is scarce, such as the location of heavy language from customer tweets. Their work reproduced an approach to word installation based on modernization. They began with a predefined model and refined it in the explicit information box.

2.5 Modeling for detecting depression

Gong et al. [42] showed how a dark location should be treated using a multimodular study. Fig. 2.1 shows the model for Twitter sentiment analysis.

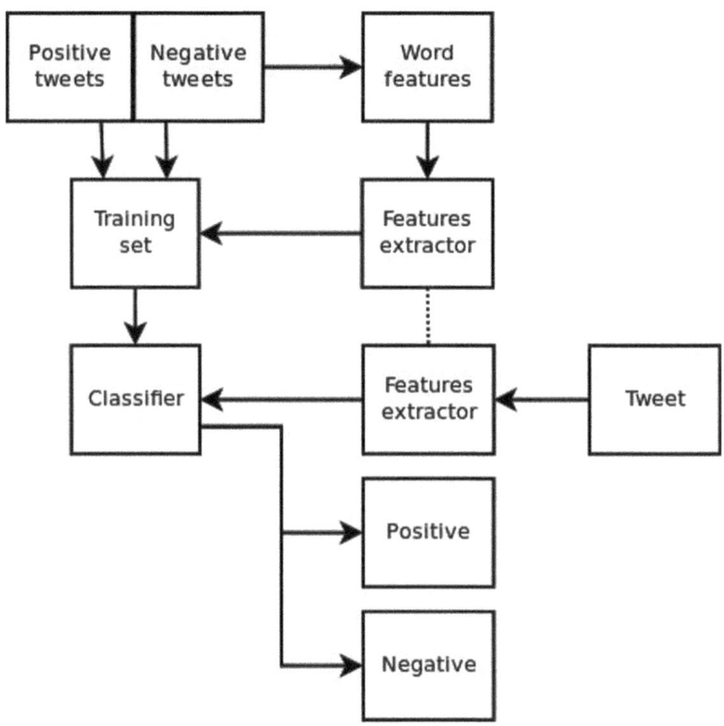

Figure 2.1 Twitter sentiment analysis model.

3. Social media data

Twitter is the social media platform which provides information as free tweets. This is why it is popular among scientists, who have extensively used Twitter for news. Tweet information can be uploaded seamlessly and efficiently through their application programming interfaces (APIs).

Normally, researchers use two approaches to analyze Twitter data. The first is to use an existing dataset openly and freely shared by other researchers. The problem with this type of dataset is that it might be old. Updated data are useful for when current trends are examined. Current scenarios can be evaluated using the current dataset of Twitter.

Creating and approving terms used in the jargon of customers with dysfunctional behaviors is tedious. A review by Shen et al. [19] gathered an enormous scope of information with reliable background information, which we intend to reuse. Information about measures can be found in Table 2.1. To embody the dataset, the authors assembled three comprehensive information collections.

Informational pain index: Each client is flagged as discouraged, in light of its tweet content in the 2009 and 2016 lineup. This includes 1402 disheartened customers and 292,564 tweets.

Uncorrelated informational index: Information from about 300 million customers' tweets was flagged as undisclosed in Dec. 2016 for collection.

Sorrow informational index requester: The authors described about depresses users, where the tweet was collected whenever content "push down." There are 36,993 depressed customers with more than 47 million tweets on Twitter.

3.1 Data cleaning and preprocessing

Data collection is tedious. Data contain lot of noise and outliers; the dataset cannot be used without preprocessing. This is especially serious when data are downloaded from online repositories. These data have lots of grammatical and spelling mistakes with other bad characters. As a result, to obtain a

Table 2.1 Statistics gathered from important dataset.

Dataset	Depressed	Not depressed
No. of users	1402	300 million
No. of tweets	292,564	10 billion

reliable predictive analysis, a preprocessing strategy must be adopted to ensure that the calculation model has satisfactory data quality.

The dataset used for the analysis was divided into two classes: depressed and not depressed. The Natural Language Processing Toolbox [43] was used to clean the data. We deleted common words such as "the," and "a" in users' tweets because they are not discriminatory against the model or useful. To enhance the quality of the text, non-ASCII characters were also removed.

Preprocessing of the data content eliminated the abundance of noisy content in the dataset. It provided reliable and good-quality data for analysis. It also reduced the complexity of algorithms used for analysis and recognition.

4. Attributes definition

Online media information conveys all of the experiences and feelings of the client reflected by the person's practices in the interpersonal organization. This information demonstrates how clients c-operate with associations. In this work, we collected data from each customer and ordered them into two kinds of traits, multimodular properties and the insertion of words.

4.1 Multimodular attributes

The purpose of this attribute is to determine how the characteristic value will be compared with each method for each client. The dimension of all types of interest is estimated to be 76. We primarily considered the four major terms recorded subsequently, and ignored two terms because of the lack of quality. These key points are:

Social knowledge and interaction. We identified some highlights of relationships with each customer profile. These are highlighted points for each customer account according to the name of each component. Most highlights are directly available in the client information, such as the number of clients who follow the persons, the best choices, and so on.

Emojis: Emojis enable clients to communicate feelings using simple symbols and nonverbal components. It is essential to distinguish between positive and negative emotional texts. Emojis shared by people can be positively, negatively, and fairly controlled. For each positive, nonpartisan, or negative category, we included these in each tweet. We then summarized the number of tweets from each customer to obtain a summary from each customer. Authors summarized the three qualities of the clients: more positive, nonpartisan and negative expressions.

In this work, we used unsupervised linear discriminant analysis (LDA) [44] to retrieve the distribution of the most latent topics from users' tweets. Although nonparametric Bayesian control strategies and strategies exist [45], we chose a simple, popular, and effective method to help us achieve results.

Symptoms features (count of depressed symptoms). This is the number of symptoms of depression that show up in a tweet. We selected some key words for various symptoms of depression. We also expanded the list of key words by integrating various words related to depression. Moreover, we counted the repetition of key words in all tweets.

5. Hybrid deep learner model

In this segment, we illustrate a 50/50 model with multinodular strengths. Although different models of in-depth mixing are offered, this technique learns multimodal highlights that incorporate effective highlights (Fig. 2.2). The joint learning component learns the boundaries of the model in a solidified bounding space where the model is diversified. The boundaries are shared during the preparation phase, which produces stronger results. Simple methods based on drop merge cause an error from one phase to the next [46].

5.1 Model overview

We obtain preparatory information as an integration network for each client addressing the customer event course. In addition, a 76-dimensionally integer vector is available for each client addressing the multimodality (MM) trait. We propose a CNN-based 50/50 model that joins the bidirectional gated recurrent unit (BiGRU) to identify poverty through online media, as shown in Fig. 2.2. The performance is related to the address of a single vector, including that which has taken care of in a sigmoid initiation layer for forecasting.

In the areas that accompany it, we will examine the two existing separate designs that will be attached, which will lead to a new calculation model to display multiple spatial constructs and modalities.

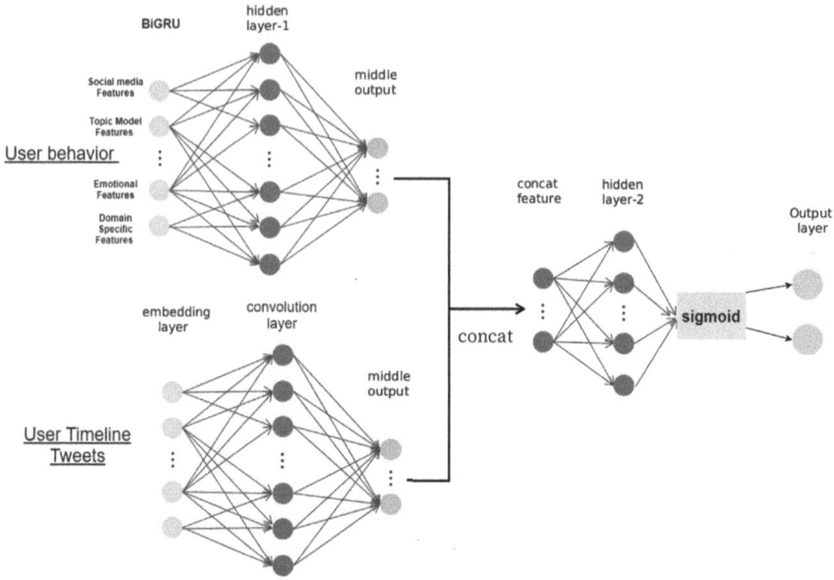

Figure 2.2 Outline of suggested model. *BiGRU,* bidirectional gated recurrent unit, *Concat,* concatenate.

5.2 Convolutional neural network

The schedule of an individual client includes semantic data and highlights in the vicinity. CNN has been used efficiently to learn strong, reasonable and durable descriptions [47]. The powerful learning abilities of NPC components enable them to make the perfect decision to remove semantic highlights from a client message. We propose to use the CNN organization to extract the strengths of customer's semantic tweets.

We set the size of each client sentence anywhere in the range of 0 and 1000 words and depict the normal of only 10 tweets for each client. This size is much bigger than what has been used in other closely related ongoing models that rely on BERT. The info layer is connected to the convolution layer through three regular layers to learn the n-gram highlights linking the word demand. Hence, catch significant semantic content which, in general, cannot be captured by a word packet based on the pattern [48].

5.3 Bidirectional gated recurrent unit neural network

The recurrent neural network (RNN) is a class of artificial neural networks where the information is fixed vectors to be measured in the arrangement regardless of whether the information is nonsuccessive. Models such as BiGRU, gated recurrent unit (GRU), and long short term memory

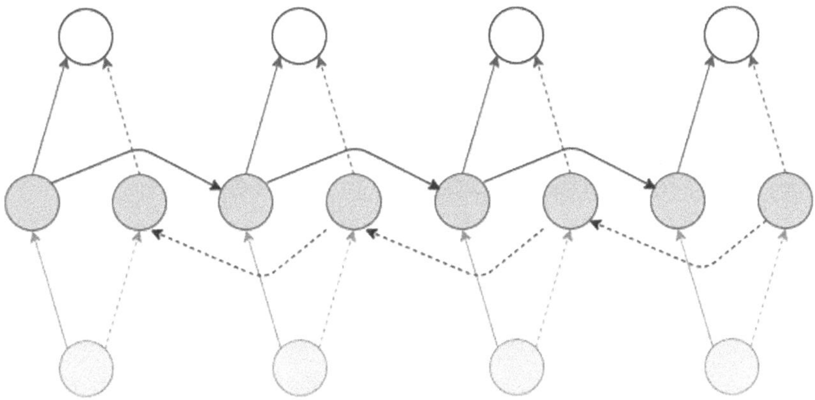

Figure 2.3 Synchronized unit 2-way structure.

(LSTM) are within the RNN class. Static appropriations are normally entered in BiGRU. It is computationally productive that a network of LSTM declines due to entryways. The GRU can capture significant data between highlights, but a one-way or other GRU might just capture the authentic data. Furthermore, for descriptive data, we might want to get data on each client's social meadia posts.

The bidirectional GRU actually consists of two layers of GRU, as shown in Fig. 2.3, and is familiar with prior and regressive data acquisition. Moreover, the secret layer has two qualities for performance: one for inverse performance and the other for advanced performance.

We compare the proposed model with the associated bundling strategies:
The multimodal dictionary learning (MDL) model distinguishes among customers not recommended for Twitter [28]. It uses a key word to determine how to extract highlights from dormant information and a thin description of a client.
Support vector machines (SVMs) are a class of AI model in text clustering that try to rationalize an unhappy job. This explains how to draw an extreme isolating hyperplan between two named information schemes (e.g., plotting the largest edge hypermap between positive and marked negative information) [49].
Naive Bayes (NB) is a group of probabilistic calculations dependent on applying the Bayes hypothesis with the innocent assumption of contingent autonomy among opportunities [50]. Although appropriate contingent freedom has been approached by various scholars, these models give scandalously predominant performance when they are contrasted, and many refined models [51].

6. Experimental setting

The dataset was using Web scraping on Twitter posts. We collected tests sets for analysis:

- The number of users identified as positive was 5899.
- The number of positive users' tweets was 508,786.
- The number of users tagged negative was 5160.
- The total number of negative user tweets was 2,299,106.

During data collection we have rejected customers with less than 10 posts, and included the customers whos have more posts with more than 5000 followers. We are left with a final dataset composed of 2500 positive and 2300 negative customers. We received an 80:20 proportion for distributing information in preparation and testing. The word2vec was prepared on the Google News corpus, which includes three billion words. We used Python 3.6.3 and TensorFlow 2.1.0 as development tools. For BiGRU organization and CNN improvement, we used the Adam advance calculation. Finally, we had a 10-cycle template with a cluster size of 32. The number of cycles was sufficient to combine the model and the test results even more concretely to defeat existing solid standard strategies.

6.1 Evaluation metrics

We used conventional data retrieval measures such as accuracy, review, F1, and accuracy based on the disarray framework to assess the model. A confusing network is a shocking framework used to evaluate execution of the arrangement; it is also referred to as an error grid (Table 2.2).

The number of inaccurate predictions was relative to the number of exact predictions in a table. Some important terminologies related to the computation of the confusion matrix include:

- P: This is a positive case that is depressed at work.
- N: The present negative state, which is not depressed by the task.

Table 2.2 Comparison of findings using various classification methods.

Features	Methods	Precision	Recall	F1	Accuracy
Multimodalities	Support vector machine	0.72	0.63	0.60	0.64
	Naive Bayes	0.72	0.62	0.59	0.64
	Multimodal dictionary learning	0.79	0.79	0.79	0.79
Multimodalities + word embedding	Bidirectional gated recurrent unit–convolutional neural network	0.89	0.82	0.85	0.85

- TN: The actual case is not depressed, as are the predictions.
- FN: The reality is not depressed, but the outlook is depressed.
- PS: The current situation is depressed, but the projections are not.
- TP: The reality is depressed, and so are the predictions.

With the help of the confusion matrix, we can calculate the accuracy, precision, recall, and F1 score.

6.2 Experimental results

The MM quality and customer price of semantic events emphasizes property; we will use these two features mutually. After assembling customer behavior in MM-owned Web media, we evaluate the exposure of the model. First, we use various classifiers to test the sustainability of using multimodal characters (MM). Second, we show how execution of the template develops when we merge implementation of the word with the MM. Next, we discuss the results shown in Table 2.2 and Fig. 2.4.

Gullible Bayes has the lowest F1 score, indicating that this model has a lower ability to group tweets compared with other existing models with

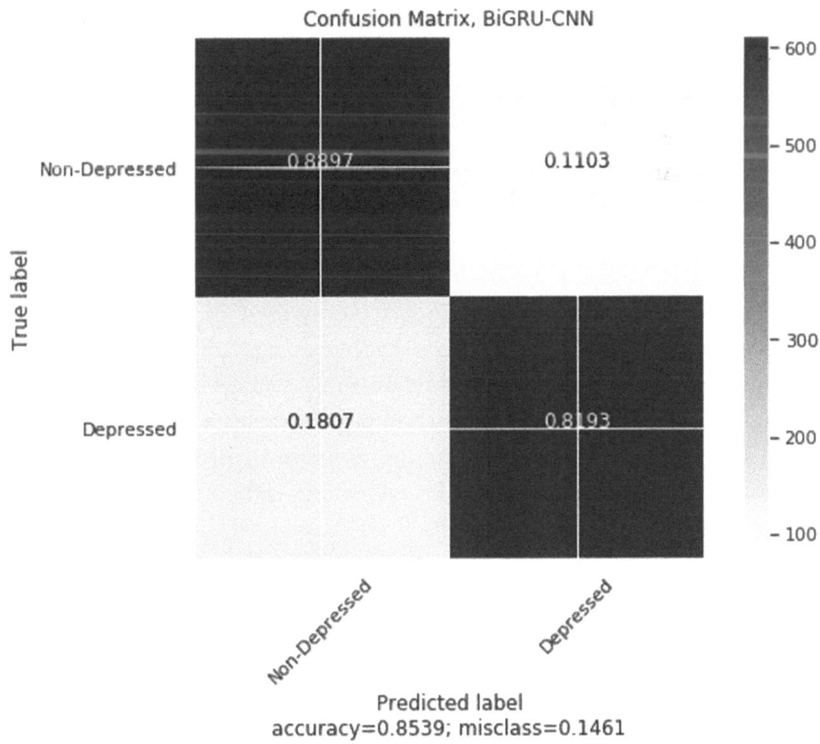

Figure 2.4 Confusion array for bidirectional gated recurrent unit–convolutional neural network (BiGRU-CNN).

obvious frustration. The reason for his argument may be that the model is not functional enough to make insufficient information and noisy.

The MDL model defeated SVM and NB and achieved better accuracy than these two technologies. Because this is a new model specifically designed to find frustrated customers, it captures the complexity of the dataset and uses its limitations to achieve better results.

We can see that the proposed model improved the location of the slowdown by up to 6% in F1 score compared with the MDL model. We therefore think that the proposed model goes further than a solid one.

Moreover, the model achieved the best layout, at 85% in F1. Fig. 2.4 is showing that joining BiGRU with CNN for the multimodal procedure for the client calendar of the semantic highlights system is enough to acknowledge the darkness in Twitter.

7. Discussion

To improve the research of the model, we used the network of confusion matrices. To do this, we imported the Sklearn Disorder Network Module, which helps us create the disorder frame. We imagine the grid of disorder, which shows how classes are associated, to demonstrate the level of examples. Fig. 2.4 shows that the model includes both undisclosed and depressed clients.

We considered the relevance of each of the two attributes of the model. We built the model to examine every property independently and see how the model works. We tested the model using only the MM feature. Fig. 2.5 shows that the model works less ideally when we used BiGRU unaltered. On the other hand the model works best when we only use CNN with the quality of words included in the post. It means that removing highlights from semantic data from customer tweets is important to discourage location.

After characterizing depressed customers, we analyzed the most widely recognized side effects of sadness among depressed customers. In Fig. 2.6, we can see that one indication (depressed feeling) is the best-known side effect displayed by depressed customers. This shows how depressed customers discover and display their heavy mindset via Web-based media over other side effects. Apart from this, various manifestations such as energy misused, sleep disorder, feelings of worthlessness, and thoughts of self-destructive have manifested themselves in over 20% of depressed clients.

To explore the five most influential signals among depressed customers, we gathered each tweet related to demorlizing words. At that time, a cloud

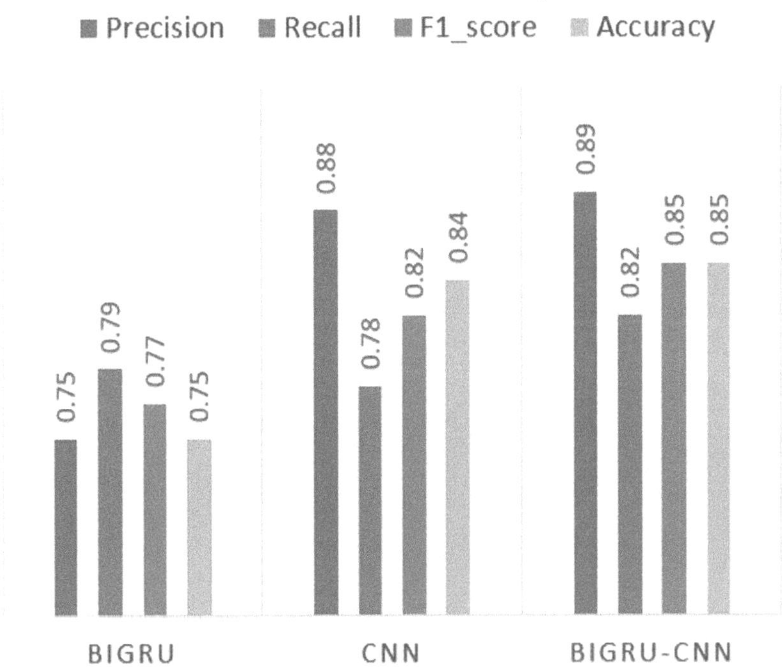

Figure 2.5 Comparing the effectiveness of the model with various attributes. *BIGRU*, bidirectional gated recurrent unit; *CNN*, convolutional neural network.

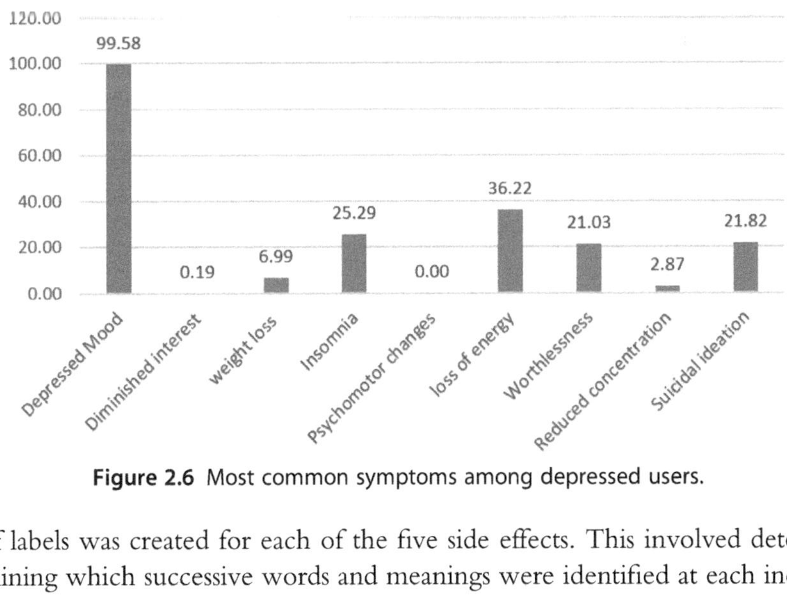

Figure 2.6 Most common symptoms among depressed users.

of labels was created for each of the five side effects. This involved determining which successive words and meanings were identified at each indication, as shown in Fig. 2.7. Coarser textual words are generally more

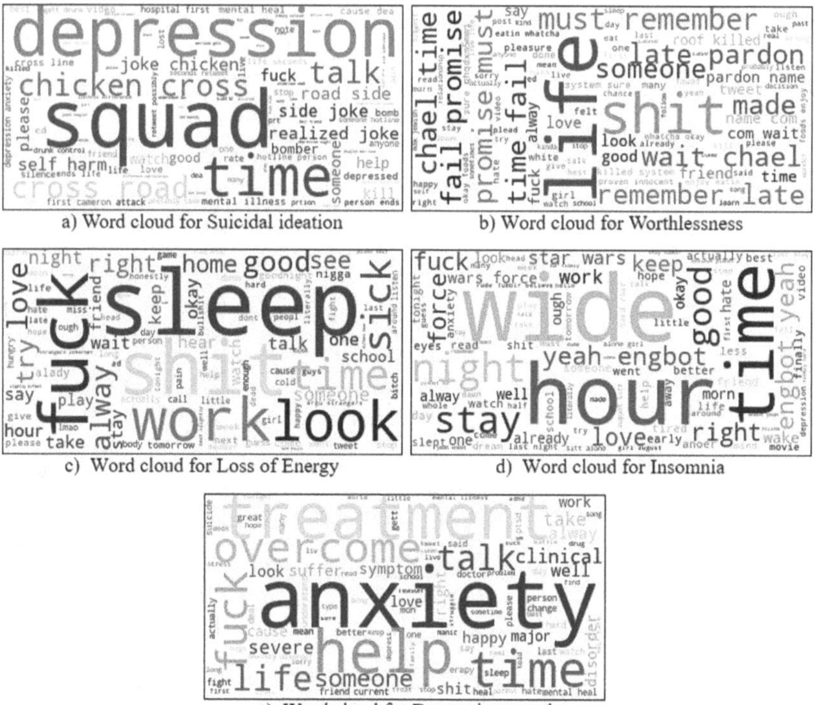

a) Word cloud for Suicidal ideation
b) Word cloud for Worthlessness
c) Word cloud for Loss of Energy
d) Word cloud for Insomnia
e) Word cloud for Depression mood

Figure 2.7 Word clouds for most influencing symptoms.

meaningful than those in a similar cloud representation. These clouds gave us a glimpse of the relative multitude of words that usually occur within each of these five indications.

8. Conclusion and future work

We discussed proposing a model to recognize depressed clients through an online media review by identifying highlights of clients' conduct and clients' online schedules (messages). We used a certifiable information index for depressed and depressed customers and applied it to the model. We proposed a mixed model represented by an interplay between the BiGRU and CNN models. We designated the most common properties that addresses the customer's conduct in BiGRU and the customer social media timeline presents to CNN on removing relevent posts. The proposed model demonstrates that preparing of this network enhances order fulfillment and distinguishes depressed customers compared with using other sound techniques.

Moreover, the use of another famous word, for representation procedure has prepared language template. Although difficulties when using such pre-prepared language models can be present owing to the limitation they force on the arrangement length, contemplating this undertaking assists in uncovering their upsides and downsides. Future work hopes to identify other psychological instability associated with melancholy, to address complex mental problems that have plagued peoples' lives.

References

[1] American Psychiatric Association, et al., Diagnostic and Statistical Manual of Mental Disorders (DSM-5®), American Psychiatric Pub, 2013.

[2] E.A. Ríssola, M. Aliannejadi, F. Crestani, Beyond modelling: understanding mental disorders in online social media, in: European Conference on Information Retrieval, Springer, 2020, pp. 296–310.

[3] M.L. Zou, M.X. Li, V. Cho, Depression and disclosure behavior via social media: a study of university students in China, Heliyon 6 (2) (2020) e03368.

[4] K.C. Bathina, M. ten Thij, L. Lorenzo-Luaces, L.A. Rutter, J. Bollen, Depressed individuals express more distorted thinking on social media, Nat. Hum. Behav. 5 (4) (2021) 458–466, https://doi.org/10.1038/s41562-021-01050-7. In this issue.

[5] M. Park, C. Cha, M. Cha, Depressive moods of users portrayed in Twitter, in: Proceedings of the ACM SIGKDD Workshop on Healthcare Informatics (HI-KDD), vol. 2012, 2012, pp. 1–8.

[6] Y. Ding, X. Chen, Q. Fu, S. Zhong, A depression recognition method for college students using deep integrated support vector algorithm, IEEE Access 8 (2020) 75616–75629.

[7] D. Lyu, Z. Wang, Y. Du, R. Kim Marjerison, R. Chen, Using social media content to identify mental health problems: the case of# depression in Sina Weibo, Rev. Integr. Bus. Econ. Res. 9 (2020) 448–464.

[8] S. Chancellor, M. De Choudhury, Methods in predictive techniques for mental health status on social media: a critical review, NPJ Digi. Med. 3 (1) (2020) 1–11.

[9] C. Hawn, Take two aspirin and tweet me in the morning: how Twitter, Facebook, and other social media are reshaping health care, Health Aff. 28 (2) (2009) 361–368.

[10] L. Neuhauser, G.L. Kreps, Rethinking communication in the e-health era, J. Health Psychol. 8 (1) (2003) 7–23.

[11] K.W. Prier, M.S. Smith, C. Giraud-Carrier, C.L. Hanson, Identifying health-related topics on twitter, in: International Conference on Social Computing, Behavioral-Cultural Modeling, and Prediction, Springer, 2011, pp. 18–25.

[12] D. Scanfeld, V. Scanfeld, E.L. Larson, Dissemination of health information through social networks: twitter and antibiotics, Am. J. Infec. Contr. 38 (3) (2010) 182–188.

[13] M. Deshpande, V. Rao, Depression detection using emotion artificial intelligence, in: 2017 International Conference on Intelligent Sustainable Systems (ICISS), 2017, pp. 858–862, https://doi.org/10.1109/ISS1.2017.8389299.

[14] M. De Choudhury, M. Gamon, C. Scott, E. Horvitz, Predicting depression via social media, in: Seventh International AAAI Conference on Weblogs and Social Media, 2013.

[15] A. Kumar, A. Sharma, A. Arora, Anxious Depression Prediction in Real-Time Social Data, 2019. Available at: SSRN 3383359 (2019).

[16] I. Fatima, H. Mukhtar, H.F. Ahmad, K. Rajpoot, Analysis of user-generated content from online social communities to characterise and predict depression degree, J. Inf. Sci. 44 (5) (2018) 683–695.

[17] T. Wang, M. Brede, A. Ianni, E. Mentzakis, Detecting and characterizing eating- disorder communities on social media, in: Proceedings of the Tenth ACM International Conference on Web Search and Data Mining, ACM, 2017, pp. 91–100.
[18] T. Simms, C. Ramstedt, M. Rich, M. Richards, T. Martinez, C. Giraud-Carrier, Detecting cognitive distortions through machine learning text analytics, in: 2017 IEEE International Conference on Healthcare Informatics (ICHI), 2017, pp. 508–512. IEEE.
[19] G. Shen, J. Jia, L. Nie, F. Feng, C. Zhang, T. Hu, T.-S. Chua, W. Zhu, Depression detection via harvesting social media: a multimodal dictionary learning solution, IJCAI (2017) 3838–3844.
[20] A.H. Orabi, P. Buddhitha, M.H. Orabi, D. Inkpen, Deep learning for depression detection of twitter users, in: Proceedings of the Fifth Workshop on Computational Linguistics and Clinical Psychology: From Keyboard to Clinic, 2018, pp. 88–97.
[21] R. Lebret, R. Collobert, Rehabilitation of count-based models for word vector representations, in: International Conference on Intelligent Text Processing and Computational Linguistics, Springer, 2015, pp. 417–429.
[22] Q. Hu, A. Li, H. Fei, J. Li, T. Zhu, Predicting depression of social media user on different observation windows, in: 2015 IEEE/WIC/ACM International Conference on Web Intelligence and Intelligent Agent Technology (WI-IAT), vol. 1, IEEE, 2015, pp. 361–364.
[23] S. Tsugawa, Y. Kikuchi, F. Kishino, K. Nakajima, Y. Itoh, H. Ohsaki, Recognizing depression from twitter activity, in: Proceedings of the 33rd Annual ACM Conference on Human Factors in Computing Systems, ACM, 2015, pp. 3187–3196.
[24] P. Resnik, W. Armstrong, L. Claudino, T. Nguyen, V.-A. Nguyen, J. Boyd-Graber, Beyond LDA: exploring supervised topic modeling for depression-related language in twitter, in: Proceedings of the 2nd Workshop on Computational Linguistics and Clinical Psychology: From Linguistic Signal to Clinical Reality, Association for Computational Linguistics, Denver, Colorado, 2015, pp. 99–107, https://doi.org/10.3115/v1/W15-1212.
[25] T. Shen, J. Jia, G. Shen, F. Feng, X. He, H. Luan, J. Tang, T. Tiropanis, T. Seng Chua, W. Hall, Cross-domain depression detection via harvesting social media, in: Proceedings of the 27th International Joint Conference on Artificial Intelligence, IJCAI, 2018, pp. 1611–1617. https://eprints.soton.ac.uk/423226/.
[26] D. Ramírez-Cifuentes, M. Mayans, A. Freire, Early risk detection of anorexia on social media, in: International Conference on Internet Science, Springer, 2018, pp. 3–14.
[27] A.H. Yazdavar, H.S. Al-Olimat, M. Ebrahimi, G. Bajaj, T. Banerjee, K. Thirunarayan, J. Pathak, S. Amit, Semi-supervised approach to monitoring clinical depressive symptoms in social media, in: Proceedings of the 2017 IEEE/ACM International Conference on Advances in Social Networks Analysis and Mining 2017, ACM, 2017, pp. 1191–1198.
[28] C. Lin, P. Hu, H. Su, S. Li, J. Mei, J. Zhou, H. Leung, SenseMood: depression detection on social media, in: Proceedings of the 2020 International Conference on Multimedia Retrieval, 2020, pp. 407–411.
[29] J. Devlin, M.-W. Chang, K. Lee, K. Toutanova, BERT: pre-training of deep bidirectional transformers for language understanding, Proceedings of the 2019 Conference of the North {A}merican Chapter of the Association for Computational Linguistics: Human Language Technologies, Volume 1 (Long and Short Papers) (2019) 4171–4186, https://doi.org/10.18653/v1/N19-1423. In this issue.
[30] C.Y. Chiu, H.Y. Lane, J.L. Koh, A.L.P. Chen, Multimodal depression detection on instagram considering time interval of posts, J. Intell. Inf. Syst. (2020) 1–23.

[31] W. Zheng, Y. Lan, C. Gou, F.-Y. Wang, Graph attention model embedded with multi-modal knowledge for depression detection, in: 2020 IEEE International Conference on Multimedia and Expo (ICME), IEEE, 2020, pp. 1–6.
[32] D. Xezonaki, G. Paraskevopoulos, A. Potamianos, S. Narayanan, Affective conditioning on hierarchical networks applied to depression detection from transcribed clinical interviews, arXiv (2020) preprint arXiv:2006.08336.
[33] J.T. Wolohan, Estimating the Effect of COVID-19 on Mental Health: Linguistic Indicators of Depression during a Global Pandemic, 2020.
[34] T. Mikolov, E. Grave, P. Bojanowski, C. Puhrsch, J. Armand, Advances in pre-training distributed word representations, Proceedings of the Eleventh International Conference on Language Resources and Evaluation (LREC 2018) (2018) preprint arXiv:1712.09405, https://aclanthology.org/L18-1008. In press.
[35] A. Shrestha, E. Serra, F. Spezzano, Multi-modal social and psycho-linguistic embedding via recurrent neural networks to identify depressed users in online forums, Net-MAHIB 9 (1) (2020) 22.
[36] M. Trotzek, S. Koitka, C.M. Friedrich, Utilizing neural networks and linguistic metadata for early detection of depression indications in text sequences, IEEE Trans. Knowl. Data Eng. (2018), https://doi.org/10.1109/TKDE.2018.2885515. In press.
[37] J. Pennington, R. Socher, C.D. Manning, Glove: global vectors for word representation, in: Proceedings of the 2014 Conference on Empirical Methods in Natural Language Processing, EMNLP), 2014, pp. 1532–1543.
[38] H. Zamani, W.B. Croft, Relevance-based word embedding, in: Proceedings of the 40th International ACM SIGIR Conference on Research and Development in Information Retrieval, 2017, pp. 505–514.
[39] M. Bahgat, S. Wilson, W. Magdy, Towards using word embedding vector space for better cohort analysis, in: Proceedings of the International AAAI Conference on Web and Social Media, vol. 14, 2020, pp. 919–923.
[40] A. Trifan, R. Antunes, S. Matos, J. Luís Oliveira, Understanding depression from psycholinguistic patterns in social media texts, in: European Conference on Information Retrieval, Springer, 2020, pp. 402–409.
[41] N. Farruque, O. Zaiane, R. Goebel, Augmenting semantic representation of depressive language: from forums to microblogs, in: Joint European Conference on Machine Learning and Knowledge Discovery in Databases, Springer, 2019, pp. 359–375.
[42] Y. Gong, C. Poellabauer, Topic modeling based multi-modal depression detection, in: Proceedings of the 7th Annual Workshop on Audio/Visual Emotion Challenge, 2017, pp. 69–76.
[43] K. Horecki, J. Mazurkiewicz, Natural language processing methods used for automatic prediction mechanism of related phenomenon, in: Lecture Notes in Artificial Intelligence (Subseries of Lecture Notes in Computer Science) 9120, 2015, pp. 13–24, https://doi.org/10.1007/978-3-319-19369-4-2.
[44] D.M. Blei, A.Y. Ng, M.I. Jordan, Latent dirichlet allocation, J. Mach. Learn. Res. 3 (2003) 993–1022.
[45] W.T. Yee, M.I. Jordan, J.B. Matthew, D.M. Blei, Sharing clusters among related groups: hierarchical Dirichlet processes, in: Advances in Neural Information Processing Systems, 2005, pp. 1385–1392.
[46] J. Zhu, A. Ahmed, E.P. Xing, MedLDA: maximum margin supervised topic models, J. Mach. Learn. Res. 13 (1) (2012) 2237–2278.
[47] B. Liu, X. Yu, P. Zhang, A. Yu, Q. Fu, X. Wei, Supervised deep feature extraction for hyperspectral image classification, IEEE Trans. Geosci. Rem. Sens. 56 (4) (2017) 1909–1921.

[48] X. Wang, A. McCallum, W. Xing, Topical n-grams: phrase and topic discovery, with an application to information retrieval, in: Seventh IEEE International Conference on Data Mining (ICDM 2007), IEEE, 2007, pp. 697–702.

[49] C.-C. Chang, C.-J. Lin, LIBSVM: a library for support vector machines, ACM Trans. Intell. Syst. Technol. 2 (3) (2011) 1–27.

[50] A.Y. Ng, M.I. Jordan, On discriminative vs. generative classifiers: a comparison of logistic regression and naive bayes, in: Advances in Neural Information Processing Systems, 2002, pp. 841–848.

[51] D. Stephens, M. Diesing, A comparison of supervised classification methods for the prediction of substrate type using multibeam acoustic and legacy grain-size data, PLoS One 9 (4) (2014) e93950.

CHAPTER THREE

A graph convolutional network based framework for mental stress prediction

Akhila Sahiti Racherla, Raj Sahu and Vandana Bhattacharjee
Department of Computer Science and Engineering, Birla Institute of Technology, Mesra, Ranchi, India

1. Introduction

A healthy person is an asset to society. And when one says healthy, it includes both physical and mental health. With the current pandemic situation where people are being faced with strange situations, unforeseen and not even thought of before, it is all the more pertinent that mental health be given special importance. With the advent of social networking platforms, people very often tend to vent out their feelings in the form of tweets, posts, etc. In this work we aim to utilize these tweets/posts as attributes to build our classification framework. The use of advancements in information technology, especially in the field of machine learning, comes to be of great help. One can think of people as points and their interrelationships as lines joining these points. This is, in mathematical terms, the definition of a graph. And to process graph data with machine learning, graph convolutional networks (GCNs) are the most natural choice. GCN is increasingly becoming popular as a technique due to its capability of solving the task of classification of nodes, graphs, or links. Following the message passing strategy, a graph neural network (GNN) learns a node's embeddings by aggregating representations of its neighbors and itself. GNNs are recently being used in health care, disease prediction, physiological impacts, etc. Modeling the problem of disease prediction using a graph where each data sample (healthy/unhealthy) is denoted as a node, and the edges are used to represent the similarity between the denoted nodes, becomes a task of classification. The success of such a classification lies in the ability of the researcher to model the problem so that the transformed features (node embeddings) also represent the real-world problem closely. The task of the node classification can be defined as its ability to learn the parameters of a function say, f_θ, which uses the

Artificial Intelligence, Machine Learning, and Mental Health in Pandemics
ISBN: 978-0-323-91196-2
https://doi.org/10.1016/B978-0-323-91196-2.00007-7

adjacency matrix and node features in the form of input, and its main aim is to determine the aggregated features for each sample and then label the unlabeled samples. The intuition behind the GCN is incorporating the features along with the relation of nodes in a graph by using some concept such as averaging the features of every node by its direct neighbors' features.

Due to huge volumes of medical datasets, the possibility of imbalance in the dataset occurs where there is a probability that the distribution of classes can be skewed. The graph classifiers tend to be inclined more toward the majority of classes. The skewness or imbalance can range from very low to very high (severe imbalance). The loss functions that are used for training a classifier aim to hike up the accuracy, so that the outputs are dealt on the datasets, which have balanced classes. But this may not work while handling imbalanced classes. This happens due to the fact that the loss function depends upon trying to achieve a high accuracy in favor of the major class. Researchers in Ref. [1] have proposed variants of GCN work to boost up the performance and efficiency of the graph-based classifier and prevent it from relying more on the samples of any particular class only.

In our research paper, a GCN-based framework for learning the node features is presented, which would be used for node classification. We have taken up a study of the graph of persons as nodes, labeled as "*Stressed*" or "*Normal*," and use GCN to label the unlabeled nodes. The goal is to build up a machine learning model that helps in predicting stress or other problems on various sets of people.

Our contributions are as follows:

- Construct a graph structure with people as nodes, and links between two nodes would depend upon the similarity of the nodes.
- Node features are created with data about people such as age, gender, occupation, history of chronic ailment, and the tweet words used by the user in a certain time frame.
- The node features are aggregated using GCNs, and final node embeddings are obtained.
- These node embeddings are used for labeling the nodes (people) as "*Stressed*" or "*Normal.*"

To perform the experiments, data was collected from a known set of people, that is, friends of authors, or their friends. The implementation was done on three sets. The first set consisted of a dataset of size 30. The second set was of length 50, and finally, the implementation was done on 100 data entries. The experiments were executed on the Tesla T4 platform.

In a general graph, the edge strengths may be taken as proportional to the people's similarity score. Which means, as the strength increases, so does the similarity in their views and their mental state. However, these being structural properties, we need to incorporate the node feature properties, so GCN is used. In particular, when generating the initial node features, we aim to include the tweet words more relevant to the pandemic situation. Also, in this research work, we have taken edge weights as constant.

The rest of the paper is organized as follows: Section 2 presents the related work for GNNs and applications related to machine learning on healthcare data. We present an extensive literature survey for the benefit of the reader and due to the relevance of the papers to our work. Section 3 presents the theoretical background of GCNs. Section 4 presents the methodology and experiments. Section 5 presents the results followed by Section 6, which concludes the paper with the future scope of the work.

2. Related work

This section covers an overview of the literature related to application of machine learning in general and GCNs in particular, focusing mostly on the healthcare data.

Ghorbani et al. in Ref. [1] propose an approach to handle imbalance in graph data. They assign a graph-based network for each and every class. Implementing a graph between each patient increases the accuracy in the training model. This imbalance is handled with the help of two approaches that are classified as data-level and cost-sensitive. In the former approach, the resampling concept is used on classes in a random way or targeting undersampling of the major classes and oversampling of the minor classes. But this is not so useful when it comes to dealing with graphs due to the use of features and the relations between each data point. The undersampling and oversampling weakness is resolved by modifying the cost function by assigning different weights to each class. Using RA-GCN, loss value is calculated automatically and dynamically for each sample, which is done to solve the class imbalance problem and improve performance of classification. Two GCNs are used where one GCN is used for node classification and the other GCN is used on the training samples in each class for learning the weights. And this is done for all the classes present. These weighting GCNs (W-GCNs) and the classifier are trained in an opposite manner. The classifier tries to update and modify itself after every iteration, whereas, on the other hand, W-GCNs try to work on classifying if the samples are correctly classified or not. Adding a self-loop for all the nodes changes the structure of the graph that is taken as input followed by the features of each node, which are replaced by average of node features and its neighbors present in the graph. The second step includes the updated features that are fed to a fully connected layer, which is then used for mapping to a latent space. The goal of the RA-GCN is to learn different weights for the samples dynamically, with respect to the decision of the classifier on samples, and these learned weights are used in cross-entropy loss. The authors have performed experiments on Synthetic Datasets for Binary Classification, Synthetic Datasets for Multi-Class Classification, and also experiments on Real Datasets and have shown the results of Macro F1, Binary F1, ROC curve. Pima Indian Diabetes (Diabetes), Haberman's survival Dataset, Parkinson's Progression Markers Initiative (PPMI), are some of the real datasets used.

The biopsychosocial medical model theory states that mental health plays an important role in treatment [2]. Hence, it has become a necessity to have the knowledge of the diseases that have high potential in causing Psychological Trauma and Social Avoidance (PTSA). Major disease survivors have more impact on their mental status. These mental problems are considered to be neurosurgical diseases. Breast cancer is one of such diseases. Researchers have found that similar molecules lead to similar diseases.

A disease network can be built up by using GCN and identifying diseases that result in PTSA by XGBoost. Experimentally, only 23 diseases contribute to PTSA; hence the use of leave-one-out cross-validation leads to the testing of the performance of GCN-XGBoost. In comparison of the experiments driven using artificial neural network (ANN), support vector machine (SVM), random forest (RF), and deep neural network (DNN), GCN-XGBoost performed the best. PTSA in patients having breast cancer is very high. Breast cancer patients experience severe Social Avoidance and Distress (SAD). Patients were categorized into four groups with respect to four phases of treatment such as before mastectomy, after mastectomy, before chemotherapy, and after chemotherapy. After experiments and analysis of breast size, self-esteem, spouse education, and willingness for contralateral prophylactic mastectomy were the factors that caused a huge difference in social avoidance and suffering.

The similarities of diseases with respect to their related genes were followed by obtaining related proteins. Then the disease network was built with respect to GCN for extracting features for each and every particular disease. After encoding, features of each disease contain relationships with other diseases along with protein information. To identify diseases that cause

PTSA, XGBoost was used to build models. Cross-validation was used to verify the method. A calculation method named gene-based similarity was used to calculate the similarities among the obtained diseases. Since most of the diseases that are based on PTSA are usually due to genes, therefore, it is reasonable to calculate the similarity of gene-based diseases. GCN aims to apply nonlinear functions to transfer the networks to the outputs. And the use of XGBoost is that the sparse matrix can be taken as input. The features that are sparse in nature are handled well by the XGBoost. Thus, XGBoost was used to identify PTSA diseases.

In Ref. [3], the authors show that a three-dimensional (3D) deep learning (DL) gGNN speeds up the differentiation of multiple datasets consisting of COVID-19-infected cases from normal cases. The inputs are 3D-CT images (computed tomography (CT) datasets). z-score standardization is used to process and evaluate the initial CT scans. The entire dataset is converted into the same size while feeding into neural network layers. Features are extracted from these input images. This is done using the help of a transfer learning method. This enhances the performance of predicting the parameters that help to segregate the samples of infected cases and normal cases. After this first step, the next step taken is building a COVID-19 graph in GCN based on the extracted features. The information consists of equipment-type, hospital, and disease status. The graph divides the samples into various clusters. The edge connection and the edge weights are dependent on the combination of the correlation distance of the score differences and extracted features obtained from the 3D-CNN structure. The edges along with the edge weights regulate the convolution operation. This graph is then used as input into GCN to achieve the diagnosis results.

Zheng et al. in Ref. [4] use CID-GCN as an effective GCN along with gating mechanism, which is incorporated for chemical—disease relation, Chemical Induced Disease (CID) relation extraction. Heterogeneous graph is constructed that contains sentence, mention, and entity nodes. Graph convolution operation is used in aggregating the interactive information onto the constructed graph. Oversmoothing problem is resolved by using the gating mechanism with the use of graph convolution operation. The oversmoothing term over here means that after multilayer graph convolution, the Laplacian smoothing effect causes the representation of node toward a space that contains distinguished information. The challenge of correlation between chemicals and diseases is overcome. This challenge includes two categories, one is Disease Named Entity Recognition (DNER) task and the other is CID relation extraction task. The former is in identifying and normalizing to Medical Subject Headings (MeSH) concept identifiers. The followed task is to check if there is association or link between chemicals and diseases which is denoted by MeSH identifier pairs. This paper focuses on the later part, that is, the CID relation extraction task. This is formulated to be a binary classification problem. The technique used for CID relation extraction is based on a graph-based approach. Words are nodes and edges are intra and intersentential relations between words, which are extracted simultaneously. Graph convolutional operations apply a nonlinear activation function after applying the linear transformation to all the neighbors of a node. Multi hop reasoning over heterogeneous graphs is obtained by stacking multiple graph convolutions one above the other. A total of three modules are used, an encoding layer that is used to learn the feature vector representation of nodes with the help of RNN with LSTM cell. The other module is the graph aggregation layer that basically deals with all the convolutional network layers of graph. Then comes the third module, which is the classifier layer. After several times of aggregation, a new set of representations is obtained for all the nodes. The stochastic gradient descent (SGD) algorithm is used to minimize the log likelihood function.

In Ref. [5], the authors built an intelligent model that can automatically recommend the medications of patients based on lab tests, which may be incomplete. The relations are read between multiple types of medical entities with their inherent features in a heterogeneous graph. A construction of a graph is done to associate or link the patients, encounters, lab tests and medications, and has conducted the two tasks: medication recommendation and lab test imputation. Heterogeneous graph, named Medical Graph (MedGraph) and a medical Graph Convolutional Networks (MedGCN), is proposed. It consists of four types of nodes: encounters, patients, labs, and medications, each of which could have their inherent features. Cross-regularization, an effective regularization technique, is used to reduce over-fitting. GCN learns node representations based on the node features and their connections. Lab test imputation is done as matrix completion where common imputation methods such as mean or median imputation will overlook the correlation between different columns. In medication recommendation, for each medication, the model should output the recommendation probability. This is tackled by many machine learning algorithms such as logistic regression.

Authors in Ref. [6] present an overview of all such machine learning computational concepts that can be useful to work on health care. A DL algorithm is considered to be a learning representation that involves feeding to a machine with some data in raw form and developing its own representation that is formed by multiple layers, which are arranged sequentially. These layers include a huge number of primitives, nonlinear operations, in such a way that the representation of one layer is fed into the next layer and is then transformed into an even better abstract representation. Clinics are beginning to employ object detection and segmentation in images using computer vision (CV). Natural language processing (NLP) mainly focuses on inferring texts and analyzing the speech as well. Another such domain that can benefit from deep reinforcement learning (RL) is robotic-assisted surgery (RAS). These computational techniques or domains impact the areas of medicine and explore how to build end-to-end systems.

In Ref. [7], Biomedicinal areas including disease diagnosis, living assistance are explored. Artificial intelligence (AI) can be a major contributor to health care in becoming more personal, predictive, preventative, and participatory. AI in biomedicine can be categorized into four categories. AI can be used in smart robotic systems that assist the living of elderly and disabled people. NLP is broadly used in the field of biomedical and in its applications. In biomedical question answering (BioQA), the aim is to find quick and precise answers. Biomedical research area is also one of the areas covered. Digital data conditioning involves band-pass filtering along with a noncausal linear-phase finite impulse response (FIR) filter. Computation of background neural activity where the background baseline is calculated by averaging of neural FR. Epilepsy, a neurodegenerative disease is characterized to be spontaneous, unpredictable, and recurrent seizures. Research has been done to predict the seizure. A genetic algorithm is used to choose the features of the preictal state.

The authors in Ref. [8] emphasized on the point that with the increase in volume of imaging information as well as the nonimaging information, researchers needed a powerful tool such as graph for modeling individuals (which are denoted as nodes) and associations or similarities between these nodes were denoted as edges. The effectiveness of GCN to collect information from neighborhoods has resulted into their applications in various different problems with respect to 2D and 3D images such as classification, image segmentation, etc. This paper worked on Autism Spectrum Disorder (ABIDE) and Alzheimer's Disease (ADNI) databases. The researchers of this paper worked on analysis of key parameters of the proposed GCN model for the ABIDE database along with exploration of some of the new feature selection strategies. While building the population model, feature vector x(v) describing each graph node and its connectivity in the graph with the help of nodes are one of the important sections that the researchers focused on. Some of the common approaches used along with the discussed strategy in the paper are Principal Component Analysis (PCA), Multilayer Perceptron (MLP), and Autoencoders. The key feature that outcasts DL from other methods is that the network learns an optimal feature representation. Another graph construction strategy, apart from the mentioned strategy in the paper, could be a pure learning-based approach, in which learning is done by a graph structure from self-attention weights and using all potential features.

In Ref. [9], GCN is applied for the analysis and prediction of comorbidity health related to patients with the help of sparse health records. This is done by formulating the health risk predictions in the form of bipartite graph matrix. GCN is used to solve the health link prediction problem. One such application where the link prediction algorithms can be applied directly on any graph structure is the recommendation system. The Graph Convolutional Matrix Completion (GCMC) performs link prediction on graphs. The main goal covered in this paper is to predict the individual's missing condition or event times such as underreported or emerging items based on existing or past adverse events. In the bipartite graph representation used, each condition node stores their corresponding category of conditions as the node features. Attributes for each patient node include entities such as gender, medicaid enrollment aid category, etc. The methods used include Graph Auto-Encoder that learns an efficient way to compress and encode data into a lower-dimensional representation. Some of the baseline methods mentioned in this paper for the evaluation purpose are related to Association Rules, K-Nearest Neighbor (KNN) graph, and Collective Matrix Factorization (MF) (where decomposition is done on the original provided sparse matrix to low-dimensional matrix with factors/features and comparatively less sparsity.)

Medical images provide valuable information especially when it is related to brain images or areas with respect to brain neurons [10]. A 11-layer deep 3-D Convolutional Neural Network is built for brain lesion segmentation. A dense training scheme is built to tackle the complexity of the computations and also overcoming the burden of computing three-dimensional medical scans. This is also helpful in easing the problems related to inherent class imbalance of segmentation issues. A dual pathway architecture is used to process the input images at multiple scales simultaneously. This pathway is used to incorporate both local and the contextual information that is larger in size. Although neural networks seem very efficient when it comes to dealing with medical image analysis, yet it is also a necessity to interpret and understand when the network fails, which was dealt nicely with in this paper. The test datasets on which the system is applied on are BRATS and ISLES datasets.

Hao Jiang along with other coauthors worked on the brain connectivity networks that are widely used for the classification of some of the neurological disorders, such as autism spectrum disorders (ASDs) or Alzheimer's disease (AD) [11]. This helps in exploring the association between underlying disruption with respect to brain disorders. The concept of network embedding learning deals with the automatic learning of low-dimensional representations of the brain networks. A GNN is built upon for producing some representations for graph classifications that are in an end-to-end fashion. This is achieved with the help of the hierarchical Graph Neural Networking system (GCN framework), which is also called hi-GCN. In this, both the network topology information and the subject's association are considered at the same time during the learning process of graph feature embedding. The dataset used to demonstrate this approach is Alzheimer's Disease Neuroimaging Initiative (ADNI) dataset and Autism Brain Imaging Data Exchange (ABIDE) dataset.

According to the survey work presented in Ref. [12], Electronic Health Record (EHR) documents deal with the process of healthcare delivery and some other functioning needs such as tracking care, billings, and payments. Clinical data is usually heterogeneous data that has various forms. Some of the technical challenges are dealing with missing data, casualties, etc. These considerations are crucial for modeling frameworks, learning targets. Learning from incomplete, or missing, data in the machine learning concept in the field of healthcare is a process that is considered to be dynamic. The input representation is also a fundamental issue that spans all kinds of machine learning frameworks. In this survey, a mixture and heterogeneous methods of DL techniques and frameworks are being applied to various types of clinical implementations including information extraction, phenotyping, representation learning, outcome prediction analysis, deidentification, etc. Repeated orders are transported from the labs and doctors to respond to previous observations. They are classified into missing completely at random, which means it deals with the probability of missingness. Second is incomplete data, which is dropped, and is called as complete case analysis, but this leads to unbiased results. Finally, data can be Missing Not At Random (MNAR), in which the probability of missing data depends on the missing variable or any other missing/unobserved variables. Since correct clinical decision-making plays a vital role in predicting and is a matter of life and death, hence it becomes important to understand and trust the predictions as well as the recommendations done by DL systems.

In the paper mentioned in Ref. [13], a smart dental health system that includes intelligent hardware, DL, and IoT devices (mobile terminal) is proposed. The main aim is for in-home dental health care. A dataset of 12,600 clinical images is collected and an automatic diagnosis model that uses MASK R-CNN (Region-Based Convolutional Neural Network) is developed. These images were collected from around 10 private dental clinics. The trained model was utilized to detect, identify, and categorize (classify) the teeth disorders such as tooth decay, dental plaque, periodontal disease, and fluorosis. A corresponding application was incorporated for both the dentist and the client. This was used to provide services of preexamination, consultation, appointment, evaluation, etc. The main arena that led to this project is cheap hardware accessibility as cheap hardware makes home usage easier.

In Ref. [14], the authors have presented the use of two paradigms, Fog and cloud computing, which have grabbed a significant attention of both industries and the academic field. The writers of this paper focused on collaborating these with health care along with the use of big data and DL. In this work, a Smart Healthcare System based on fog computation for Automatic Diagnosis of Heart Diseases using DL and Internet of Things (IoT) named Health-Fog has been proposed. Fog computing fetches the resources and deploys it onto DL models. An automatic heart-patient-based diagnosis system that is using a DL ensemble called Health-Fog has been developed. Deployment of Health-Fog has been done using Fog Bus framework for integrating with the IoT-Edge-Cloud for real-time data analysis. Fog Bus is basically a framework that is a structured and organized communication and execution of applications that is independent of the platform. It links numerous IoT sensors (referred to as healthcare sensors) to gateway devices for sending the data. Some of the hardware components used are Electro Cardio Gram (ECG) sensor, oxygen level sensor, Electro Encephalo Gram (EEG) sensor, Electro MyoGraphy (EMG) sensor, gateways such as mobile phones, laptops, tablets, cloud data center, etc. Software components include resource manager, DL module where neural network is used to classify the data points, which are the feature vectors that are obtained from the Body Area Sensor Network. The dataset is divided into training set, validation set, and testing set in the ratio of 70:10:20. Ensemble module is used to predict the results from different models and uses the concept of a voting system for decision-making for obtaining the output class that states whether the patient has heart disease or not. This module resides in the fog-bus node.

The writers of the paper mentioned in Ref. [15] proposed their work on building a single network trained according to pixel-to-label format with the help of DL to focus on the issue of automatic multiple organ segmentation in three-dimensional (3D) computed tomography (CT) images. These CT images that provide some necessary and vital internal information about the human anatomy are used to support surgery, therapy, etc. The methodology used can be summed up as multiple 2D followed by 3D integration. To model the huge and big amount of 2D sectional image appearances, a deep CNN is trained to incorporate the encoding of the anatomical structures that are obtained from 3D CT images and accomplish CT image segmentation using pixel-wise labeling followed by decoding of the input image data that is based on the deep trained CNN. This segmentation process is repeated to sample two-dimensional sections from a three-dimensional computed tomography image data. This is then passed on to the deep FCN and then stacking of 2D labeled results back into 3D takes place. In an overall sense, this can be explained in the form of 3D-2D-3D transformations. The database used consisted of 240 3D CT scans where 95% were used up for training and 5% for testing.

In Ref. [16], the work was based on segmentation using multimodality that consists of fusion of multiinformation. This is done to improve and enhance the segmentation. Multimodality is widely spread in the field of medic as it can provide multiinformation about a desired output/target (tissue or organ). Due to the ability of self-learning and generalization over huge volumes of data, DL has been used in medical image segmentation. Because of the varying size or shape or location of targeted tissue(or organ), medical image segmentation requires a DL algorithm to tackle these difficulties. The BraTs dataset is used for presenting this technique. The pipeline of the model proposed in this paper consists of data preparation where the data dimension is adjusted to lower the change between images. It also includes data augmentation to avoid overfitting. Then the pipeline consists of network architecture followed by a fusion strategy where the strategies are presented to train the segmentation network. These fusion strategies are divided into groups of input-level fusion, layer-level fusion, and decision-level fusion. And the last process in the model is the data postprocessing.

The paper in Ref. [17] proposes an intelligent medicine recognition system based upon DL concept. The proposed system monitors or assists the chronic patients for choosing the appropriate medications and thus avoiding wrong medications. This includes an application running on any Android mobile device along with a DL training server and a cloud platform. This system can automatically identify the pills a particular patient needs with respect to the disease the patient is suffering. Through android device logging and fetching details of the medical information of the patient/user, the cloud-based management platform transmits this medication data to the presented intelligent medicine recognition device with the help of a Wi-Fi network. In this proposed intelligent medicine recognition device, the DL method (Google TensorFlow is adopted along with RCNN) collects the drug images that are used by patients suffering from chronic diseases, then inputs them into the adjusted parameterized module for training onto the cloud server, and then transfers this trained module to the embedded computing system module for testing process, that is, drug image recognition. After fetching the results, it is returned back to the android app device and displayed on the screen.

3. Overview of graph neural networks

GNNs are neural networks that are categorized under DL, which deal with data described by graphs. GNNs are the tool of choice for machine learning on graphs. Adjacency matrices represent graphs without any loss of information. There are other matrix representations of graphs that have useful mathematical properties. These matrix representations are called Laplacians and are formed by various transformations of the adjacency matrix. The most basic Laplacian matrix is the unnormalized Laplacian, defined as follows: $L = D - A$, where A is the adjacency matrix and D is the degree matrix. The Laplacian matrix of a simple graph has a number of important properties: It is positive, semidefinite, has $|V|$ nonnegative eigenvalues, and the following vector identity holds.

A person graph $G = (V, E, X, L)$ is a graph that describes the relations within a set of persons. Each node $v_i \in V$ represents a person and each edge $e_{ij} \in E$ is directed from v_i to v_j if person v_i is similar to person v_j. This similarity was computed as the Jaccard similarity between the node features. Additionally, $x_i \in X$ and $l_i \in L$ are the feature vectors and label associated with node v_i. The dimension of matrix X is $m \times n$ where m is the number of documents and n is the length of the feature vector. The adjacency matrix A is of dimension $n \times n$, and its (i, j)th entry a_{ij} is 1 if there is certain level (above a threshold) of similarity between node v_i to node v_j.

Let us consider the node feature update rule as follows. For a node v_i, its feature x_i is updated to be the sum of $a[i,j]$ over all the nodes v_j to which v_i has an edge. This rule can be written as, $x_{i'} \leftarrow a_{i1}x_1 + a_{i2}x_2 + \cdots + a_{in}x_n$. Considering the new updated feature as an intermediate (hidden) representation, we name the corresponding matrix as H and write the above update rule as: $H = A^*X$. Multiplying a feature vector by the adjacency matrix propagates the feature vectors from node to node. In an arbitrary graph there may be multiple nodes propagating signals to each other, depending on the structure of the adjacency matrix. Thus, convolutional filters can be defined on general graphs as matrices that commute with the adjacency matrix. Intuitively, this gives a spatial construction of a convolutional filter on graphs. In particular, if we multiply a node feature vector x by such a convolution matrix, the convolved feature at each node corresponds to some mixture of the information in the node's n-hop neighborhood. The weight terms control the strength of the information coming from different hops.

Fig. 3.1 shows the node classification task. For example, in a communication network we may consider black nodes as malicious and green ones are nonmalicious, and the classification task is to find whether a white colored node is malicious or not. In our research work, a black node in a graph may represent a "stressed" person and a green node stands for a "normal" person, and we wish to find the label of unlabeled white nodes. Fig. 3.2 shows how the node embeddings are generated based by aggregating the local network neighbourhoods.

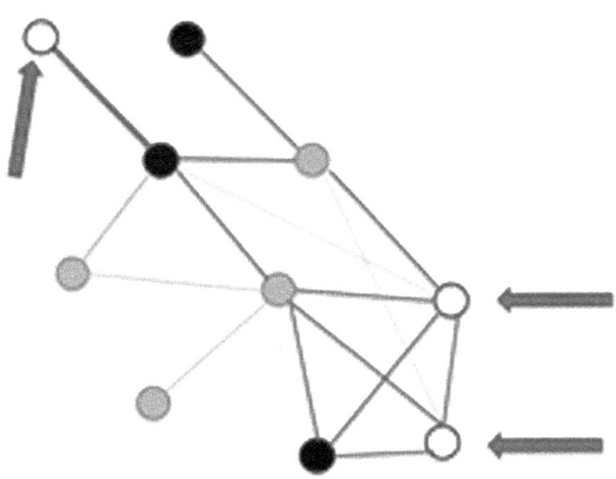

Figure 3.1 Node classification task.

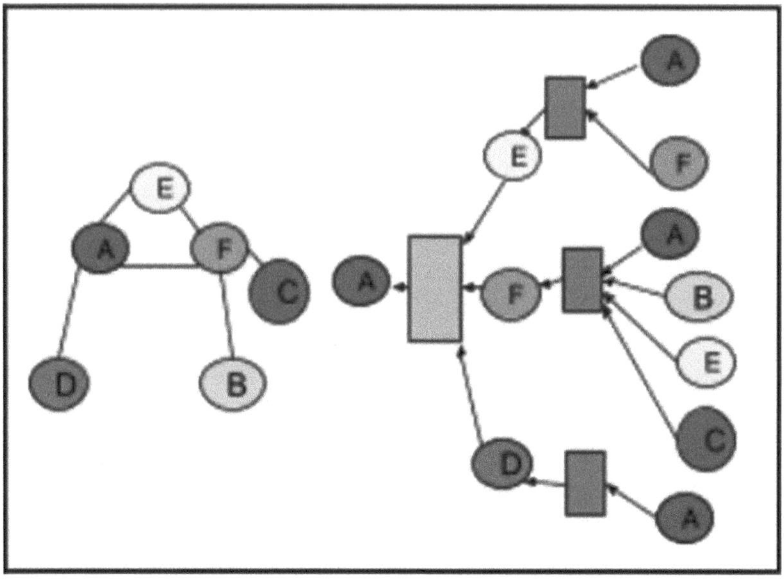

Figure 3.2 Aggregate the neighboring nodes.

In the next section, we present the methodology of the research work, and an overview of the dataset. The detailed steps of the working of a graph convolutional network model are also given for the sake of completeness and for the interested reader.

4. Methodology

In this section, the methodology of this research is shown in Fig. 3.3 and then briefly explained.

In the first step, the data was collected by following the tweets of persons who were the friends of authors on any social networking platform. This was done to make sure that the demographic features and other health-related information would be available to us. For this study, the other attributes

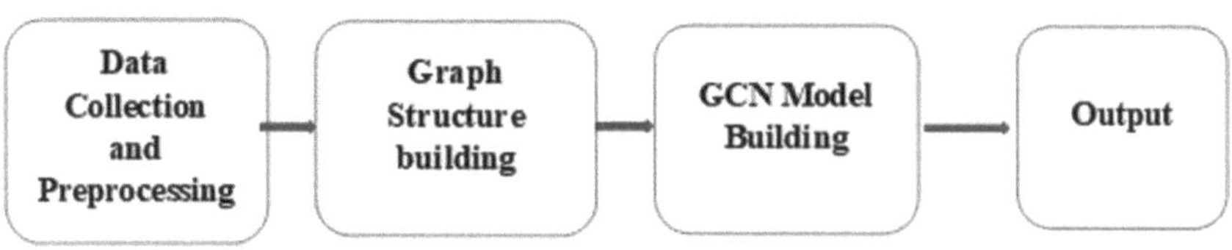

Figure 3.3 Workflow of the MSP - GCN.

used were age, gender, occupation, and history of past ailment. The tweet words were treated as a Bag of Words. The occurrence of a word was considered only if it was used in more than 50% of the posts, in a 15-day window. The labeling of records was done manually, with the help of domain experts. After this, preprocessing was done to remove noisy data such as missing values, which may have occurred during data collection.

In the second step, we build the graph structure. This graph structure has people as nodes, and links between two nodes depend upon the similarity of the nodes. The features age, gender, occupation, history of chronic ailment, and the tweet words used by the user were taken as the input node features, say $X0$. The distance between the nodes was calculated using Jaccard Similarity, and node pairs having distance less than a threshold value ϵ were connected. This threshold parameter is chosen empirically. Mathematically,

$$a_{ij} = 1 \quad \text{if } \operatorname{dist}(i, j) < \epsilon, 0 \quad \text{otherwise.}$$

Here, a_{ij} is the (i,j)th element in the Adjacency Matrix of the graph. Now, the mental stress prediction problem is equivalent to the problem of node classification.

In the third step, the graph from step 2 is fed into the GCN model. This model is built with 80% of the nodes that are used for training and 20% of them for testing. It should be noted that, even though the experiment subjects were a known group of people, their friendship relation was not considered while forming the edges. The intuition was to only model their collected node features with the classification problem.

The overall method of mental stress prediction via GCN feature representation is as follows:

1. The node features are built by the individual person features and the tweet words converted into Bag of words.
2. To convert each person node and its features into a graph, edges are inserted based on the similarity between the nodes.
3. Create node vector matrix X of the graph with node features values.
4. Obtain the adjacency matrix A.
5. The adjacency and feature matrices are input to the GCN to generate feature representations, which have the same dimensions.
6. To propagate the feature representation to the next layer (forward pass), the equation is

$$H^{[i+1]} = \sigma\left(W^{[i]}H^{[i]} + b^{[i]}\right.$$

Where,
$H^{[i+1]}$ is feature representation at layer $i + 1$
σ is the activation function
$W^{[i]}H^{[i]}$ is the weight and feature representation at layer i
$b^{[i]}$ is the bias at layer i

7. Perform dot product of A and X, which represents the sum of neighboring node features, and then perform normalization.
8. Build a GCN layer by adding weights and activation functions. For our work we set eight neurons in the hidden layer and two neurons in the output layer, and Relu as the activation function. The output layer finally predicts the unlabeled node as "stressed" or "normal."

4.1 Experiments

The implementation was done on three sets. The first set consisted of a dataset of size 30. The second set was of length 50, and finally, the implementation was done on 100 data entries. The experiments were executed on the Tesla T4 platform.

5. Results

Implementation on different sizes of dataset leads to checking the variation obtained in terms of loss, accuracy, time computation. With the increase in the volume of dataset, the number of epochs has also been increased to achieve better performance and transparent results.

Figs. 3.4 and 3.5 present the accuracy and loss curves; and the labeling of nodes is given in Fig. 3.6. The accuracy values have been presented in

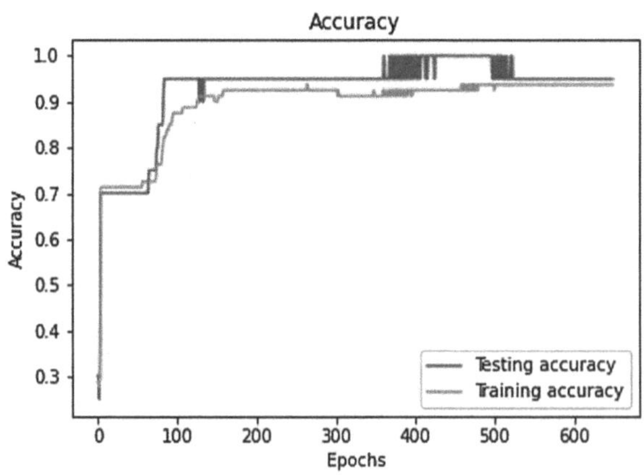

Figure 3.4 Accuracy curves for 100 nodes.

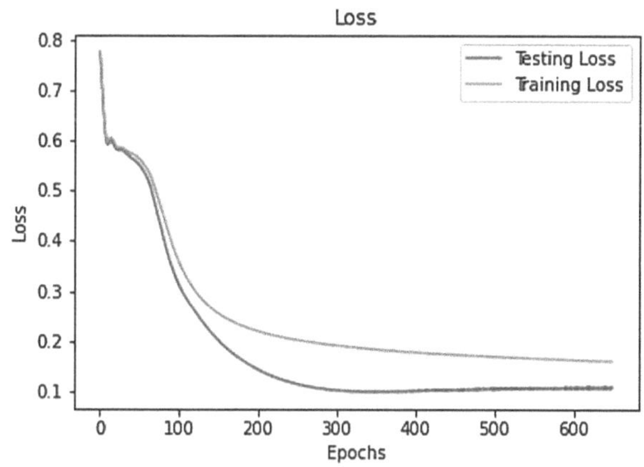

Figure 3.5 Loss curves for 100 nodes.

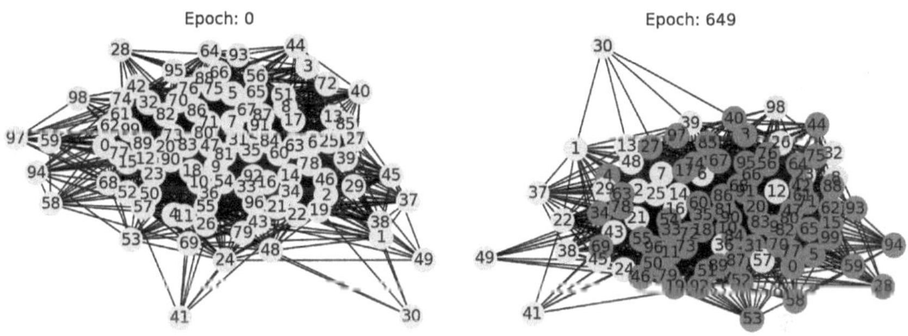

Figure 3.6 Labeling of nodes by GCN for 100 nodes at different epochs.

Table 3.1. It is observed through the curves presented and also some other observations that can be made from the obtained results, plots, and graphs is that, when the dataset size is 30, the training and testing accuracy were 87% and 83%, respectively. As the dataset size increased from 30 entries to 50 entries, the training accuracy increased by 5%, thus turning to 92.50%. And in

Table 3.1 Accuracy values for varying dataset sizes.

	Size 30	Size 50	Size 100
Epochs	135	250	650
Train accuracy %	87.50	92.50	95.00
Test accuracy %	83.30	90.00	93.75
Train time (s)	1.0843	2.2093	5.3867
Edge computation time (ms)	10.8	19.9	87.8

the case of the test dataset, the accuracy hiked up even at a better pace by covering around 7%, that is, moving from 83.30% to 90% accuracy.

Though the edge computation time and the training time increased with increase in dataset entries, which is majorly due to a greater number of calculations of edge linking, yet it can be noted that the transparent and better results were achieved with the dataset size of 100. That is, training set and testing set accuracy both were 95.0% and 93.75%.

It is seen in the present work that increasing the number of entries (that is increasing the dataset volume) that are used as input to build a graph, which is then fed into convolutional layers, and by tuning the epochs higher, the model performance as well as the efficiency turned out to be improvising and optimizing. However, for experiments with much larger datasets, more parameters need to be conducted to affirm this fact.

6. Conclusion

The use of GCNs is growing at a very high speed at present. And that is evident because of its uniqueness in fetching a transparent output. The creation of neural networks with the help of graphs and its respective nodes and edges enables a clear representation of any given problem. The building of these convolutional networks along with graphs is very useful in solving most of the ongoing challenging issues. This is possible only if this GNNs are utilized judiciously and aptly. One such arena has already been covered in this paper, that is, health care with respect to mental stress prediction of a person. Health care as a service is a huge task and responsibility, which each and every person has full right to access. The accessing of medical care or any kind of medical help should be affordable as well as effortlessly. This is because the foremost and prime need of any person is fit and sound health. With the high demand in technologies and evolving of people along with these technologies, focusing on this field of health and its development is like a bestowing of blessings onto this mankind. Some of the trending technologies, which boost up and help in advancement of health care, are such as IoT, Android Application, Cloud-based Computing, Big Data, Machine Learning, DL, Computer Vision, etc., people in this field hold a massive power to build a powerful tool that can change the entire view and scenario of healthcare department all across the globe. All the tech-brains working in all the mentioned fields and many more could collaborate and succeed to reach the target of improvising healthcare.

As per proposed framework, the work is confined to the file-based input data where the data can be either synthetic data or authenticated data. The dataset of people can be further segregated as senior citizens, kids, ladies, pregnant women, disabled people, doctors, nurses, medical students, etc., and the impact on each class can be studied separately. This, however, is part of the future scope of this work. This work could also be extended, and it could be reachable to every person in need by connecting it with the help of IoT. Android developers collaborating with the IoT developers can improvise this work and take it to another level. In a broader sense, an App can be created, which could have a format similar to "google form." In this way, every user can download this from the App Store. Based on the access provided by the user, this App can access the necessary information such as medication details, location of the user and nearby hospitals/pharmacies, medicinal history of the user, suitable and affordable protocol that can be followed to reach out the person in case of emergency, etc. This information that is provided by the user can then be transferred from the IoT devices (such as Android-based phones or any other device that installed this App) to a cloud. Cloud is a massive workspace where all this data can be dumped in an organized manner. This cloud-based database is responsible for collecting and holding all these details from each user operating or filling the data, which is then followed by providing this informative data as an input to the GCNs where the convolutional layers process and filter to reach the final required result.

As part of our ongoing work, we aim to make a more robust, efficient, and highly powerful tool to enable the access of Smart health care to a large number of people. The advancement in Biomedical research can be an add-on to this abovementioned idea of future work.

References

[1] M. Ghorbani, A. Kazi, M.S. Baghshah, H.R. Rabiee, N. Navab, RA-GCN: Graph Convolutional Network for Disease Prediction Problems with Imbalanced Data, arXiv preprint arXiv:2103.00221.

[2] H. Xu, H. Wang, C. Yuan, Q. Zhai, X. Tian, L. Wu, Y. Mi, GCN-Xgboost: identifying diseases that cause psychological trauma and social avoidance, BMC Bioinf. 21 (2020). Article number: 504.

[3] X. Liang, Y. Zhang, J. Wang, Q. Ye, Y. Liu and J. Tong, Diagnosis of COVID-19 Pneumonia Based on Graph Convolutional Network 2020. PubMed ID: 33585511, PubMedCentral ID: PMC7875085, https://doi.org/10.3389/fmed.2020.612962.

[4] D. Zeng, C. Zhao, Z. Quan, CID-GCN: An effective graph convolutional networks for chemical-induced disease relation extraction, Front. Genet. 12 (2021) 624307, https://doi.org/10.3389/fgene.2021.624307.

[5] C. Mao, L. Yao, Y. Luo, MedGCN: Graph Convolutional Networks for Multiple Medical Tasks, arXiv preprint arXiv:1904.00326v1, 2019.
[6] A. Esteva, A. Robicquet, B. Ramsundar, V. Kuleshov, M. DePristo, K. Chou, C. Cui, G. Corrado, S. Thrun, J. Dean, A guide to deep learning in healthcare, Nat. Med. 25 (1) (January 2019).
[7] G. Rong, A. Mendez, E.B. Assi, B. Zhao, M. Sawan, Artificial intelligence in healthcare: review and prediction case studies, Engineering 6 (3) (March 2020) 291–301.
[8] S. Parisotb, S.I. Ktenaa, E. Ferrantec, M. Leea, R. Guerrerod, B. Glockera, D. Rueckerta, Disease prediction using graph convolutional networks: application to autism spectrum disorder and Alzheimer's disease, Med. Image Anal. 48 (August 2018) 117–130.
[9] R. Wang, M.-C. wang, M. Radigan, Modeling latent comorbidity for health risk prediction using graph convolutional network, in: The Thirty Third International FLAIRS Conference (FLAIRS – 33), 2020, pp. 341–346.
[10] K. Kamnitsasa, C. Lediga, V.F.J. Newcombe, J.P. Simpson, A.D. Kane, D.K. Menon, D. Rueckert, B. Glocker, Efficient Multi-scale 3D CNN With Fully Connected CRF for Accurate Brain Lesion Segmentation, arXiv preprint arXiv:1603.05959v3, January 2017.
[11] H. Jiang, P. Cao, M.Y. Xu, J. Yang, O. Zaiane, Hi-GCN: a hierarchical graph convolution network for graph embedding learning of brain network and brain disorders prediction, Comput. Biol. Med. 127 (December) (2020) 104096.
[12] B. Shickel, P. James Tighe, A. Bihora, P. Rashidi, Deep EHR: A Survey of Recent Advances in Deep Learning Techniques for Electronic Health Record (EHR) Analysis, arXiv preprint arXiv:1706.03446v2, February 2018.
[13] L. Liu, J. Xu, Y. Huan, Z. Zou, S.-C. Yeh, L.-R. Zheng, A smart dental health-IoT platform based on intelligent hardware, deep learning, and mobile terminal, IEEE J. Biomed. Health Inform. 24 (June 2019).
[14] S. Tuli, N. Basumatary, S.S. Gill, M. Kahani1, R.C. Arya, G.S. Wander, R. Buyya, HealthFog: an ensemble deep learning based smart healthcare system for automatic diagnosis of heart diseases in integrated IoT and fog computing environments, Fut. Gener. Comput. Syst. 104 (March 2020) 187–200, https://doi.org/10.1016/j.future.2019.10.043.
[15] X. Zhou, R. Takayama, S. Wang, T. Hara, H. Fujita, Deep learning of the sectional appearances of 3D CT images for anatomical structure segmentation based on an FCN voting method, Med. Phys. 44 (10) (October 2017).
[16] T. Zhou, S. Ruan, S. Canu, A review: deep learning for medical image segmentation using multi-modality fusion, Array 3–4 (2019) 100004.
[17] W.-J. Chang, L.-B. Chen, C.-H. Hsu, C.-P. Lin, T.-C. Yang, Digital Object Identifier 10.1109/ACCESS.2019.2908843, A Deep Learning-Based Intelligent Medicine Recognition System for Chronic Patients, vol. 7, April 2019.

CHAPTER FOUR

Women working in healthcare sector during COVID-19 in the National Capital Region of India: a case study

Veenus Jain and Senu Mary Skariah
Amity University, Noida, Uttar Pradesh, India

1. Introduction

Women globally make up over 70% of workers in health, including those working in care institutions [1]. It is rightly said—if you educate a man, you educate an individual but if you educate a woman, you educate a nation. In the 21st century, although being in a patriarchal society, women managed to get themselves educated, prove their potential but what still stands as a challenge is managing the balance of responsibilities at the workplace and home happily. Women in all the spectrum of work go through innumerable issues such as gender bias, unequal pay, lack of maternity leaves, etc., and the arrival of pandemics created havoc in the nation and increased the problems of women in multifold.

Women are the forerunner of society and play an important role in society, in all fields of life, without their contribution no society can nurture properly. Industrialization, improved level of education, urbanization and awareness about rights, and media impact have significantly changed the status of women in society [2]. The changing roles of women in India have led to their greater contribution in the employment sector and changes in many aspects of Indian life [3]. Even though more and more women are engaging themselves in employment to be independent and financially contribute to their families. The mindset of society has still not completely changed [2]. Working mothers of today fulfill family responsibilities and try to remain fully involved in their careers, coping with the competing demands of their multiple roles. The caring responsibilities that working mothers have lay heavy stress on them when it is combined with their professional duties.

Artificial Intelligence, Machine Learning, and Mental Health in Pandemics
ISBN: 978-0-323-91196-2
https://doi.org/10.1016/B978-0-323-91196-2.00015-6

The attempt of working women to integrate, organize, and balance the various problems and activities in their different roles simultaneously puts them under tremendous pressure [4].

Coronavirus outbreak came with the onset of different uncertainties. The deadly virus, which was new to the world, with no medication or vaccination, curtailed fear among the people and resulted in lockdown, financial crises, and stress knowing the uncertainty about this virus. Healthcare workers faced more challenges as they had to maintain a balance between their personal and professional life while treating both COVID patients and non-COVID patients without getting infected by this virus [5].

Health workers are people whose job is to protect and improve the health of the communities. Together these health workers, in all their diversity, make up the global health workforce [6]. The pandemic COVID-19 increased the burden of women working in all walks of life, but the health workers were most affected as they were in primary contact with virus-affected people. Healthcare workers being the frontline to handle the pandemic faced major issues while working, being quarantined, and managing it during the lockdown. It not only drained them physically but also emotionally.

2. Research methodology

(i) This research paper will mainly focus on the qualitative method of research.

(ii) Authentic data directly from doctors and nurses working in both private and government sector institutions have been collected.

(iii) Authentic data from private and government sector institutions will be obtained.

(iv) A review of books and articles by reputed authors on the subject will be carried out.

(v) Published research work done by other universities in India and abroad on this subject will be reviewed.

(vi) Papers published in indexed journals will be consulted.

(vii) During this pandemic, when the whole world came to standstill with complete lockdown, it was healthcare workers who struggled most to manage the balance between work and life. Hence, they will be interviewed as the objective of this study is to analyze the experience they had, issues they faced, and the coping mechanism they developed to counter the pandemics.

(viii) The study will cover a study of diversified age groups, different marital statuses, and varied responsibilities at home and the workplace.

(ix) The parameters considered during the research include the type of organization (public/private), age of the participant, relationship status, number of children under care, working hours at the COVID ward, number of days of work, and the kind of stressful situations faced during work hours.

3. Literature review

India's nearly 50% of working women reported an increase in stress during the pandemic. LinkedIn Workforce Index suggests 31% of working mothers gave full attention to childcare compared to 17% of working fathers. Based on this survey conducted among 2254 professionals, during the period of July 27—August 23, showed the effect of the pandemic among India's working mothers and working women, freelancers toward personal finances and career prospects. The data uncovered that 47% of working women stated that the anxiety due to pandemics increased the stress in personal and professional life. The study revealed that 42% of working women reported that they were unable to give complete attention to household chores and children and 46% were working late at night to complete the work. Data also highlighted that 20% of working women depended on their family or friends to look after their children as they struggled to juggle between personal and professional life [7].

Several studies conducted highlighted that pandemics increased the workload among the people leading to more stress. Most of the research conducted suggested that frontline and healthcare workers were more likely to experience anxiety, insomnia, depression, and other psychological issues. Evidence proves that the COVID-19 pandemic affected the sleep cycle and stress led to suicidal thoughts in healthcare workers [8]. The results of the qualitative research revealed that the underlying causes for suicide were due to the fear of COVID-19 infection, fear of being positive for coronavirus, financial trouble due to loss of job, hopelessness, lack of support from peers, and stress related to work before and after the lockdown [9].

Healthcare workers faced an increase in stress due to certain common factors: Lack of access to the personal protective unit, being exposed to virus leading to bringing the virus home, lack of support for families if the health care worker gets infected by the virus, being unable to give proper time to children and other personal needs due to the increased working hours, financial instability. Workers prone to psychological issues are at higher risk of being more vulnerable to the stress faced by the pandemic. Improvements to workplace infrastructures, providing high-quality safety materials, including regular personal protective equipment (PPE) provision, regular breaks from long working hours, enhancing team support are all possible initiatives that will lessen the psychological impact of the pandemic on workers' mental health [10].

Different categories of healthcare workers experienced varied mental health problems owing to their heterogeneous sociodemographic backgrounds. Among the healthcare workers, doctors had the highest level of anxiety. A greater level of irritability was perceived in both doctors and nurses compared to other healthcare workers. Other healthcare workers faced a lack of sleep [11]. Anxiety, Depression, Posttraumatic Stress Disorder were common in healthcare workers, lack of social support, daily quarantine after work led to an increase in stress. Women in the healthcare sector were at more risk for developing stress [12]. The risk of depression and anxiety was more among young, unmarried healthcare workers. Further, it was found that the healthcare workers who were affected by anxiety and depression from moderate to severe had a negative impact on their quality of life [13].

Nurses are the world's largest population/manpower in healthcare services; they are known as the hospital's backbone and nucleus; however, in most countries, nurses do not have adequate/sufficient facilities. The condition of nurses in India, both in the public and private sectors of health care, is in serious decline [14].

G. Delina and Dr. R. Prabhakara Raya in their study analyzed that work–life balance pressure is high in women, and it affects their quality of life. They were able to find out that married women were not happy or satisfied with their life. Working women found it difficult to find time for themselves, for hobbies, or other leisure activities. In their questionnaire, the highest mean score of 2.67 was of healthcare workers, which showed that healthcare workers wanted to reduce the working hours but had no control over it. She even pointed out that work–life balance even depended upon the number of children. Women with no children have a better work–life balance compared to the ones with children [4].

Maithreyi Krishna Raj in his paper talks about the framework where the situation of the educated employed women is that the family role and occupational role place a conflicting demand, which leads to a stressful situation. He analyzes the problems faced by working women with small children is that they are forced to leave their children to daycare or in the hands of the maid, which gives them more stress in their life [15]. Demands on both fronts at home and work lead to stress in women, the stereotypical role of women comes with the norms that only females will look after the child and household responsibilities. The societal pressure accompanied with juggle between personal and professional life often leads to more stress. This stress indeed takes a toll and decreases their work skills and affects them in all aspects [16]. Rinku Rani, in her study, addresses marital adjustment problems faced by married working women. It highlights that employed married women face more difficulties compared to unemployed married women, thus stressing the insignificant contribution of working married women to the well-being of their families. Their attention to their marital life gets diverted because of two main reasons. First, working women with added responsibilities from their professional life can have severe problems of maladjustment at home, in turn affecting their job. Second, their domestic duties toward children, husband, and in-laws consumes a lot of time, which diverts them from the essence of a healthy marriage [17]. Women members are not able to attend family meetings due to no proper leaves and are not able to give proper care to family members. This creates stress and leads to health problems. Long-term exposure of workers to excessive work hours and job demands elevates the risk of mental and physical health problems [18].

Manju Chhugani and Merlin Mary James highlight the violence faced by workers in healthcare sectors. The possible sources of violence include patients' visitors, intruders, and even coworkers. In their study, they analyze that the workplace violence from the year 2000 to 13 was more in healthcare setting than in private industry [19].

The Caravan reported that scarcity of medical workers has also plagued countries that are struggling with the COVID-19 pandemic. It points out an interview of a female resident doctor, speaking on condition of fear of losing her job, she reveals that she was terrified—she and her husband worked in the hospital and had a newborn baby at home. They decided, only one of them should take the risk of infection. Her husband would work on the frontline, while she stayed home and supported the hospital's administrative work remotely. She feared that she may not see her husband again and she also claims that she was not only the one thinking this way but the entire community of resident doctors was equally worried [20].

Reports suggested that the increase in the number of cases in COVID-19 during the second wave led to an increase in psychological stress. The officials of the Kerala State of Mental Health Authority suggested that nearly 25%–50% of workers required help to overcome anxiety and fear. As during the second wave, many lost their parents, children, and other family members, the fear led to sleepless nights and dreadful dreams among the workers. To help the healthcare workers to cope with the psychological stress, the state provided free counseling services for health care. As during the second wave many lost their parents, children, and other family members, it was noted that most of the healthcare workers complained of lack of sleep and posttraumatic stress [21].

Not only did the frontline workers face immense stress but workers from all sectors faced burnout. Even though the number of journalist deaths was not highlighted, India was third in Journalist death due to COVID. Many journalists quit their jobs as reporting the endless number of deaths every day led to sleepless nights and negative thoughts among them [22].

The impact of COVID-19 not only affected the healthcare workers but also alarmed the country to realize the importance of the healthcare industry. The news article "Covid-19 shows why we need a healthcare reboot for India" brings the attention that even though the highest death rates in India are due to communicable respiratory diseases, the Indian Healthcare system lags in providing efficient public healthcare facilities. The writer addresses the need to revive health care in India by providing better public health infrastructure, involving things such as sanitation, water, waste management, food safety, etc. It highlighted that India in the 2019 Global Health Security Index measures at 57 out of 195 countries, indicating that India may be more vulnerable than Italy (at 31) and China (at 51), which have seen the highest number of COVID-19-related deaths, which states that there is a need to improve the healthcare facilities in India [23]. In another news article, "A chance to rejuvenate India's healthcare sector," the writer indicates that the Indian healthcare industry needs to raise an efficient pharmaceutical and biotechnology sector. Focus on providing health equipment and services would help the Indian healthcare industry and economy in providing healthcare facilities to the rest of the world. The writer points out that COVID-19 has given a chance to the Indian Healthcare industry to make uniform and structural changes in the pattern of health services in India. This improvement would strengthen the healthcare industry and decrease the import of medical devices [24].

Anu Sharma, Pankaj Gupta, and Rishabh Jha in their paper highlight that the new health supply chain is the need of the hour. The new supply chain technology will help the healthcare industry to resist the shock. They recommend four steps to combat the problem of supply chain management risk, i.e., Identity→ Quantify→ Mitigate→ Respond. According to them forecasting the predictions based on the data analysis, of previous pandemics and diseases will help in preparedness for the demand. These steps will help in balancing the demand and supply chain and would also increase employment opportunities [25].

4. Problems

Healthcare facilities around the world employ over 59 million workers who are exposed to a complex variety of health and safety hazards [26]. Stress is the feeling when the person is not able to cope with mental or emotional pressure [27]. On the emotional front, stress can cause anger, sadness, or frustration, change in appetite, difficulty in making decisions and concentrating on work. Physically, it can lead to a lack of energy, frequent headaches, and stomach ache [28].

It is important to identify the stress faced by the healthcare workers. Problems faced by working women in the healthcare sector can be classified into the following categories.

4.1 Emotional stress

According to the American Psychological Association [29], women are more likely to report physical and emotional symptoms of stress than men, such as having a headache or having an upset stomach, or indigestion. Married women report higher levels of stress than single women, one-third reported that they have experienced a great deal of stress compared to a single woman. Similarly, significantly more married women report that their stress has increased over the past 5 years (56% vs. 41% of single women).

The emotional stress faced by women working in the healthcare sector during COVID-19 was immense. It was observed in the interview that the amount of stress during COVID-19 is more than the routine days as being in hospital healthcare workers are at more risk-taking care of the patient with COVID-19.

Joymala Bagchi in the news article published in Heath World.com from Economic Times says, the lack of a definite cure for the infection makes their work extra tough and there is also the added pressure of calming the nerves of the patients and their families. The threat of catching the disease and infecting own families also worried them, due to which most of the doctors have given up going home and have shifted to solitary accommodations, where they go to take rest after completing their duty hours, which could stretch to 15 or even 18 h in a day [30].

Healthcare workers worked for a minimum of 8—12 h of shift and one doctor and one nurse were responsible for looking after at least 13 patients, which added more pressure on them as they were solely responsible for all these patients. The added challenge was to make the patient understand the gravity of the situation and request them to help in the treatment and make their relatives feel comfortable with the healthcare services.

The survey showed that emotional stress was increased due to the noncooperation of the patients and their relatives as the patient would get frustrated and not cooperate with the medicines and the relatives fail to understand the gravity of reason in not being allowed to see their loved ones.

4.1.1 Pre-COVID

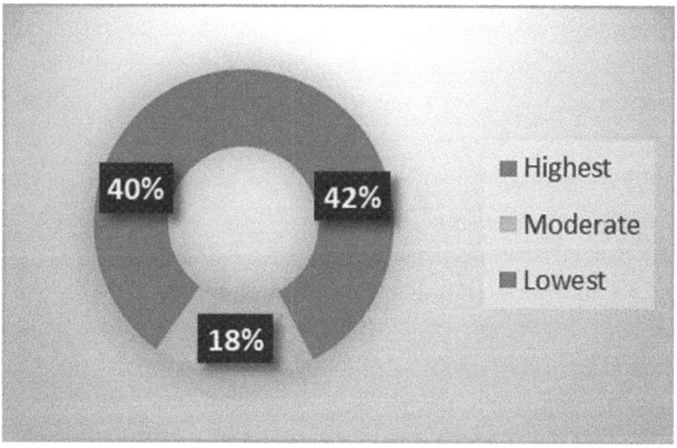

Figure 4.1 Personal life.

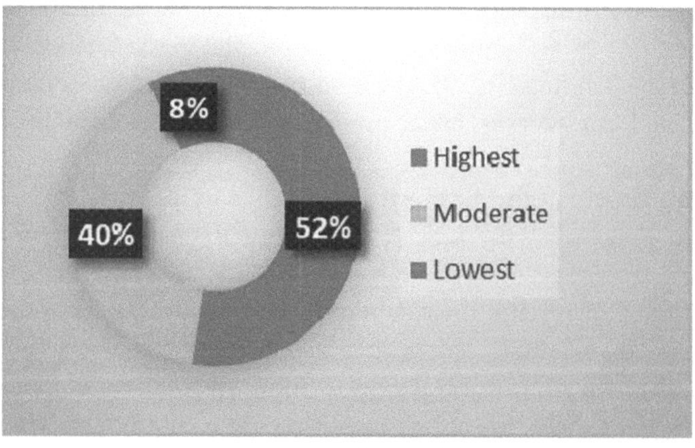

Figure 4.2 Professional life.

4.1.2 During COVID time

Figs. 4.1 and 4.2 show the intensity of emotional stress faced by healthcare workers in personal life and professional life, respectively. Figs. 4.3 and 4.4. show the intensity of emotional stress faced by healthcare workers while working in the COVID wards in personal life and professional life, respectively. The graphs indicate that there was a significant rise in emotional stress faced by the female healthcare workers in professional life in comparison to the situation before COVID-19.

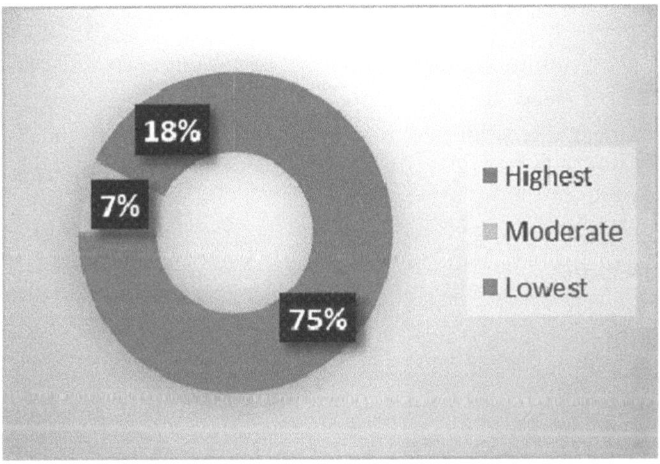

Figure 4.3 Personal life.

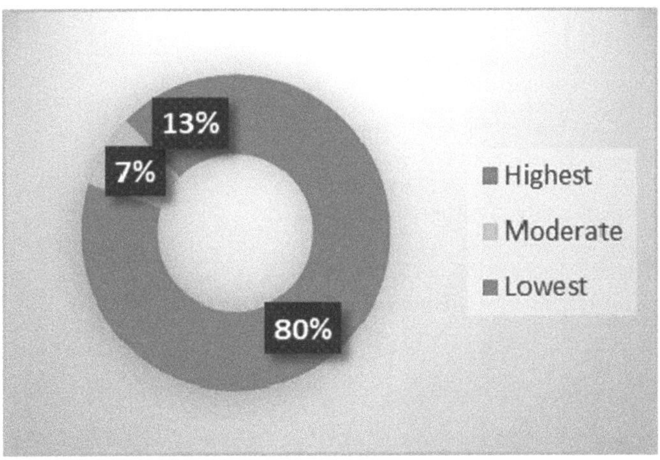

Figure 4.4 Professional life.

4.2 Mental stress

The study conducted on "Mental Health and Depression among Working and Non-Working Women" showed that nonworking women tend to face less stress compared to working women [31]. The mental stress among healthcare workers increased as the fear of the virus made people less helpful to the healthcare workers. The news from various parts of the country of medical staff being attacked and ill-treated added to their fear of being attacked while commuting or the landlord might ask them to leave the accommodation.

Shreya Shrivastava in her news report published in The Print reported that five nurses and one doctor committed suicide due to stress and the stigma of contracting COVID-19. The major mental stress they faced was due to lack of sleep, as this led to less concentration in work and turn more headaches and other health issues. It was important to be always alert as the sole responsibility of every patient was on them and any mistake may result fatally [32].

4.2.1 Pre-COVID

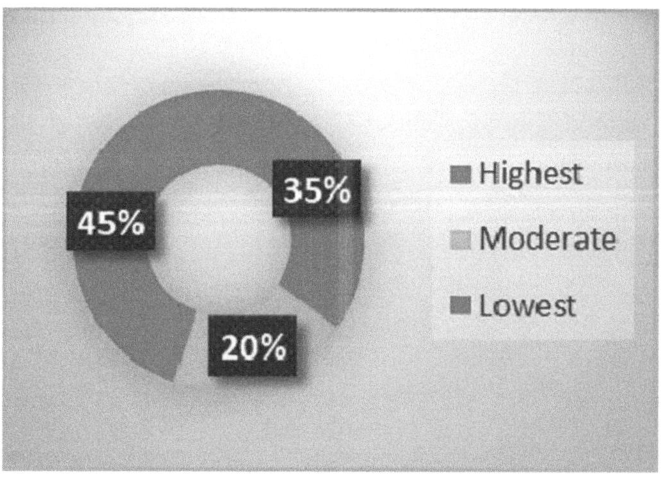

Figure 4.5 Personal life.

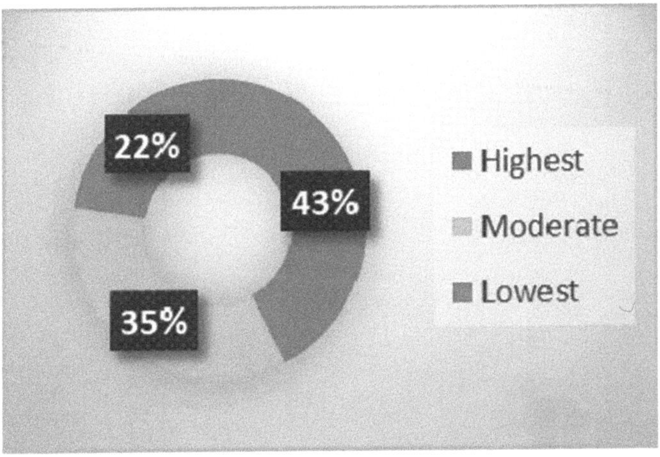

Figure 4.6 Professional life.

4.2.2 During COVID time

Figs. 4.5 and 4.6 show the intensity of Mental Stress faced by healthcare workers in personal life and professional life, respectively. Figs. 4.7 and 4.8 show the intensity of Mental Stress faced by healthcare workers while working in the COVID ward in personal life and professional life, respectively. The survey showed there was a significant rise in the Mental stress faced by a healthcare worker, 80% of the participants felt the high intensity of Mental Stress in Professional Life.

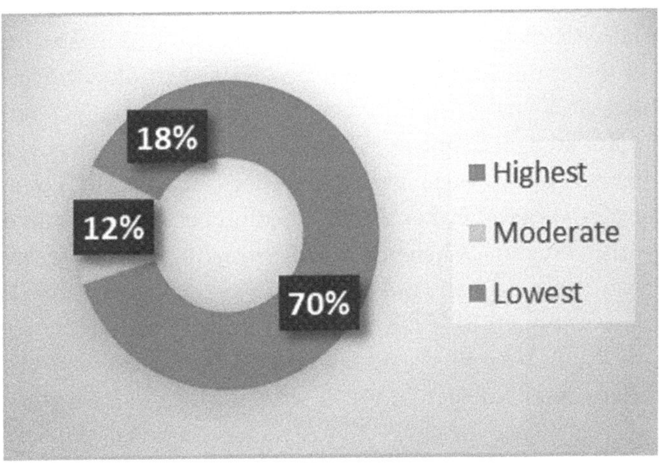

Figure 4.7 Personal life.

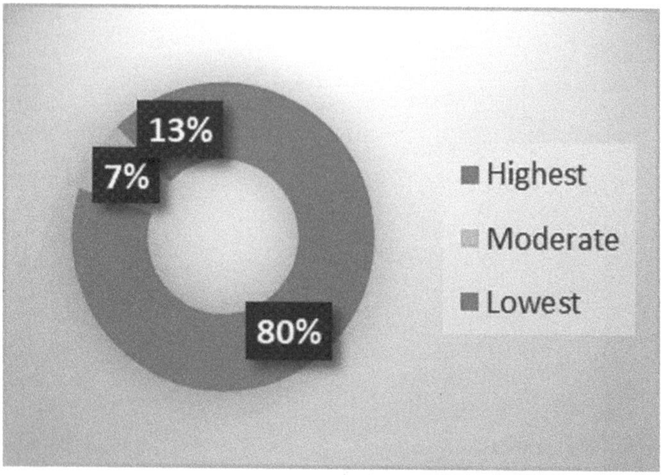

Figure 4.8 Professional life.

4.3 Physical stress

Physical stress comes from a long-standing condition or overuse, which is also known as chronic stress. The accumulation of standing for long hours, sitting in bad posture daily, or conditions such as arthritis, create stress on the body that can be just as harmful as any injury [33]. As the number of working hours was 8—14 h/day, the long-standing hours in the PPE kit drained the healthcare workers physically as the PPE would make them sweat. They wore two N-95 masks, which created scars on their faces and even behind their ears. It was difficult for women who were going through their menstrual cycle, as going to the toilet in PPE Kit was a very difficult process.

Disha Roy Choudhury in her news report published in The Indian Express writes the testimony of Dr. Jaslovleen Kaur, neurologist, Paras Hospital, Panchkula, "We usually wear a diaper for passing urine," who must wear a PPE for 8 h straight regularly. While this is a challenge for all health workers, female professionals perhaps need to make more compromises, given their physiological makeup. The situation becomes difficult especially when they menstruate. "When you are menstruating, you are wearing a sanitary pad along with a diaper, and you cannot even change it for 8 h. So, we take extra precautions. I have never used XL sanitary pads or tampons in my life but now I must wear them. With a tampon particularly, it is a little more comfortable to wear a diaper." [34].

4.3.1 Pre-COVID

Figs. 4.9 and 4.10 show the Physical Stress faced by healthcare workers in personal life and professional life, respectively.

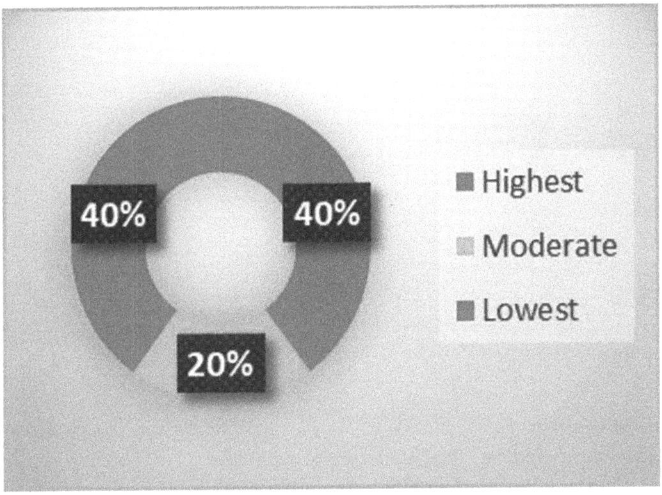

Figure 4.9 Personal life.

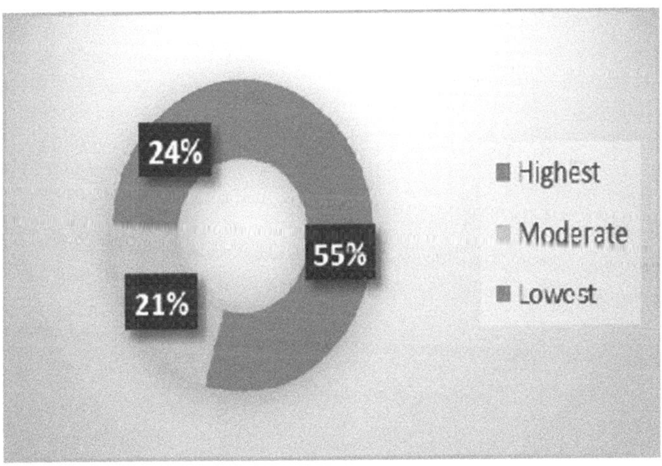

Figure 4.10 Professional life.

4.3.2 During COVID time

Figs. 4.11 and 4.12 show the Physical Stress faced by healthcare workers while working in the COVID-19 ward in personal life and professional life, respectively.

The survey highlighted that the physical stress during the COVID-19 period was more, as before COVID-19 only 55% felt the high intensity of physical stress in Professional life, whereas working during COVID-19, 75% of the participants felt high stress.

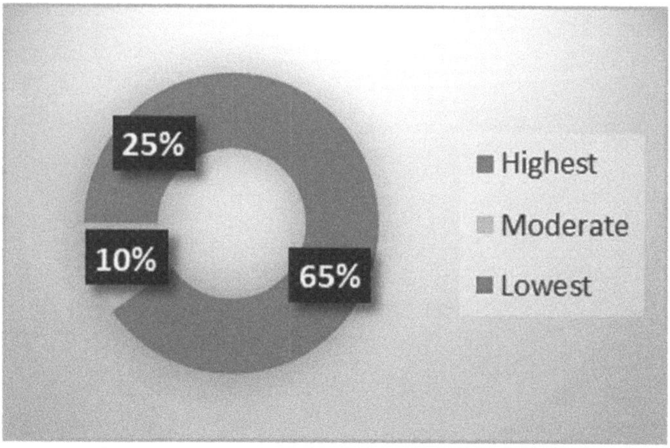

Figure 4.11 Personal life.

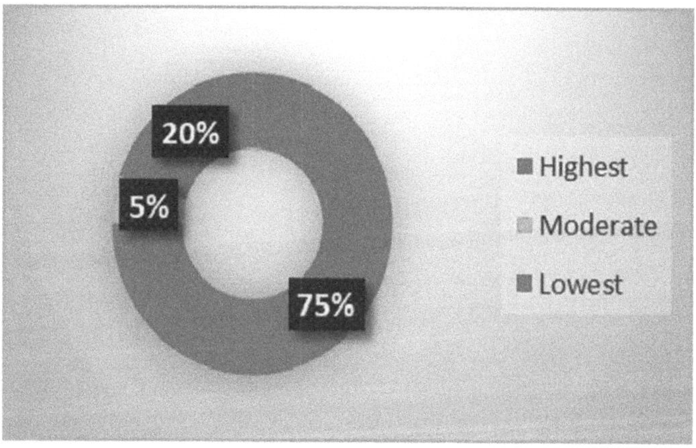

Figure 4.12 Professional life.

4.4 Lack of resources

The healthcare sector of Delhi came to the edge during the second wave, and one of the main reasons for the city is in the top five in the mortality list was lack of resources. BBC in the news article "Covid-19 in India: Patients Struggle at Home as Hospitals Choke" said, the hospitals in Delhi and many other cities ran out of beds, and due to this people were forced to find ways to get treatment for sick patients at home. Many turned to the black market, where prices of essential medicines, oxygen cylinders, and concentrators were much costlier than the original price [35]. The number of deaths and the increasing number of cases in the hospitals added to more stress among doctors and nurses. Due to the increased number of patients, many workers had to work double the time and were mentally and physically exhausted.

The emergent outbreak of COVID-19 created a sudden lack of resources. The major setback that turned out to be a challenge for both private and public institutions was the lack of nurses and doctors. The FEDERAL in a news article focuses on the lack of resources in the hospitals. One of the doctor's responses in the article was, "There is a shortage of doctors. Our hospital has a cardiac unit and our doctors are trained to handle those cases. But with a hitherto unknown disease, you need many kinds of specialists, like internal medicine, respiratory medicine specialists, etc." It shows how healthcare workers were the most vulnerable in this situation. Further, the news article shows that "At the Delhi Heart and Lung Institute (DHLI), a quarter of nurses had quit even before the hospital was converted into a COVID facility while another 15% nurses quit after it was turned into a coronavirus facility, citing reasons like parental pressure, lack of transportation and personal fears and anxieties, according to hospital officials." [36].

It was observed during the study that they had to do extra work because there was a shortage of nurses and doctors and scarcity of the PPE kit and mask added to more difficulties.

4.5 Work–life balance

Work–life balance is a term used to describe the balance between an individual's personal life and professional life. A healthy work life balance assumes great significance for working women particularly in the current context in which both the family and the workplace have posed several challenges and problems for women [37]. Workplaces often place a disproportionate burden on female workers that includes workload as well as emotional and relational labor within the workplace. Historically, women have also been responsible for the majority of work at home [38]. It can be noted that the pandemics have had a considerable impact on the lives of women, as they are required to manage the household while juggling their professional responsibilities. Moreover, in the present circumstances, women are more likely to develop professional anxieties and mental disorders as quarantine due to the pandemic leaves little room for any personal escape when compared to men in society [39].

The emotional, physical, and mental stress disrupted maintaining work–life balance. The healthcare workers were not able to spend time with their family members as due to working in the COVID ward most of them were getting quarantined. It was stressful to manage everything without having any kind of domestic help during the lockdown. Workers with children and old parents faced more issues, as they had to make sure household things were reaching their loved ones and their daily routine was also managed. It was observed that healthcare workers who lived alone or were unmarried faced less stress as compared to the ones who had children and parents to look after.

5. Findings

The parameters considered during the research included: the type of organization (public/private), age of the participant, relationship status, number of children under care, working hours in the COVID ward, number of days of work, and the kind of stressful situations faced during work hours.

The findings reached through this survey brought forward the following facts.

Fig. 4.13. shows the age group of surveyed women out of which, 43% of participants age lied between 20% and 30%, 35% of participants age lied between 30% and 40%, 12% of participants age lied between 40% and 50%, and 10% of the participants were of the age group of 50 and above category.

Fig. 4.14 highlights the occupation of the surveyed women, 65% of the participants worked as nurses, 15% as doctors, and 20% were of the other category, which included social workers, counselors, etc.

Fig. 4.15 shows the type of organization the participants worked in, 65% worked in the private sector and 35% worked in the government sector.

Fig. 4.16 highlights the marital status of the participants, 65% of the participants were married, and the rest 35% were unmarried. Fig. 4.17 points out that 58% have children and 43% do not have children.

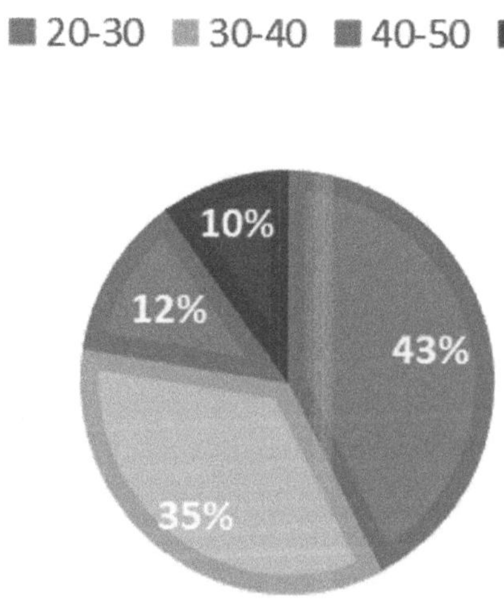

Figure 4.13 Age.

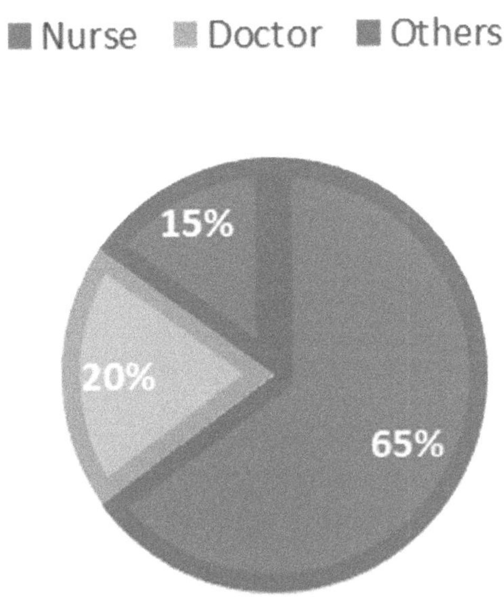

Figure 4.14 Occupation.

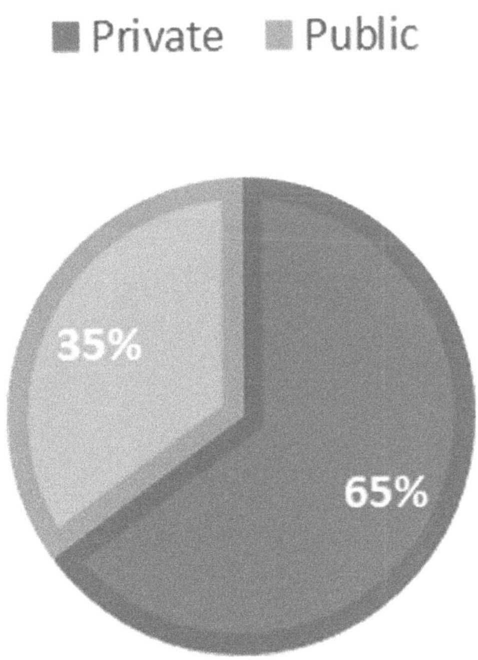

Figure 4.15 Organization.

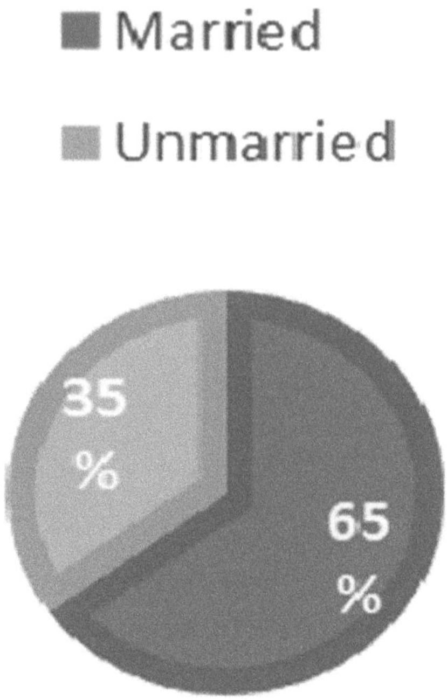

Figure 4.16 Marital status.

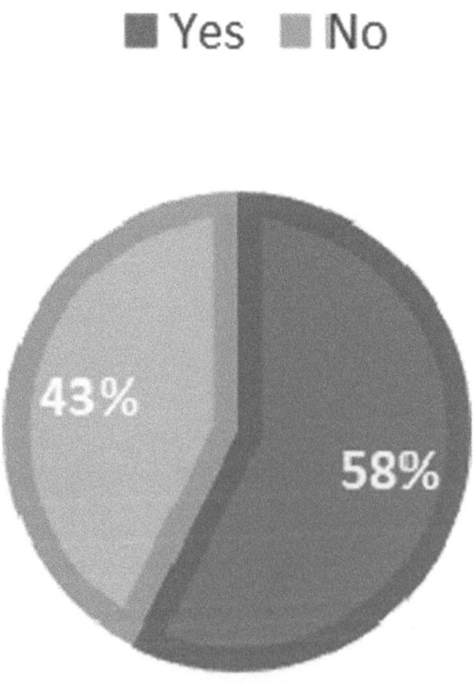

Figure 4.17 Women having children.

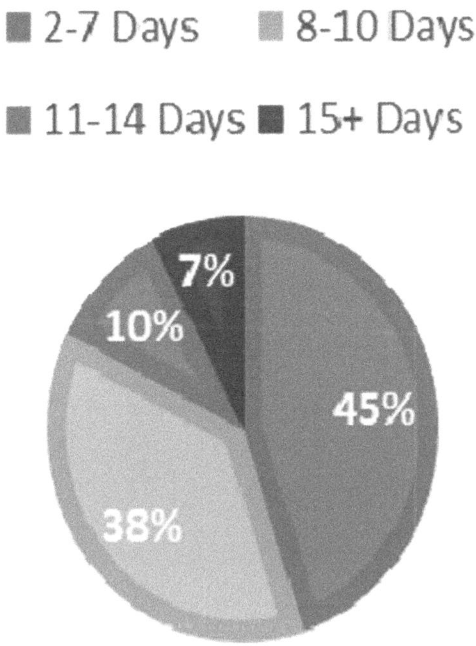

Figure 4.18 Days working in COVID ward.

As the stress was increased during the pandemic COVID-19, the number of days and working hours before COVID-19 and during COVID-19 were also studied. Fig. 4.18 indicates the number of working days working in COVID ward in one shift, 45% of participants worked for 2–7 days, 38% of participants worked for 8–10 days, and 10% of participants worked for 11–14days, and rest 7% worked for more than 15 days.

As the new work conditions required healthcare workers working in the COVID ward to work for a greater number of days, get quarantined, and take necessary precautions.

Fig. 4.19 indicates the number of working hours in a day before COVID-19. 53% of participants worked for 5–8 h, 35% of participants worked for 9–12 h, and 12% of participants worked for 2–4 h.

Fig. 4.20 shows the number of hours working in the COVID ward, 52% of the participants worked for 9–12 h, 35% of the participants worked for 12–14 h, 13% of participants worked for 4–8 h.

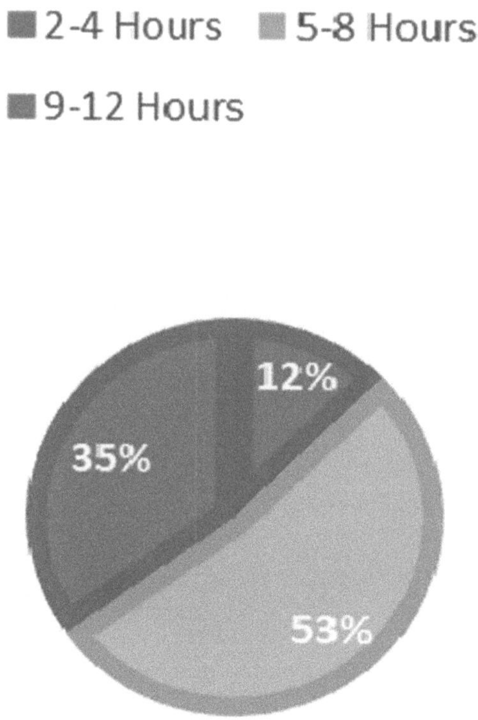

Figure 4.19 Hours working before COVID.

Fig. 4.21 highlights the number of days the healthcare workers were quarantined after working in the COVID ward, 65% of the participants were quarantined for 2–5days, 20% of the participants were quarantined for 6–9 days, and 15% participants were quarantined for 10–14 days.

This clearly shows that the number of working hours of healthcare workers in the COVID ward was increased from 6 to 8 h/day to 8–14 h/day. combined with three quarantine days in private hospitals, while nurses in public hospitals required 14 days of work combined with 14 days of quarantine.

The hospital staff was required to wear PPE during work, which was extremely uncomfortable and irritable to wear due to the mix of plastic that is used to make the equipment. The seven continuous days of duty did not allow nurses to visit home and were instead provided with accommodation such as a hostel or a hotel, wherein they were quarantined for

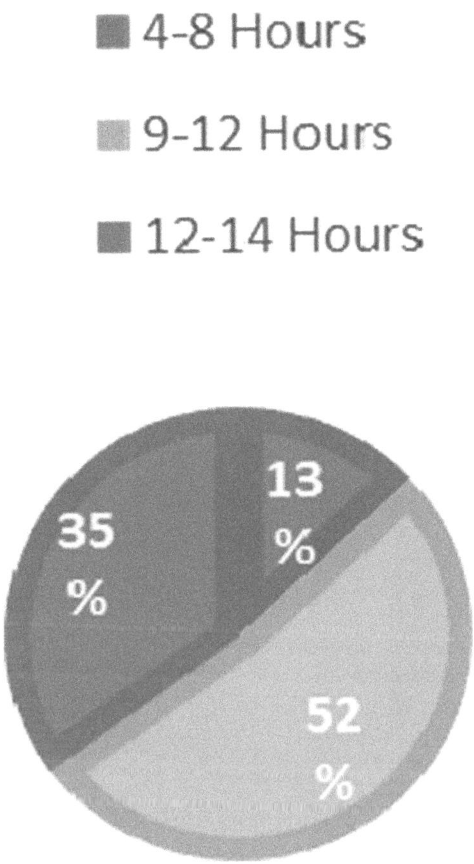

Figure 4.20 Hours working in COVID ward.

another 3 days, which resulted in severe anxiety among them and their family members. Nurses also reported that the facilities provided to handle COVID patients were insufficient and were also improper to cater to the needs of the patients, causing the need to adjust with substandard equipment. The nurses also came across false allegations by the patients of misusing their personal belongings, which were difficult for them to take but were ignored to continue to work in such challenging times. These healthcare workers also came across various health problems such as muscle pain, frequent headaches, varicose vein, various kinds of infections as were not able to maintain hygiene during menstrual cycles being in PPE kits for very long hours.

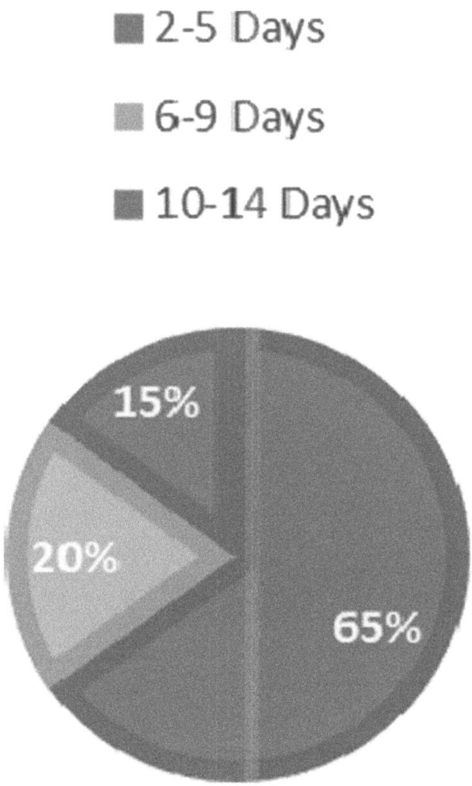

Figure 4.21 Quarantine days.

6. Suggestions

Based on the information obtained from the study, there are few suggestions:

(a) Hospitals may come up with a team of counselors who would help the healthcare workers specifically the ones working in the COVID ward with mental and emotional support. The counselors can offer them mental comfort and techniques to deal with different kinds of situations.

(b) Effective breaks in during long hours will help the healthcare worker to regain energy.

(c) To reduce the panic at the last moment, an efficient way to allocate scarce resources needs to be developed.

(d) A system that automates queries and addresses issues can help hospitals identify operational inefficiencies, thus finding solutions to run their administration.

(e) A feedback mechanism would help the hospitals to come up with solutions to get the administration to work more efficiently.
(f) During these prolonged working hours, a backup of people working in other sectors and were having no work during a pandemic could be provided who could help these warriors with nonmedical backhand support.
(g) A positive environment both at home and workplace can reduce the stress faced them.

7. Limitations

This research had certain limitations, due to social distance regulations caused by the global pandemic. The interviews were carried out through phone and video call interaction and observations were noted accordingly. However, no observations could be made about the condition of the place they were working in. The data analysis of the number of hours working and days being quarantined differed from hospital to hospital.

8. Implications

(a) The appointment of counselors to deal with such pandemics will mentally and emotionally prepare the healthcare workers.
(b) The mental health and emotional support will help to reduce panic at the last moment and resources will be allocated efficiently.
(c) Operational efficiency will be identified and addressed to give solutions to improve administration successfully.
(d) By giving a backup of people during these working hours, better mental health and the workplace will be created. This will give them the strength to combat the situation effectively.
(e) The collective measures taken by the administration, management, and government authorities will help in reducing the stress and will create an environment for better support.

9. Conclusion

The position of women has significantly changed over the years, from getting the right to vote to be financially independent. Even though modernity has come to its play, the situation of women has not yet completely changed. Women have secured their position in all sectors but, still goes through innumerable issues related to gender basis, unequal pay, discrimination, etc. Health care is one of the vulnerable sectors, where the job of an individual is to take care and cure the patient, which comes with added stress.

COVID-19 pandemic came with its own set of problems; the healthcare sector was affected adversely as they were in primary contact with people affected by this virus. As there was no definite cure or medicine, the healthcare workers went through psychological and physical stress due to their work environment. Even though the new vaccination brought some relief, the fear of catching the virus has always been there. Women while carrying out their duty as healthcare workers do come across various kinds of problems because they play different roles in their professional as well as their personal life, which affects them emotionally and mentally in their personal life, which in turn affects their professional performance too.

Pandemic increased the stress in all sectors of work for both men and women. But, working women faced more stress as they were expected to look after the children and do other daily chores compared to the men. It is important to highlight the stress faced by working women, as the increase in stress often leads to negative and suicidal thoughts. Healthcare workers who are a part of frontline workers faced the major part of the stress as their professionals required them to look after the coronavirus-affected patients.

The research showed that women healthcare workers faced more emotional, mental, and physical stress during the pandemic. The increase in stress was due to the shortage of staff, lack of resources, long working hours, fear of catching the virus, increase in the number of deaths, uncertainty about the virus, and no authentic way to cure. The long-standing hours in Personal Protective Kit with triple-layer masks brought more stress among the female workers who were going through the monthly cycle, were pregnant, had children, or had old parents to look after. The added responsibilities in personal life led to an increase in stress, which exhausted the female healthcare workers. Working in hot and humid conditions with no proper food also brought different health issues.

Helping hand is important in every sector, healthcare is no less, during these trying times a backup of people ready to offer social service could have provided the healthcare worker's necessary support. Moreover, a team of counselors to relieve their stress would have helped them to perform their duties diligently. A caring work environment would have made them emotionally strong, which helps in bring better results.

This research traced that due to the pandemic, the amount of stress faced by the healthcare workers rose tremendously, which has been showcased in the form of graphs. Therefore, the emotional, mental, and physical stress of a healthcare worker should be considered a matter of concern for all including the state. The state should introduce policies keeping in mind the needs of these workers during emergency times and these warriors should be accorded with high respect for their selfless and exemplary hard work.

It is also important for one to understand the seriousness of psychological stress. Being aware of one's stress and being able to understand when someone else is going through it, will help an individual to look for help and other ways to cope up with stress.

References

[1] Emanuela Pozzan Umberto Cattaneo, Women Health Workers: Working Relentlessly in Hospitals and at Home, April 7, 2020. Available: https://www.ilo.org/global/about-the-ilo/newsroom/news/WCMS_741060/lang–en/index.htm.

[2] A. Panigrahi, A.P. Padhy, M. Panigrahi, Mental health status among married working women residing in Bhubaneswar city, India: a psychosocial survey, BioMed Res. Int. (2014), https://doi.org/10.1088/1757-899X/949/1/012075. PMC3988941.

[3] M. Darji, P. Panchal, S. Belani, The challenges faced by Indian working women to balance professional and social life IN 21 ST century, in: International Conference Women in Science & Technology : Creating Sustainable Career, 2016.

[4] G. Delina, R.P. Raya, A study on work-life balance in working women, Int. J. Commer. Bus. Manag. (2016) 8–9.

[5] J. Shreffler, J. Petrey, M. Huecker, The impact of COVID-19 on healthcare worker, West. J. Emerg. Med. (2020) 1059–1066.

[6] World Health Organisation, [Online]. Available: https://www.who.int/occupational_health/topics/hcworkers/en/.

[7] N. Mathur, Nearly 50% of India's Working Women More Stressed Due to Pandemic: LinkedIn, September 10, 2020. Available: https://www.livemint.com/companies/news/nearly-50-of-india-s-working-women-more-stressed-due-to-pandemic-linked in-11599722943378.html.

[8] D. Jeng Li, N. Ying Ko, Y.-L. Chen, P.-W. Wang, Y.-P. Chang, C.-F. Yen, W.-H. Lu, COVID-19-Related factors associated with sleep disturbance and suicidal thoughts among the Taiwanese public: a facebook survey, Int. J. Environ. Res. Publ. Health (2020), https://doi.org/10.3390/ijerph17124479.

[9] D.D. Dsouza, S. Quadros, Z.J. Hyderabadwala, M.A. Mamun, Aggregated COVID-19 suicide incidences in India: fear of COVID-19 infection is the prominent causative factor, Psychiatr. Res. (2020), https://doi.org/10.1016/j.psychres.2020.113145.

[10] G. Giorgi, L.I. Lecca, F. Alessio, G.L. Finstad, G. Bondanini, L.G. Lulli, G. Arcangeli, N. Mucci, COVID-19-Related mental health effects in the, Int. J. Environ. Res. Publ. Health (2020), https://doi.org/10.3390/ijerph17217857.

[11] S.S. Chatterjee, M. Chakrabarty, D. Banerjee, S. Grover, S. Chatterjee, U. Dan, Stress, sleep and psychological impact in healthcare workers during the early phase of COVID-19 in India: a factor Analysis, Front. Psychol. (2021), https://doi.org/10.3389/fpsyg.2021.611314.

[12] B.G. Jagiasi, G. Chanchalani, P. Nasa, S. Tekwani, Impact of COVID-19 pandemic on the emotional well-being of healthcare workers: a multinational cross-sectional survey,

in: Indian Journal of Critical Care Medicine : Peer-Reviewed, Official Publication of Indian Society of Critical Care Medicine, 2021.

[13] N. Suryavanshi, A. Kadam, G. Dhumal, S. Nimkar, V. Mave, A. Gupta, S.R. Cox, N. Gupte, Mental health and quality of life among healthcare professionals during the COVID-19 pandemic in India, Brain Behav. (2020), https://doi.org/10.1002/brb3.1837.

[14] V. Vijayaraddi, Challenges faced by nurses in India - the largest manpower in of healthcare in trouble, J. Phram. Nurs. (2020) 10−11.

[15] M.K. Raj, Research on Women and Career: Issues of Methodology, October 25, 1986. Available: https://www.jstor.org/stable/4376265?seq=3.

[16] S.M. Freedman, M. Bisesi, Women and workplace stress, AAOHN J. (1998) 271−275.

[17] R. Rani, Marital adjustment problems of working and NonWorking women in contrast of their husband, Int. J. Relig. Educ. (July 2013) 1−5.

[18] G. Shiva, A study on work family balance and challenges faced by working women, IOSR J. Bus. Manag. (2013) 1−4.

[19] M. Chhugani, M.M. James, Challenges faced by nurses in India-the major, Nurs. Care Open Access J. (2017) 1−3.

[20] L. PAGE, India's under-supported force of healthcare professionals is crumbling under the pressure of COVID-19, Available: https://caravanmagazine.in/health/india-under-supported-health-care-workers-crumbling-pressure-covid-19, March 29, 2020.

[21] S. Mohan, At Wits' End: Healthcare Workers in Kerala Reel under COVID Fear as Second Wave Rages, June 1, 2021. Available: https://www.newindianexpress.com/states/kerala/2021/jun/01/at-wits-end-healthcare-workers-in-kerala-reel-under-covid-fear-as-second-wave-rages-2309986.html.

[22] N. Kwatra, S. Imad, Covid-19: Trauma from India's Second Wave May Have Lingering Effects on its Frontline Workers, July 4, 2021. Available: https://scroll.in/article/998947/covid-19-trauma-from-indias-second-wave-may-have-lingering-effects-on-its-frontline-workers.

[23] S.A. Surbhi Bhatia, Covid-19 Shows Why We Need a Healthcare Reboot for India, March 2020, 2020. Available: https://www.livemint.com/politics/policy/will-covid-19-prompt-health-reboot-11585497828527.html.

[24] K. Reddy, D. Singhania, S. Sasidharan, J. Nabar, A chance to rejuvenate India's healthcare sector, Indian Exp. (May 22, 2020). Available: https://indianexpress.com/article/opinion/coronavirus-a-chance-to-rejuvenate-indias-healthcare-sector6422865/.

[25] P.G.R.J. Anu Sharma, COVID-19: impact on health supply chain and lessons to Be learnt, J. Health Manag. (2020), https://doi.org/10.1177/0972063420935653.

[26] World Health Organisation, [Online]. Available: https://www.who.int/whr/2006/chapter1/en/.

[27] Mental Health Foundation, Stress, March 26, 2021. Available: https://www.mentalhealth.org.uk/a-to-z/s/stress.

[28] National Center for Chronic Disease Prevention and Health Promotion, Coping with Stress, [Online]. Available: https://www.cdc.gov/mentalhealth/stress-coping/cope-with-stress/index.html.

[29] Stress and Gender, Available: https://www.apa.org/news/press/releases/stress/2011/gender, 2011.

[30] J. Bagchi, Doctors, Healthcare Workers Deputed at COVID-19 Wards Share Their Challenges, Apprehensions as Crisis Deepens, April 14, 2020. Available: https://health.economictimes.indiatimes.com/news/industry/doctors-healthcare-workers-deputed-at-covid-19-wards-share-their-challenges-apprehensions-as-crisis-deepens/75135702.

[31] R.R. Dudhatra, Y.A. Jogsan, Mental health and depression among working and NonWorking women, Int. J. Sci. Res. Pub. 2 (8) (2012).
[32] S. Shrivastava, India's Healthcare Workers Are the Most Vulnerable, but There Is No Framework for Their Health, July 14 , 2020. Available: https://theprint.in/opinion/indias-healthcare-workers-most-vulnerable-but-no-framework-for-their-health/459827/.
[33] Randy, Physical Stress – Part One of the Three Forms of Stress, March 28, 2012. Available: https://moyerwellness.com/physical-stress-part-one-of-the-three-forms-of-stress/.
[34] D.R. Choudhury, Have to Wear Sanitary Pad with Diaper for Hours: Female Doctors on Challenges of Wearing PPE, August 27, 2020. Available: https://indianexpress.com/article/lifestyle/health/female-health-workers-ppe-challenges-periods-coronavirus-6563136/.
[35] V. Pandey, Covid-19 in India: Patients Struggle at Home as Hospitals Choke, April 26, 2021. Available: https://www.bbc.com/news/world-asia-india-56882167.
[36] Hospitals Face Shortage of Doctors, Nurses; Govt Focused on Increasing Beds, June 25, 2020. Available: https://thefederal.com/covid-19/hospitals-face-shortage-of-doctors-nurses-govt-focused-on-increasing-beds/.
[37] S. Sundaresan, Work-life balance – implications, Oida Int. J. Sustain. Dev. 7 (2014).
[38] APA Committee on Women in Psychology, How Working Women Can Manage Work-Life Balance during COVID-19, October 9, 2020. Available: https://www.apa.org/topics/covid-19/working-women-balance.
[39] V. Jain, P. Mohanan, Work and personal life during COVID-19, J. Human. Soc. Sci. Res. (2020) 67–76.

CHAPTER FIVE

Impact of COVID-19 on women educators

Veenus Jain and Meher Chopra
Amity University, Noida, Uttar Pradesh, India

1. Introduction

"Educator" itself is a very powerful term. She/he is the one who helps in making a child's whole future. Teachers give their whole life to their students, yet in today's world, they are facing so many issues in their day-to-day lives. Talking about women educators, which is the focus of this paper, there are more than 50% women educators in primary education [1] and 42.2% in higher education [2] in India, which means that more than half of the population of teachers are facing severe issues. Major issues faced by women in general and during this pandemic phase can be divided into two categories:

- Professional
- Personal

Family is said to be the backbone of a person. Sometimes problems and opinions arising within the family can be a hindrance to the growth of a person. Girls are often advised by their parents to join the teaching profession as this profession will help them in carrying out their personal life comfortably, as the education sector is not a sector where women are out till late, moreover, it gives you holidays whenever children have holidays. Whereas teachers and especially women educators are working around the clock, as this profession in real life is very demanding and with it taking care of your household and family without any support from your spouse or family increases the pressure. Professional issues that women educators face in general can be identified as:

- Gender differentiation and
- Lack of adequate infrastructure.

Women Educators during this pandemic have gone through different levels of problems. Women with newborn babies, school-going children, and college-going children have been facing different issues in their lives during this very challenging phase. With this also came two major problems, lack of security of job, and technological issues.

Artificial Intelligence, Machine Learning, and Mental Health in Pandemics
ISBN: 978-0-323-91196-2
https://doi.org/10.1016/B978-0-323-91196-2.00006-5

2. Research methodology

The major focus in terms of methodology will be quantitative in nature. Surveys will be filled by teachers of various institutions, which will give an insight into their problems and experiences with online teaching. Interviews will be carried out with teachers having children of various age groups to know about the problems being faced in different phases of their lives. The study has been divided among different age groups of women, the age groups of children, the family environment, and the working hours.

3. Literature review

The role of women in Indian society during the ages has been confined to the household. Taking care of the children, taking care of husband and his family, the role is confined to four walls of the houses. During the era of Dharmashastra and Manusmriti, there were many restrictions placed on women, and they were seen to be created just to give birth to a son. "According to Kautilya, a man may marry any number of women; for women are created for the sake of sons" [3]. "In the laws of Manusmriti it is said that, in childhood a female must be subject to her father, in youth to her husband, when her lord is dead to her sons; an women must never be independent" [3]. This is how the ancient people viewed women, someone who can never be independent, the one who will always need a shoulder to lean on. Coming to modern times, the scenario has changed, women are going out of their homes for jobs, are free, independent, but this is not the case everywhere. Women may be working outside their households, but they are still facing major problems in their lives. Taking the case of rural schools, one study says that, "Even though there is an increase in female teachers, there is few lady teachers in rural areas. Lack of security, material amenities like hostel, quarters, transport, medical facilities and lack of support from the families. In short they are facing problems related to social, political, economic and service matter etc. These problems are not only concerned with woman teachers in rural but urban as well" [4].

The career of women has been seen as secondary to those of men. "In a working environment, actions of women are more scrutinized than those of her male colleagues. It is possible that a criticism directed at a woman leader may take a personal tone than that for a man" [5]. There are various prejudices in the minds of people regarding working women. Their work is thoroughly checked as even if people don't outwardly show it, they do have an inkling that there must be some mistake in the work presented by women.

As per the 2019 data, there is less participation of women in the workforce. The female labor force participation rate (FLFPR) in the country has fallen from 30.27% in 1990 to 20.8% in 2019, as per data from the World Bank [6]. Many reasons can be attributed to this decline. The female labor force participation rate takes into consideration participation from the age group of 15–29 years. One of the reasons for this decline is said to be the involvement of women in higher education. According to the report of Gross Enrollment Ratio (GER), the year 2019–20 has seen more female participation in higher education than male participation. The percentage has gone up to 27.3% [7].

Besides other reasons, the standard set for women by society is one of the main reasons for the low participation. Many restrictions are put on women by their families. On average women spend 5 hours per day taking care of household duties, which is much more than a man. Mobility restrictions are also one that stops women from working. Families don't feel safe sending women to faraway places to work thinking they cannot handle themselves. These constant sacrifices made by women have resulted in their low participation in the workforce [8].

Ginette Azcona, in her report regarding the effects of the pandemic on women, points out that the pandemic has been hard for both men and women. The difference is that women more than men came under the effects of economic depression. "For the last 22 years, extreme poverty globally had been declining. Then came COVID-19, and with it, massive job losses, shrinking of economies and loss of livelihoods, particularly for women. Weakened social protection systems have left many of the poorest in society unprotected, with no safeguards to weather the storm" [9].

Women suffering more than men from the loss of jobs also widen the gender poverty gap. "In 2021, it is expected there will be 118 women aged 25 to 34 in extreme poverty for every 100 men aged 25 to 34 in extreme poverty globally, and this ratio could rise to 121 poor women for every 100 poor men by 2030" [10].

One fatal increase that can be seen during the pandemic phase is the increase in domestic violence. Loss of employment and livelihoods is not the only problem women are suffering from. Locked inside their households with their abusers without any regular support is another problem they are facing. Domestic violence cases have always been high, but during

COVID-19 they have reached a new level. Kanika Arora and Shubham Kumar in a report about Domestic violence during COVID say that "On 24 March 2020, the Prime Minister of India announced a nationwide lockdown to contain the spread of the Novel Coronavirus. Within a fortnight, the National Commission of Women (NCW) reported a 100% rise in complaints of domestic violence cases." The situation was becoming so unacceptable that a Whatsapp number was launched nationwide by the NCW so that women had another way to report the abuse [11].

On the situation of women during the pandemic, Phumzile Mlambo-Ngcuka, the Executive Director of UN Women, says that "COVID-19 is already testing us in ways most of us have never previously experienced, providing emotional and economic shocks that we are struggling to rise above. The violence that is emerging now as a dark feature of this pandemic is a mirror and a challenge to our values, our resilience and shared humanity. We must not only survive the coronavirus, but emerge renewed, with women as a powerful force at the centre of recovery" [12].

The education of girl children has also taken a back seat during the pandemic phase. According to a recent study by UNESCO, more than 11 million girls would not be going back to resume their education in schools after the end of COVID. Besides the gender biases, another reason that highlights this is the economic burden. With the fall of economies, the poor are becoming poorer. In this situation, their priority is educating a boy rather than a girl. Even where education is free, the value of uniforms and supplies for school is unaffordable [13].

Educators have also been facing a lot of issues during this pandemic phase right from the start. It was reported that while educational institutions were closed for students, teachers still had to continue their work from institutions. Their safety during the initial phase of the lockdown was not taken care of. In response to these adverse measures, a petition called "KeepTeachersSafe" was started. Ananya Parekh, who started this petition, believes that closing the educational institutions for students was a good plan, but questions the government regarding the safety of teachers. She says, "But about the teachers? Why are educational institutions asking their teachers and staff to come to work? They are as prone to COVID-19 as students are. By asking them to commute (most of us take public transport) and work in the staff rooms, where they encounter many more individuals - they are being put at risk" [14].

Talking about women educators, in a study, it was shown that a strong female teacher may be seen as rigid and controlling rather than intellectually rigorous and challenging [15]. Strong, this has always been associated more with a man than with a woman, here the question comes on our mentality why do we only see a man as strong and a woman as weak. According to these lines, a female teacher who wants to maintain discipline in class is seen as rigid and controlling rather than intellectually sound. Many times we have seen in our school lives the attitude of students toward male and female teachers. This mentality of students having no respect for female teachers has to change. This is an everyday thing for them, even during this pandemic when teachers are working overtime so that studies of students do not get affected, students are misbehaving with teachers especially the female ones taking them lightly and not turning up in their classes.

According to one article, an 11th-grade Mathematics teacher said that her students kept misbehaving with her and a lot of other teachers by cutting her from the meeting in class and blocking her ID [16]. This shows that nothing has changed, student's mentality is still the same, in offline teaching they used to disrespect teachers (especially females), and in online classes too they are doing the same thing.

A report by European Trade Union Committee for Education on its report during the pandemic phase says that "Women education workers are more likely to be placed on temporary unemployment schemes with lower remuneration and risk losing their jobs altogether. The COVID-19 outbreak and the economic crisis risk further increasing gender inequality in the education sector in all its forms: pay and pension gaps, horizontal and vertical gender segregation" [17]. Gender equality has always been existent in every society, whether Indian or foreign, this pandemic phase has increased this equality gap further. With schools cutting their losses by firing teachers, we can see the trend of female teachers facing this issue more as it is believed by almost everyone that the job of a man is more important than that of women. Hence women are being subjected to firing, pay gaps, and many other problems hindering their growth. This pandemic has badly affected the progress made by women in the workforce. "the COVID-19 pandemic has come as a shock, resulting in massive job losses for women, especially informal workers, and slower recovery of women-led microbusinesses. It has also increased domestic work, deepened gender digital divides, disrupted girls schooling and placed millions of female health workers at risk" [8]. "Many educators looked for alternative jobs to sustain their families as they lost their teaching jobs or their salaries were withheld. Now former teachers are now trying to fit into any job that they can get" [18].

In a study, it is also mentioned that "Workers in female-dominated professions like teaching are already more exposed to adverse social behavior such as bullying, harassment and violence" [17]. Bullying, harassment are now seen as a common occurrence in classes for female teachers. Students are now so accustomed to this kind of behavior that it is now becoming a big issue. Such students are waiting for online classes to be over and classroom teaching to resume so that they can bully and harass female teachers.

The most important aspect during this time was the mental health of teachers as they without any training were pushed into the virtual world overnight. Teachers have been working overtime to engage learners in virtual classes; they have been supporting learners in whatever way possible. They are expected to be a mentor, a friend, and a teacher to normalize the atmosphere for their learners. Rashmi Chari in an article points out how teachers just like doctors are expected to hide their feeling and always keep a smile on their faces. She says, "While other professionals need not go to great lengths to hide their grief at personal loss, however, teachers, just like doctors, have to mask their personal grief and worries and maintain an optimistic façade before the learners" [19].

The article titled, "Stress Topped the Reasons Why Public School Teachers Quit, Even Before COVID-19," informs us the condition of teachers during this pandemic phase. It tells us how they have quit their jobs because of an increase in stress levels, low pay, and taking care of their children. With more working hours and increased responsibilities both personally and professionally, stress and anxiety levels have increased significantly in teachers resulting in affecting their emotional, physical, and mental health. It also says that older teachers have left their jobs due to health conditions and would only join again if everyone is properly vaccinated [20].

COVID-19 has shifted the world into an online mode of communication. From shopping for clothes, groceries to the education system everything has shifted to the virtual platform. This has also brought into focus the technological gaps faced by educators. Not all teachers are computer-savvy, which has led to many problems in the teaching-learning experience. Issues faced by teachers regarding technological gaps can be divided into three groups; access gap, pedagogical skills, and digital literacy gap, and usage gap [21]. Online teaching and offline teaching require different types of teaching modes. While offline is more dominated by lecture methods, online teaching requires the use of more audio-visual aids. In a survey conducted by researchers on teachers, it was noted that around 69% of teachers faced a technological gap and 22% believe that the online method of teaching is different from the traditional method [22].

In another survey conducted on teachers, it was noted that a good majority of teachers (84%) have faced technical issues such as signals and data expenses, which hampers the teaching-learning experience. It also came to notice that two out of every five teachers lacked the necessary equipment for online teaching [23].

Online teaching during the pandemic phase has been categorized into two types: Synchronous and Asynchronous [24]. Synchronous involves giving students a real classroom feel. Teaching students by giving live classes through online video conferencing applications such as Zoom or Microsoft Teams. Asynchronous allows students to learn at their own pace. They are given prerecorded lessons and assignments, and communications between students and teachers are done through emails or discussion forums.

In yet another survey on technological issues conducted by QS I.GAUGE, it was revealed that technology advancement in the country is still not up to the mark to give uninterrupted delivery of lectures. According to it, "Only a few HEIs are using Moodle, Blackboard (teaching app), Microsoft Teams and Google meet for teaching but most of the HEIs are dependent on open-source platforms such as WhatsApp, YouTube, Skype, Google hangout, Zoom, etc. for online teaching" [25].

Teachers having different kinds of personal circumstances faced different types of issues as teachers with newborn babies had different problems, whereas the problems faced by teachers with school-going children were different, and teachers with college going children were different apart from the technical issues faced by almost all of them.

3.1 Teachers with newborn babies

When it comes to working from home, difficulties arise when one has a newborn baby. As newborn babies need utmost care and their mother's full attention, it becomes tricky working in this kind of situation. The situation is different for offline teaching, as mostly female teachers leave their babies in a crèche or with an older member in the family till the time they are in schools, whereas during online teaching, the situation is different. As the mothers are at home, it goes without saying that the child will be their responsibility, even if there is full support from the family members, the responsibility ultimately comes down to the mothers. The case in a joint family in this matter is better as there are people who can help if they want, whereas in a nuclear family where only a husband, a wife, and a newborn baby reside, it becomes extremely difficult. All the duties come on the head of the woman; she takes care of her husband, her small child, and her job, which often leads to not having any time for herself. Therefore, woman educators having newborn babies were serious victims of no alternative arrangements to look after their babies when they work.

3.2 Teachers with school-going children

The condition of teachers having school-going children is very different from the ones having newborn babies, though it doesn't mean that the problems are any less, it means that the problems are entirely different.

Taking the case of school-going children in primary classes, a teacher teaching class first in a Delhi school says that, "the students have to have one parent with them during online classes, as the students are too small to understand anything themselves." In the offline mode of teaching, teachers having school-going children in the primary class have a carefree mind as they know their children are well taken care of by other teachers. But, in online teaching mode, this doesn't happen. One parent has to be present in the class to see if their child understands anything or not. The situation is worse when both parents are working. A school teacher teaching online classes in this pandemic phase has classes right from the morning till afternoon and then has to work extra after-school hours to plan the classes for the next day. There is no doubt that the pressure on teachers to perform has increased in these trying times, and having to worry about the classes of their children is more worrisome. In these kinds of situations, the mindset of families also plays an important role. In many households, a man's job is taken more seriously than a woman's job; hence the responsibility of the children is in the hands of women even with a demanding job as teaching.

The situation of teachers having school-going children in senior classes is very different. Senior school children can mostly handle their studies with parents watching over them from time to time. They don't have to sit through their classes all the time like with primary class children. The senior school children are on their way to stepping into their adulthood so their behavior needs to be checked. Mostly the responsibility is to check their concentration in studies and their seriousness toward online teaching mode. Therefore, teachers having school-going children in different age groups have different kinds of problems that they have to face each day while teaching online.

3.3 Teachers with college-going children

Here the children are also facing problems. Online teaching means keeping pace with technology. A college student having a teacher as their mother said that it's very difficult. The balance between professional time and personal time has dwindled very much. Along with her college work, she has to help her mother during online classes to make her conversant with technology results in her work being slightly delayed. The demands for being technological sound these days to make classes more interesting and engaging has taken a toll on all the teachers be it male or female. Female teachers are getting more burdened as they have to take care of their household also, even when they have college-going children, in this pandemic phase doing household chores without maids in most of the houses have added the burden on female teachers and using more technology in online classes by someone who is not used to it has become very difficult for both the children and their mother.

3.4 Mental health of women educators during COVID-19

This pandemic has seen educators adapting to online teaching, which is very different from the traditional way of teaching. This change in the environment and the responsibilities and difficulties it came with affected the mental health of educators. Online teaching came with the responsibility of making the class more interesting to engage learners by using various methods of teaching such as audio-visual aids. It became difficult for teachers to cope with the technological needs of learners. Added to this stress were the increase in workload and working hours. Handling their professional and personal life has become very troublesome for women educators.

Rashmi Chari in an article for Times of India points out how a continuous observation by parents and school management regarding online classes is further affecting the mental health of educators. In the article, she says, "Teachers are in a completely unfamiliar zone with learners as remote spectators and parents as unwanted intruders. The stress of being under constant observation while teaching through an unfamiliar medium with totally new tools is least to say challenging and stressful. Several cases have also been reported in media about unwarranted comments by parents on the teacher's appearance and pronunciation which are shocking and disgraceful to say the least and interference which is unacceptable as teachers are trained professionals" [26].

Another incident seen during online classes is the attitude of learners toward their teachers. Women educators have been victims of cyber bullying wherein during classes students post some off seen pictures or messages directed toward teachers. Such incidents can be frightening for a teacher, which directly affects their mental health. Rashmi Chari in her article says, "I can clearly recall the incidents of zoom bombing in a few classes I was observing and how the teacher was left totally shaken up and shattered by the emotional violence and indignity of experiencing a cyber-attack which is usually in the form of sexually explicit language and images" [26].

During this phase, teachers are also seen taking care of their student's mental health. Asking for updates on their family situations, becoming a counselor for solving their problems and not letting learners feel alone or distant has become the daily routine of teachers. Taking care of everything from family to job requirements, teachers have forgotten to take care of themselves. Self-care among teachers is depleting every day, which is making them stressed, anxious, and affecting their mental, physical, and emotional health.

3.5 Technological issues

Transitioning the teaching-learning experience from traditional methods to virtual methods has not been easy for educators. The educators were not prepared for this change that happened overnight. Although the technology was slowly becoming a part of everyday teaching, traditional methods were still dominant. The shift brought the whole education system into the hands of technology. Another problem that came to the forefront was engaging students toward online teaching. In traditional classrooms when the students and teachers are face to face, the attention of students is always on the teacher and the teacher can regulate the classroom, whereas, in online teaching, teachers have to find different ways to keep engaging the learners. They have to make their lessons interesting by using audio-visual methods such as presentations, showing videos, and other creative ideas. In these situations, those who are not computer-savvy have faced many difficulties to keep up with digital classrooms.

The government from their side has also taken initiatives to enhance teaching-learning experiences. E-learning platforms such as the DIKSHA portal by the government have learning resources such as videos based on the curriculum for students and teachers. It provides learning opportunities for educators also in their subject matter and also on how to enhance teaching during online classes.

Fig. 5.1 suggests the age group of the surveyed women and shows that 51% of the women surveyed lied between the age group of 40 and 50 years, 26% lied between the age group of 20 and 30 years, 13% lied between the age group of 30 and 40 years, and 60 and above category were nearly 10%.

Fig. 5.2 shows that 77.3% of the surveyed women have children, whereas 22.7% of women surveyed do not have children.

Out of 77.3% of women who had children, Fig. 5.3 depicts that 79% have two children, 15% have one child, and 6% have three children.

Fig. 5.4 informs the age group of children, 44.4% of children lie in the age group of 10–20 years, 41.7% of children lie between the age group of 20 and 30 years, 30.6% of children lie in the age group of 0–10 years,

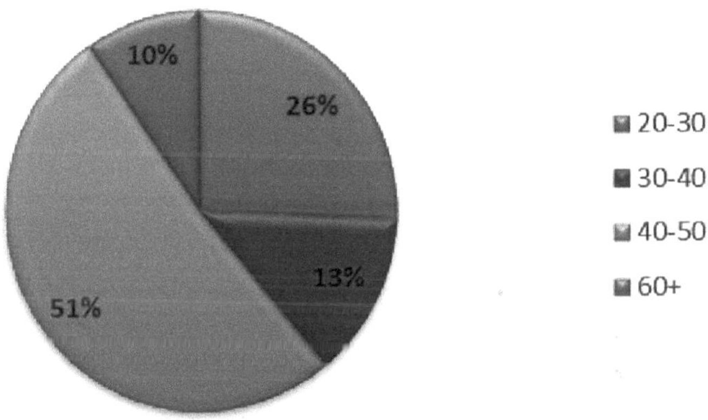

Figure 5.1 Age group.

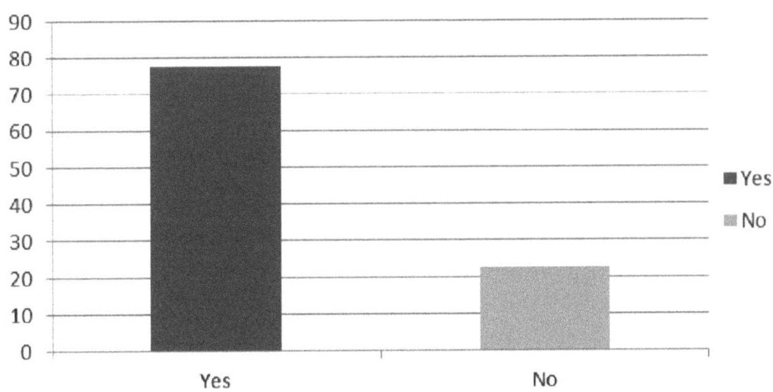

Figure 5.2 Women with children.

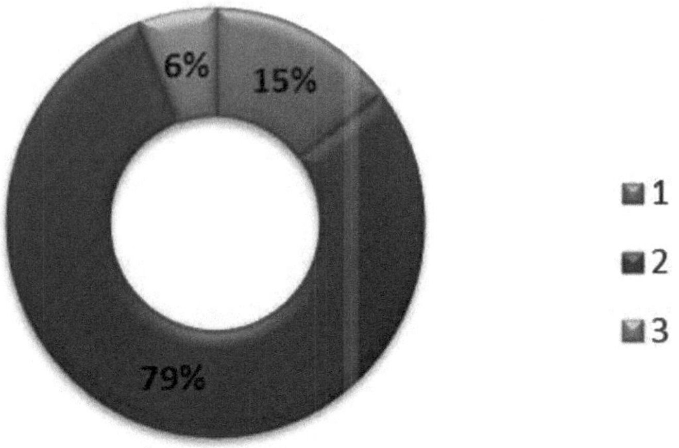

Figure 5.3 No. of children.

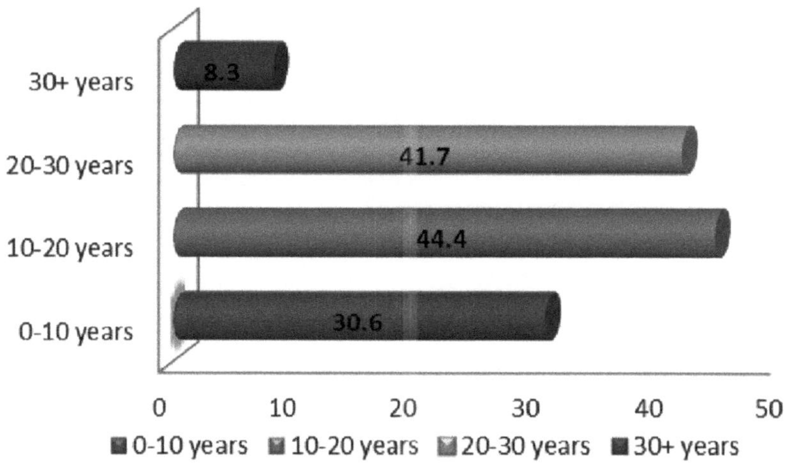

Figure 5.4 Age group of children.

and 8.3% of children are of 30+ years. Through this data, we came to know about the different problems the women educators are facing with different age groups of children.

Fig. 5.5 tells us whether the surveyed women had any domestic help during this pandemic phase or not. 75% of the women surveyed said that they had no domestic help during this pandemic and 25% said that yes they had domestic help. Through this analysis, we got to know about the extra work that women were doing, which in normal circumstances their domestic help handled.

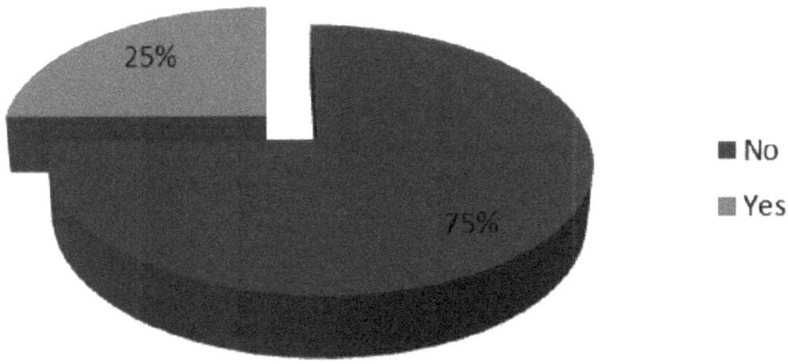

Figure 5.5 Availability of domestic help.

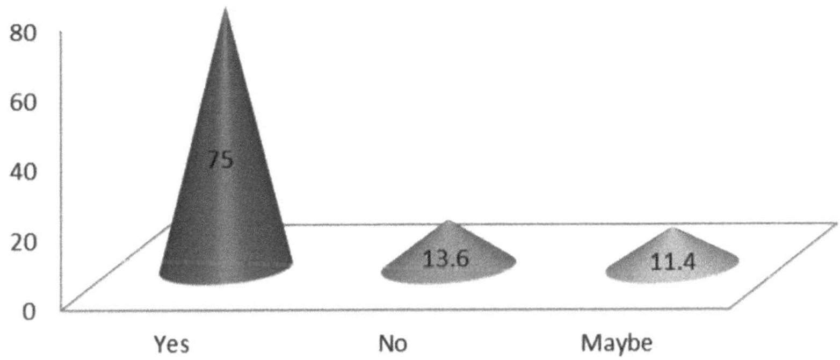

Figure 5.6 Family support.

Fig. 5.6 tells about the family support a women educator got during these trying times. 75% of surveyed women believe that they got an adequate amount of family support, 13.6% believe that they did not get any family support, and 11.4% believe that they sometimes got family support but not always.

Fig. 5.7 depicts the number of working hours of surveyed women. 31.8% of women are spending 8–10 h daily on their job, 29.5% of women are spending 6–8 h, 22.7% are spending more than 10 h in a day, 9.1% are spending 2–4 h, and lastly, 6.8% of women surveyed are spending 4–6 h. This data shows the increase of working hours of educators, and handling these extra hours with household work is very challenging for women educators.

As virtual classes have become the new norm of the education sector, it is important to know if the educators were familiar with taking virtual classes or not. It was discovered that more than half of the surveyed women, i.e., 52% were not familiar with it, 25% were a little bit familiar, and 23% were not at all familiar with how to take virtual classes. This data shows the difficulty a teacher might have had when they had to take virtual classes on short notice (Fig. 5.8).

With online classes come the technological issues that one faces in virtual teaching. Fig. 5.9 shows that more than half, i.e., 54.5% of women said that

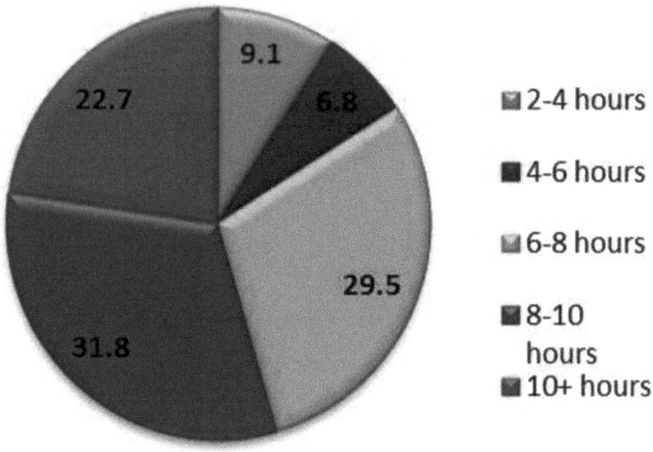

Figure 5.7 Working hours per day.

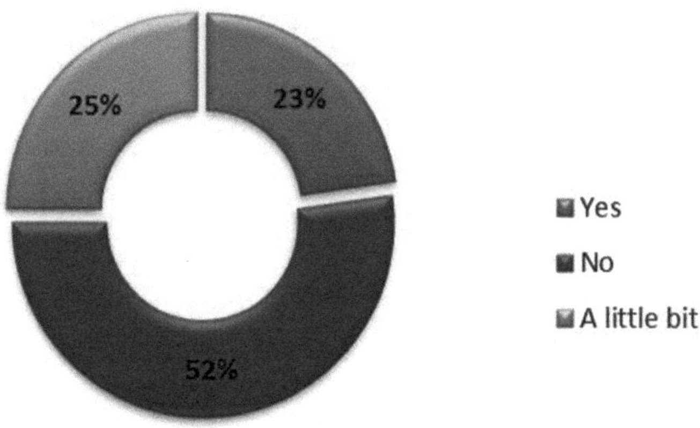

Figure 5.8 Familiarity with virtual classes.

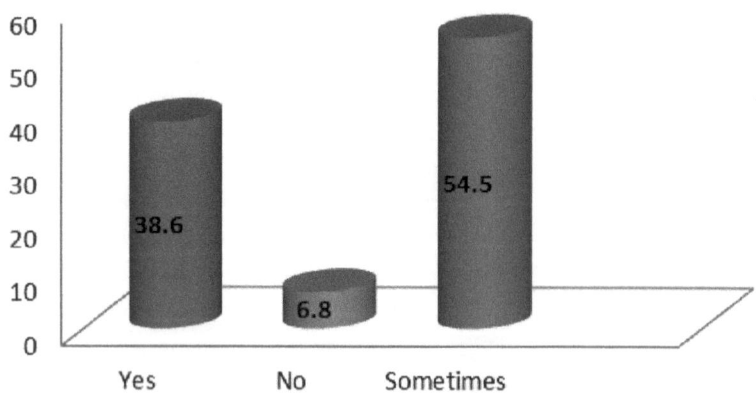

Figure 5.9 Technological issues.

they sometimes faced such issues while teaching, 38.6% said that they face these issues almost every time, and only a few percentages of women, i.e., 6.8% said that they did not face any issue.

Fig. 5.10 states the problems that the surveyed women faced while teaching during this pandemic phase.The majority of women, i.e., 77.3% find the extra work that institutions have given to them during these online classes to be the most problematic.

45.5% of women are unable to do household chores.

34.1% believe that they are not giving sufficient attention to the studies of their children.

27.3% are unable to look after aged people in their families.

18.2% of women are unable to attend the online classes of their children, out of these 18.2%; 15.9% had their kids in primary classes and 2.3% had kids in senior classes, 4.5% are facing problems while teaching online because of having newborn babies.

Rest 6.9% of women find that they are not getting time for themselves or that the teaching job has become boring for them due to online classes as teaching has now become a full-day tiring job.

Fig. 5.11 shows that 38.6% of women do not prefer teaching online, whereas 36.4% are not sure if they prefer or not hence said maybe, and 25% do prefer teaching online.

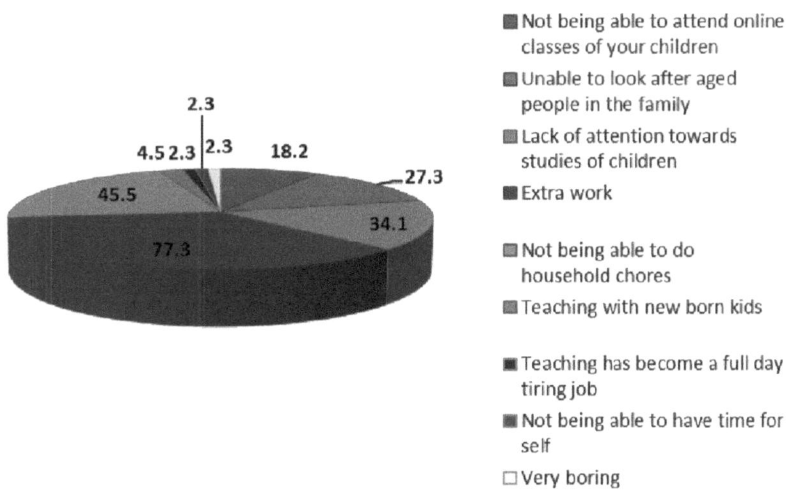

Figure 5.10 Types of problems.

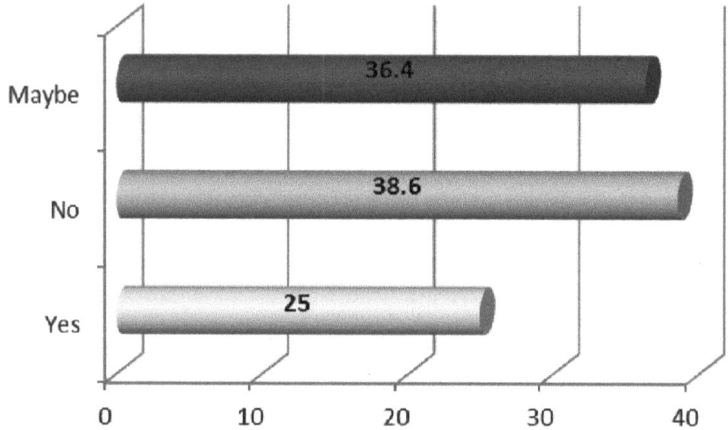

Figure 5.11 Preference for virtual classes.

4. Findings

The virtual working environment has proven to be more demanding than the offline environment. With teachers having to put more hours on their job, it is disrupting their personal and professional life balance. Another major problem that came into the picture was the problem of not being able to attend online classes of their primary school children. A positive thing that came out was the family support; ample of women got the support of their families during these difficult times, which proved very helpful for them and showcased the joint effort made by the family to cope with the situation. Even after all the difficulties, the women educators are facing; be it in their professional or personal field, a big percentage of them now feel that taking online classes is not a bad idea, as they have now managed the situation, which came to them as an emergency, and they have also crossed the technological hurdles by constantly training themselves, so they can manage it, whereas a good percentage of them also feel that online classes are a big no, and they would like to go back to normal circumstances with offline teaching as the medium of education.

5. Conclusion

The problems faced by women educators during the COVID-19 pandemic are many. It laid serious effects on different parts of society especially women who have witnessed a history of suppression at the hands of society. With the depleting economic conditions, there is an increase in gender inequality in the education sector although 50% of educators are women. Even in modern times where people are learned, there are still some households that believe that the first job of a woman is taking care of her family and her household. They think that the job of a man is more important than that of a woman, which creates more problems in the lives of women educators with such a demanding job especially during the pandemic phase where they carried out all domestic work without any hired help.

No doubt teachers are a very important part of our society, and they needed extra support during these turbulent times. As it is said, "change begins at home," the improvement in conditions of women educators was more required at home, their family although helped but was helpless in helping them as more manpower was required to look after the sick, small babies, elderly people, and more demanding and very difficult work situations. All the prejudices that people have in their minds regarding the inefficiency of women educators posed a big question mark as it was only women's multitasking inbuilt talent that sailed them through the situation. The institutions should have been empathetic in understanding the problems of making teachers work for extra hours. Their demands could have been realistic and not more than what is achievable. Every teacher is trying her best to make virtual learning effective for children in these testing times, institutions should not burden them more than what they actually can do. After all the future of mankind lies in the hands of teachers.

References

[1] Trading Economics, India - Primary education, teachers (% female), Trading Economics. [Online]. Available: https://tradingeconomics.com/india/primary-education-teachers-percent-female-wb-data.html.

[2] R.P. Nishank, Enhancing Gender Equality in India's Higher Education, Hindustan Times, March 6, 2020 [Online]. Available, https://www.hindustantimes.com/analysis/enhancing-gender-equality-in-india-s-higher-education-opinion/story-CuQKoLDc4ujMGPScy4ejJI.html.

[3] B. Pal, The saga of women's status in ancient Indian civilization, Misc. Geogr. 23 (3) (2019) 180–184 [Online]. Available: https://www.sciendo.com/article/10.2478/mgrsd-2019-0012.

[4] Problems Faced by Women Teachers, A Critical Study on the problems Faced by Women Teachers of, Voiceofresearch.org. [Online]. Available: http://www.voiceofresearch.org/doc/Jun-2017/Jun-2017_1.pdf.

[5] Women Administrators, Ksu.edu. [Online]. Available: https://nacada.ksu.edu/Resources/Clearinghouse/View-Articles/Women-Administrators.aspx.

[6] Financial Express Online, Where Are Women in India's Workforce? Slipping Female LFPR Is Worrying Trend, Financial Express, March 8, 2021 [Online]. Available:

https://www.financialexpress.com/opinion/where-are-women-in-indias-workforce-slipping-female-lfpr-is-worrying-trend/2208828/.
[7] K. Sharma, More Indian Women Enrolled for Higher Education in 2019-20, Report Shows, Theprint.in, June 10, 2021. [Online]. Available: https://theprint.in/india/education/more-indian-women-enrolled-for-higher-education-in-2019-20-report-shows/675413/.
[8] Financial Express Online, Unseen Reasons for the Fall in Women's Labour Force Participation in India, Financial Express, March 2, 2021 [Online]. Available, https://www.financialexpress.com/lifestyle/unseen-reasons-for-the-fall-in-womens-labour-force-participation-in-india/2204686/.
[9] Unwomen.org. [Online]. Available: https://www.unwomen.org/-/media/headquarters/attachments/sections/library/publications/2020/gender-equality-in-the-wake-of-covid-19-en.pdf?la=en&vs=5142.
[10] COVID-19 and Its Economic Toll on Women: The Story Behind the Numbers, Unwomen.org. [Online]. Available: https://www.unwomen.org/en/news/stories/2020/9/feature-covid-19-economic-impacts-on-women.
[11] K.A.A.S. Jain, Locked-down: Domestic Violence Reporting in India during COVID-19, Oxfamindia.org. [Online]. Available: https://www.oxfamindia.org/blog/locked-down-domestic-violence-reporting-india-during-covid-19.
[12] Violence Against Women and Girls: the Shadow Pandemic, Unwomen.org. [Online]. Available: https://www.unwomen.org/en/news/stories/2020/4/statement-ed-phumzile-violence-against-women-during-pandemic.
[13] A. Chaves, COVID-19 Has Added to the Educational Barriers Girls and Women Face Around the World, CBC, March 8, 2021 [Online]. Available, https://www.cbc.ca/news/opinion/opinion-women-equality-education-1.5935791.
[14] Close All Educational Institutions for Teachers and Other Staff #KeepTeachersSafe, Change.org. [Online]. Available: https://www.change.org/p/drharshvardhan-drrpnishank-mohfw-india-close-alleducationalinstitutions-for-teachers-and-other-staff-keepteacherssaferecruiter1022789424sourcesharepetitioncampaignpsfcombosharein itialmedium=whatsapp.
[15] F. Islahi, Who Make Effective Teachers, Men or Women? An Indian Perspective, Researchgate.net. [Online]. Available: https://www.researchgate.net/publication/323585621_Who_Make_Effective_Teachers_Men_or_Women_An_Indian_Perspective.
[16] I.S. Punit, qzcom, For Many of India's Teachers, Online Classes amid Lockdown Have Been an Awful Experience, Scroll.in, May 13, 2020. [Online]. Available: https://scroll.in/article/961738/for-many-of-indias-teachers-online-classes-amid-lockdown-have-been-an-awful-experience.
[17] B. Watkins, European Trade Union Committee for Education, Csee-etuce.org. [Online]. Available: https://www.csee-etuce.org/en/policy-issues/covid-19/3712-the-covid-19-pandemic-must-not-set-the-clock-back-on-gender-equality.
[18] V.M. Pothula, COVID-19's Impact on Education in India: It's Not All Bad News, Globalsistersreport.org, February 4, 2021. [Online]. Available: https://www.globalsistersreport.org/news/ministry/column/covid-19s-impact-education-india-its-not-all-bad-news.
[19] R. Chari, Teacher Stress, Burnout & Compassion Fatigue: Covids Continuing Legacy, Times of India, May 19, 2021 [Online]. Available, https://timesofindia.indiatimes.com/blogs/edutrends-india/teacher-stress-burnout-compassion-fatigue-covids-continuing-legacy/.
[20] M.K. Diliberti, H.L. Schwartz, D. Grant, Stress Topped the Reasons Why Public School Teachers Quit, Even before COVID-19, Rand Corporation, 2021 [Online]. Available, https://www.rand.org/pubs/research_reports/RRA1121-2.html.

[21] S. Jain, M. Lall, A. Singh, Teachers' voices on the impact of COVID-19 on school education: Are Ed-Tech companies really the panacea? SAGE J. (2021) https://doi.org/10.1177/0973184920976433.
[22] H.K. Tyagi, Online Teaching in Delhi-NCR Schools in India During COVID-19 Pandemic, Researchgate.net. [Online]. Available: https://www.researchgate.net/publication/346846054_Online_teaching_in_Delhi-NCR_schools_in_India_during_Covid-19_pandemic.
[23] India Today Web Desk, "84% of Teachers Facing Challenges During Online Classes: Survey," Indiatoday.in, March 18, 2021. [Online]. Available: https://www.indiatoday.in/education-today/latest-studies/story/84-of-teachers-facing-challenges-during-online-classes-survey-1780816-2021-03-18.
[24] R. Khalil, et al., The Sudden Transition to Synchronized Online Learning during the COVID-19 Pandemic in Saudi Arabia: A Qualitative Study Exploring Medical Students' Perspectives, BMC Medical Education, 2020 [Online]. Available, https://www.ncbi.nlm.nih.gov/pubmed/32859188.
[25] A. Joshi, M. Vinay, P. Bhaskar, Online Teaching Amidst COVID-19 in India: An Outlook, 2020 [Online]. Available, https://files.eric.ed.gov/fulltext/EJ1285307.pdf.
[26] R. Chari, Teacher Wellbeing & Self-Care in Covid Times, Times of India, July 3, 2020 [Online]. Available, https://timesofindia.indiatimes.com/blogs/edutrends-india/teacher-wellbeing-self-care-in-covid-times/.

CHAPTER SIX

A deep learning approach toward prediction of mental health of Indians

V. Kavitha[1] and C. Akila[2]
[1]Department of Computer Science and Engineering University College of Engineering, Kanchipuram, Tamilnadu, India
[2]Department of Computer Science and Engineering Anna University Regional Campus, Tirunelveli, Tamilnadu, India

1. COVID-19 and its impact

1.1 Introduction

The COVID-19 pandemic has shaken the entire planet as a terrible human disaster. As of mid-March, 2021, this disease caused by a novel coronavirus, SARS-CoV-2, resulted in 122,436,927 cases, 2,704,442 deaths, and 98,723,498 patients who have recovered worldwide. It was found in all nations and affected the globe in terms of economics, social lifestyle, mental health, industry, and education.

The name COVID-19 means coronavirus 2019, the year it was first identified in Wuhan, China. Coronaviruses cause respiratory illness ranging from the common cold to more severe disease such as Middle East respiratory syndrome and severe acute respiratory syndrome. The structure of a coronavirus is depicted in Fig. 6.1.

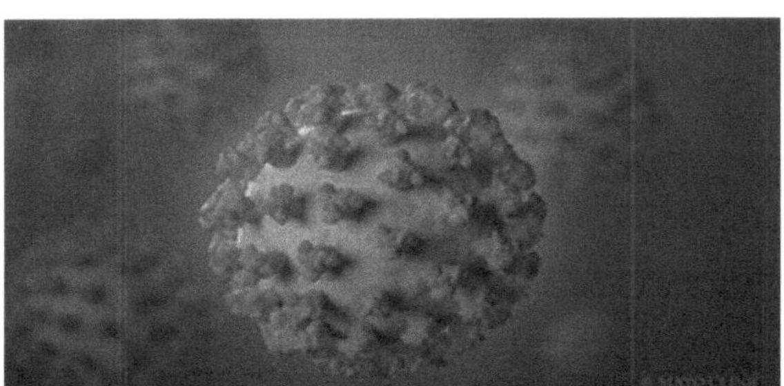

Figure 6.1 Source structure of coronavirus, from Mayo Clinic.

Artificial Intelligence, Machine Learning, and Mental Health in Pandemics
ISBN: 978-0-323-91196-2
https://doi.org/10.1016/B978-0-323-91196-2.00009-0

This virus and disease were unknown before the outbreak began in Wuhan, China. COVID-19 became a pandemic affecting many countries globally. It significantly affects health services for noncommunicable disease, such as cancer, cardiovascular disease, diabetics, mental health, and respiratory disease. The impact of COVID-19 related to health issues is depicted in Fig. 6.2.

Many nations imposed a strict lockdown during the pandemic to reduce the spread of COVID-19 that had resulted in a remarkable loss of life. As the coronavirus pandemic rapidly swept across the world, the main psychological impact to date has been elevated rates of stress and anxiety and considerable degrees of fear and worry, particularly in older adults. Anxiety refers to muscle tension and avoidance behavior. Fear is an emotional response to threat [1].

How COVID-19 affects the human body: The virus enters through the nose and finds a host cell in the respiratory system. The host cell bursts and affects other cells. Then it slowly spreads and damages human parts already infected with other diseases, and kills the person with a multifunction disorder.

Spread of COVID-19: The spread of COVID-19 occurs when people breathe out or cough. They expel tiny droplets that contain the virus, spreading it to other people. Close contact with someone infected spreads the infection around 6 ft. This infection often exhibits no symptoms.

COVID-19 symptoms: Symptoms experienced are fever, dry cough, and tiredness. Serious symptoms are difficulty breathing or shortness of breath, chest pain or pressure, loss of speech or movement, muscle ache, and sore of throat.

Preventive measures for COVID-19: Preventive measures advised by the World Health Organization (WHO) include avoiding close contact by maintaining social distancing, keeping hands clean by washing with sanitizer frequently, and wearing a mask.

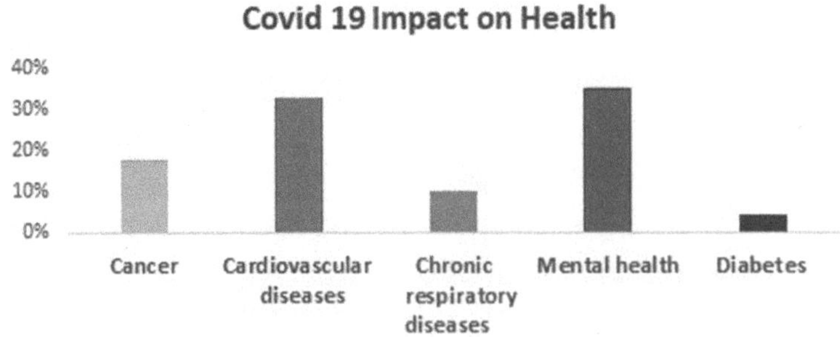

Figure 6.2 Impact of COVID-19 on health.

2. Impact of COVID-19

COVID-19 has resulted in a widespread change in the lifestyle of people. Since its outbreak, the virus has affected people physically, financially, and economically. People have attempted suicide or homicide, there is much unhappiness and conflict in families, problems have emerged related to legal and financial concerns, and there is an increase in scams owing to the loss of income, especially in online. Major areas in which consequences of COVID-19 are severe are discussed next.

Economic impact: The entire globe was deeply affected economically. The survival of each individual of the Nations faced struggle in their day-to-day life and the countries laid down many strategies and standard operating procedures from time to time to nullify the effect of loss of people and to uphold the economic status of the country. The most important sectors affected are manufacturing, information technology (IT), petroleum and diesel, agriculture, and transportation.

The economic sector decreased owing to a slowdown in the manufacture of essential goods, disruption of the supply chain, losses in national and international business, and poor cash flow in the market that directly suppressed revenue growth in all sectors.

In the IT sector, Apple revenue of $63—67 billion ended up with $58.3 billion. Amazon revenues rising from 26% to $75.5 Billion, fell from $2.5 Billion to $3 Billion. TCS expected to see revenue drop by 6%, Infosys by 5%. HCL Technologies by 8%. The rate of petroleum and diesel saw a 3-year drop; no sign of increase was found until Jun. 2020.

In agriculture, Indian farmers face risks such as low rainfall and price fluctuations. but risk from COVID-19 threatened the sector globally; the Food and Agriculture Organization expected shifts in the supply of and demand for food. The World Food Program noted that the COVID-19 crisis threatened to affect millions of people already vulnerable to food insecurity and malnutrition [2] and to poor mental health affected by economic factors.

Mental health: The impact on the economy caused to COVID-19 resulted in significant mental health problems in normal people [3,4], who experienced anxiety, loneliness, fear, stress, depression, addiction to drugs, and self-harm. Common responses related to mental health are depicted in Fig. 6.3.

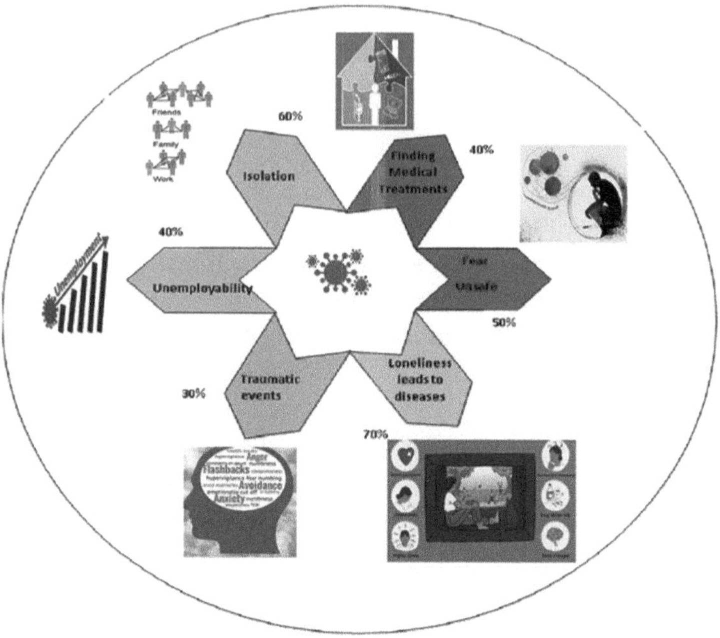

Figure 6.3 Common responses to COVID-19.

3. Mental health

Mental health contributes 80% to total positive health. Physical ailment has a mental component, and vice versa. The WHO defines mental health as the ability of an individual to form harmonious relations with others and to participate in or contribute constructively to change in the social and physical environment.

These are main characteristics of mental wellness are:

1. When one feels secure, he or she feels comfortable; one never underestimates or overestimates his own ability, one must be ready to accept his shortcomings; one has self-respect.
2. She or he feels right toward others. She or he can accept others and love them. She or he has good friendships that are long-lasting. She or he has the mindset to take responsibility of neighbors and fellows.
3. The person able to meet the demands of life. One can solve problems, think for oneself and make one's own decisions, and set reasonable goals for oneself. One is not bowled over by one's own emotions of fear, anger, love, or guilt.

Warning signs of mental illness: Signs of mental illness are always worrying, being unable to concentrate, being unhappy without a cause, having a quick temper, having wide fluctuations in moods, disliking people, being upset, dissatisfied and frightened etc.

Types of mental illness: According to the International Classification of Diseases, mental and behavioral disorders are classified as organic, including symptomatic, mental disorders, mental and behavioral disorders due to psychoactive substances, schizophrenia and delusional disorders, mood disorders, neurosis, stress-related, and somatoform disorders. Behavioral syndromes associated with psychological disturbances and physical factors, disorders of adult personality and behavior, mental retardation, disorders of psychological development, behavioral and emotional disorders, unspecified mental disorder. The major illness is schizophrenia (split personality) [5] deals with how a person thinks, feels, and behaves, manic depressive psychosis due to excitement or depression. Paranoia is associated with undue or extreme suspension. A minor illness is neurosis or psychoneuroses with symptoms such as morbid fears, compulsions, and obsessions. Personality and character disorders are a group of disorders that are the legacy of unfortunate childhood experiences and perceptions. Mental illness and serious mental illness are briefly reported in the National Institute of Mental Health Information Resource Center [6].

Causes of mental illness: Factors affecting mental health are organic conditions such as cerebral arteriosclerosis, neoplasm, metabolic disease, tuberculosis, leprosy, and epilepsy. Heredity is a major factor. Social pathologic causes are common worry, anxiety, emotional stress, tension, frustration, a broken home, poverty, and insecurity. Environmental factors include inhalation of toxic substances, addiction to psychotropic drugs, nutritional factors, and mineral deficiency.

Infectious disease such as measles or rubella before, during, and after childbirth may cause mental illness. Traumatic incidents such as road and occupational accidents and radiation to the nervous system can lead to mental issues. Critical points in the life cycle of humans that cause mental illness are prenatally, during the first 5 years of life, the school lifestyle a child undergoes, adolescence, and old age with a lack of affection, belongings, independence, and achievement.

The experience undergone by the students in school and adolescence period has a vital role in mental illness, where in school age, the school has not satisfied or she/he might have gone frustrated in emotional needs of the child, lack of guidance or psychiatric services. The child's mental health and his effectiveness in learning, the proper teacher—pupil relationship, and classroom climate are incredibly important to prevent dropouts.

Preventive measures: A primary preventive measure is improving the social environment. A secondary aspect is the early diagnosis of mental illness and social and emotional disturbances through screening programs in school, universities, industry, recreation centers, family counseling, and so on. Tertiary prevention reduces stress. The goal in this step is to prevent further breakdowns and disruptions.

4. Impact of mental health in education sector

The COVID-19 pandemic affected the educational system worldwide, leading to the near-total closures of schools, universities, and colleges, and to online technology learning. The American Psychiatric Association warned that the extreme use of e-learning leads to social isolation [7].

Online learning: Electronic learning can lead to a wide range of health risks, including muscle and joint injuries, an increased mortality rate associated with excessive sitting, and eye strain from computer use. During online learning, sitting for the long period in the same position and to overcome physical (body) stress, suggestion to get relaxed was advised by the dos and don'ts. Students and faculty were asked to exercise, sleep well, have nutritious food, develop hobbies, practice deep breathing, be positive, simplify information to students, place socializing phone calls and use social media to get the right information, schedule and follow a routine, practice exercise and yoga, engage in family activities, and take the time to relax.

People in the education sector were advised:

- Do not believe false information and rumors that might increase anxiety. Avid risk-taking behaviors. When going out, do not refuse to follow the rules imposed by the government. Do not isolate yourself socially; this can lead to boredom and loneliness. Do not become addicted to alcohol and drugs and get into bad habits and behavior.
- Electronic learning was an emergency technology that experienced a boom during the pandemic. Some of the electronic learning platforms are Google Meet, Zoom, and Microsoft Teams; these have pros and cons. Students from economically weaker sections who were not offered with Wi-Fi access and gadgets struggled to attend online classes conducted by educational institutions.

Drawbacks to online teaching methodologies are less eye-to-eye contact, less direct monitoring of students, less interactiveness, conduct of internal and external examinations exams on online mode. A mental condition marked by alternating periods of elation and depression (bipolar disorder) that affects the mood, energy, activity levels, concentration and the ability to carry out day-to-day tasks as demonstrated [8] and intern it may affect the staff and students in their daily routine.

5. Artificial intelligence

Artificial intelligence (AI) is a branch of computer science that is extended to daily applications of human life. Most fields employ AI techniques for effectiveness and efficiency to predict people's minds and promote business in all sectors.

In AI, intelligence is the capacity to learn and solve problems. Artificial means the simulation of the human brain using machines. Basic principles adapted in AI are reasoning, knowledge, planning, and learning. Major areas that contribute to building an intelligent system are computer science, psychology, neuron science, biology, mathematics, sociology, and philosophy.

History: The history of AI started in 1950. The term "AI" was coined by John McCarty in 1955. Since there was a high demand of computer applications with AI approach, the utilization of computer speed experienced an exponential growth, from 1980 the era of AI took its birth and from 2000 onwards a landmark of AI was achieved. AI has been used in health care, music, telecommunications, robotics, gaming, banking, etc.

Types and applications of artificial intelligence: AI is broadly classified as artificial narrow intelligence or weak intelligence: It is nonsentient machine intelligence typically focused on a narrow task. In artificial general intelligence or strong AI, artificial narrow intelligence algorithms are used to solve problems. In artificial superintelligence, machine learning and deep learning algorithms are used for analysis and prediction.

AI has widespread implementation in gaming, natural language processing, expert systems, vision systems, speech recognition, handwriting recognition, and intelligent robots. Current trends of AI are in the robotic process automation, accurate health care predictions, data modeling, B2B, chat bots, business, advanced cybersecurity, media and entertainment analysis, retail, and aerospace and flight operations.

Artificial intelligence in health care: In health care, AI is used for training, wellness, early detection, diagnosis, decision making, treatment, end of life care, and research. AI in medical and biological engineering has been explored for various medical devices and pharmaceutical products including human tissue. The integration of biological sciences, nanotechnology, cognitive sciences, material sciences, and IT has combined for the fast development of gene therapy and the use of smart materials in computer-assisted surgery, as well as the production of artificial organs, and in medical imaging. Analyzing one's gene using Genetic Engineering, the mental health of an individual can be predicted and it is discussed [9].

In the 1950s, artificial kidneys X-rays, electrocardiograms, and cardiac pacemakers were recent discoveries. In 1960s, ultrasound made a major contribution to the field of medicine. In the 1970s, computer-assisted tomography, biologically engineered food was developed. In the 1980s, laser surgery and magnetic resonance imaging made a drastic change to medical diagnosis and treatment. Now, computer technology has a vital role in genomic sequencing and microarrays, positron emission tomography, and image-guided surgery. The application of AI in medicine has two branches: virtual and physical.

The virtual component is represented by machine learning (also called deep learning), in which mathematical algorithms are used to improve learning through experience. The unsupervised algorithms have the ability to find patterns. Supervised algorithms classify and predict objects based on previous examples. Reinforcement learning algorithms use sequences of rewards and punishments to form a strategy for operation in a specific problem state.

AI in medicine assists physicians in making better clinical decision and provides up-to-date medical information. It is like the 24/7 availability of experts. AI also helps in early diagnosis and in predicting the outcome of disease as well as giving feedback on treatment. The physical branch of AI includes physical objects, medical devices, and sophisticated robot delivery of care and surgical robots.

6. Machine learning

Machine learning is the subset of AI that uses abstruse statistical techniques enabling systems to improve tasks and performance with experience. The subset of machine learning composed of algorithms has an inbuilt capacity to allow software to train itself to perform tasks such as speech and image recognition by exposing multilayered neural networks to learn a vast amount of data. This has led to tremendous growth in the field of AI.

Machine learning algorithms learn from data and deliver predictive models. They do not depend on explicit programming, but depend purely on data fed into them. The predictive algorithm creates the predictive model.

Deep learning is a subfield of machine learning with algorithms inspired by the brain structure; its function is known as the artificial neural network. Deep learning algorithms run classification using pictures, texts, or even sounds as input.

The basic difference between traditional programming and machine learning is that program and data are fed as input to an algorithm, whereas the output is generated in traditional programming. When input data and expected outcomes are given to a machine learning algorithm, it gives a model for prediction. The working methodology of a traditional algorithm in shown in Fig. 6.4.

Seven steps in a machine learning algorithm are (1) data collection, (2) data preprocessing, (3) model selection, (4) learning phase, (5) checking performance, (6) optimization, and (7) testing for prediction analysis.

With rapid advancements in machine learning and deep learning, immersive prediction in wide range of technical areas such as the supply chain, customer experience, human resources, fraud detection, research, and development has radically transformed.

Phases of machine learning are preprocessing in which normalization, dimension reduction, and image processing are performed. In the learning phase, supervised or unsupervised algorithms are used to train and test the domain inputs. In the error analysis phase, error is calculated using precision/recall values. Overfitting is also analyzed and test/cross-validation of data is done. The working principle of machine learning algorithm is shown in Fig. 6.5.

Machine learning algorithms are classified as supervised, unsupervised, and reinforced learning [10]. Major algorithms under the supervised category are regression with linear and polynomial, decision tree, random forest, and classification algorithms with K-Nearest Neighbor (KNN), trees, logistic regression, naive-Bayes, and Support Vector Machine (SVM).

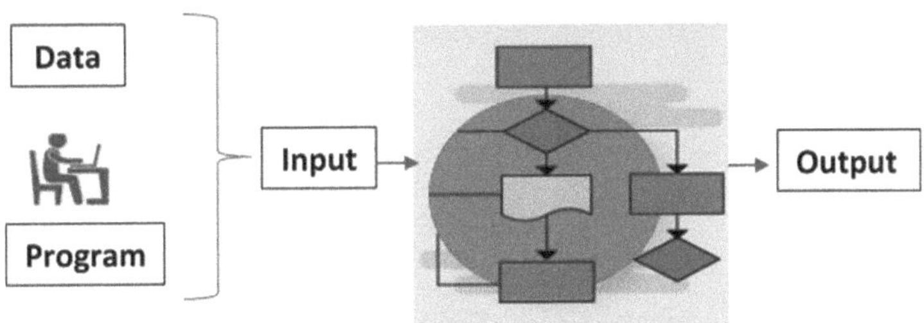

Figure 6.4 Traditional algorithm.

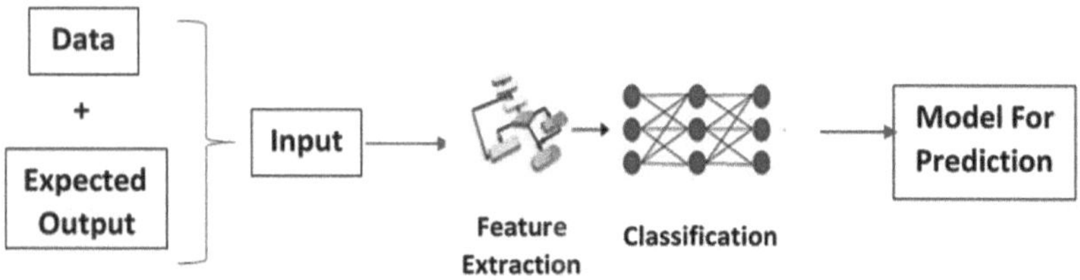

Figure 6.5 Machine learning.

Unsupervised algorithms are clustered with Singular Value Decomposition (SVD), Principal Component Analysis (PCA), and K-means. Association analysis algorithms use a priori and Frequent Pattern (FP)-growth. Reinforced learning algorithms are Convolutional Neural Networks (CNNs), in which feature extraction and classification are done automatically and a predicted model is obtained. In these, some algorithms are continuous and some are categorical.

7. Deep learning

Deep learning simulates the functionality of the human brain and performs the task of what the human brain can do in terms of information processing. It even creates the environment of decision-making, as demonstrated by Beńgio et al. [11].

Deep learning is a more confined process of machine learning under AI that has the ability to learn more events from the output data or predicted data even if they are not fed to the system (i.e., the output data are unlabeled). The other term for this is deep neural network. The deep learning algorithm has the flow of input features fed to the input layer; the hidden layer processes the input features and the output layer helps classify the input of test data once the network has learned the trained data. The working principle of deep learning is depicted in Fig. 6.6.

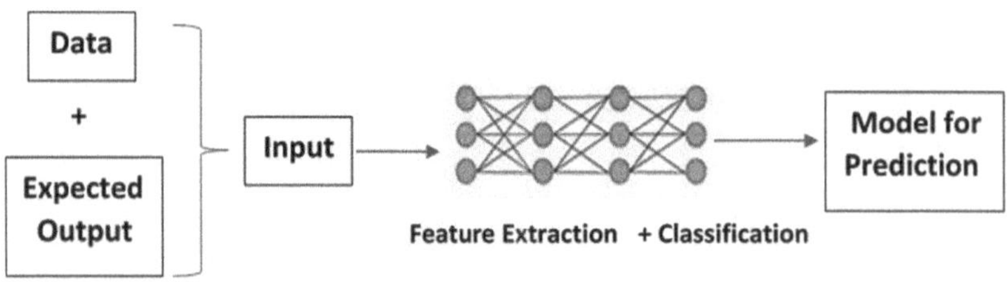

Figure 6.6 Deep learning.

7.1 Convolutional neural network

The demands of the IT industry are for skills in deep learning. Deep learning algorithms make learning much easier by extracting features required for learning using convolution, and the make the functionality of learning as accurate as that of the human brain. An existing learning algorithm such as Artificial Neural Network (ANN), reinforcement learning can be more effectively used for predictive purposes.

Yann LeCun built the first CNN in 1989. The basic idea of CNNs is that of a backpropagation neural network with a change in the implementation methodology. Processes involved in CNN are convolution and pooling layers that involve convolution and nonlinearity and do maximum pooling. In a fully connected layer after flattening, the two-dimensional (2D) arranged inputs become a 1D vector and the rest of the network functions as a backpropagation neural network. CNNs are a class of deep neural networks by Krizhevsky et al. [12] that can recognize and classify particular features from images; they are widely used to analyze visual images.

7.2 Basic architecture

The CNN architecture operates in two ways. Feature extraction is a process in which required essential features are extracted automatically to enhance the learning process. The fully connected layer helps in learning the features and predicting the class required as output. The three hidden layers of CNN are the convolution layer, pooling layer, and fully connected layer. Stacking these layers together, the CNN architecture is formed. The convolution layer helps extract the exact features required for the application to be predicted (Fig. 6.7).

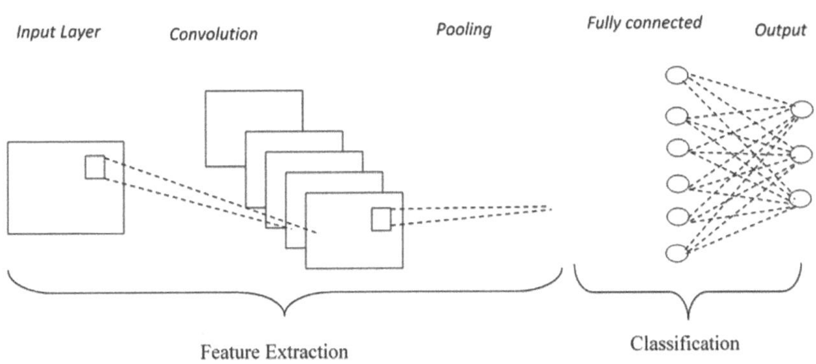

Figure 6.7 Convolution layer.

A CNN is a feed-forward neural network with a grid-like topology, referred to as a ConvNet. The convolution operation is done in the form of an array of pixel values. The convolution layer has a lot of layers; it slides the filter matrix over the image and the computed dot product generates patterns. The matrix output is of the same size as the filter.

The major task of the pooling layer is to reduce the size of the vector by violating excess features, reducing the cost of the process. The pooling layer usually serves as a bridge between the convolutional layer and the FC layer, as demonstrated by Mitchell [10].

The activation function performs an element-wise operation converting negative pixels to zero and introducing nonlinearity to the network. The output is a rectified feature map. Multiple filters can be applied to locate features. The fully connected layer helps in adjust the weight of the neural network, which enhances the learning process of the input and predicts when the unknown test data are provided. The dropout layer and activation function are two more layers that make the CNN most predictive. Overfitting of the data set is managed by the dropout layer, and the activation function helps to approximate the continuous and complex relationship among variables of the input data. Flattening is the process of converting 2D from pooled data to a single long convolution linear vector. The flattened matrix from the pooling layer is fed to the fully connected layer to classify data.

In a CNN network, the input layer accepts the pixel of the image as input and the hidden layer extracts the features and calculates and manipulates the data for classification. There are multiple hidden layers, such as the convolution layer, rectified linear unit (ReLU) layer, and pooling layer, which perform feature extraction and coin or twist and alter input data to generate new patterns. The convolution layer manipulates data in a matrix or array form. Filters are applied to extract relevant features for learning and classification. ReLU is an activation function that adds nonlinearity to the networks.

There are many other activation functions, such as Softmax, tanH, and Sigmoid for specific functionality; they are preferred for multiclass classification. The pooling layer extracts features such as edges, corners, and bodies. The Pooling layer performs down-sampling, which reduces the dimensionality of the feature map. Max pooling extracts the largest element of the feature map. Thus, feature extraction is multiple hidden layers with convolution plus the activation function and maximum pooling and the classification of the output layer is done by the fully connected layer.

8. Survey of online versus offline modes of teaching

To end the crisis of COVID-19, India imposed a strict lockdown. Standard operating guidelines were issued by the central and state government from time to time. Because of social distancing, many restrictions were imposed on public movement [13].

In the education sector, the method of handling classes switched from offline to online, as described by Kapasia et al. [14], and Adnan and Anwar [15]. Online learning was the only alternative method to teach students during the lockdown.

Cook reported that online learning is better than offline learning. Government guidelines were adapted to implement online teaching, as suggested by Aucejo et al. [16]. Five high-impact guidelines were adopted by Bao [17] for the efficient conduct of online education: (1) high interaction between the online teaching design and student observation; (2) content delivery over online media; (3) high reachability of faculty insight into the subject for students; (4) increased involvement of both faculty and students to fulfill learning and efficiently in the online mode of teaching; and (5) the support to handle unexpected events and activities to be targeted toward completing learning in the online mode.

Students adapted to this online methodology. Hasan and Bao [18] reported the level of impact of COVID-19 in the educational, social life, economic, industrial growth, and mental health of students and very depth analysis on the above factors is performed by Odriozolo-gonzalez et al., [19]. College students often report mental health issues such as anxiety and depression after academic work. They report general mental health issues and suicide attempts. The frequency of suicide attempts is 12% and 32% in general mental health and 56% result in death by suicide, as analyzed by Son et al. [20]. An online survey to understand daily activities, learning styles, and the mental health of young students in India during the crisis was analyzed using an a priori algorithm by Khattar et al. [21].

Students from rural places were unable to cope with the implementation of technology is for online education, as reported by Aucejo et al. [16]. Students at the primary school level were unable to afford online education requirements to attend the online classes students that might lead to stress and depression and it was identified by Lee [22]. Anxiety and depression go in hand to hand; most of the adults face them today [23]. In a survey conducted in the United States, of 195 students, 138 (71%) expressed increased stress and anxiety owing to the COVID-19 outbreak, as reported by Son et al. [20]. Concentration, listening, and attending classes using mobile phones, laptop, and tablets; the lack of physical movement; and stress on the eyes and brain affected students mentally.

This chapter analyses the pros and cons of offline versus online modes of education system. The survey collected from students was analyzed using a deep learning algorithm, which helped us predict whether students underwent mental stress or depression when studying using the online method of teaching.

8.1 Design of questionnaires for survey

The reachability of the online mode and comfortableness of attending classes online in higher education was determined by conducting a survey among staff and students in higher education institutions.

A set of multiple choice questions was collected from students and staff using the Google Forms platform, which had a general section, student section, and faculty section.

General section: The questionnaire in the general section was related to demographic data including name, age, gender, analysing the tendancy of staff or student and the region to which they belonged, to determine the reachability of online classes across Tamil Nadu. The authentication of the candidate was confirmed via the valid email ID.

A total of 770 students and staff respondents from across Tamil Nadu described their experience of online mode of teaching. We received 91.3% responses from students and 8.7% from faculty. Google Forms representations of total respondents are depicted in Figs. 6.8–6.12.

About 52.3% of respondents were male and 47.7% were female. Male candidature actively participated in response to the queries.

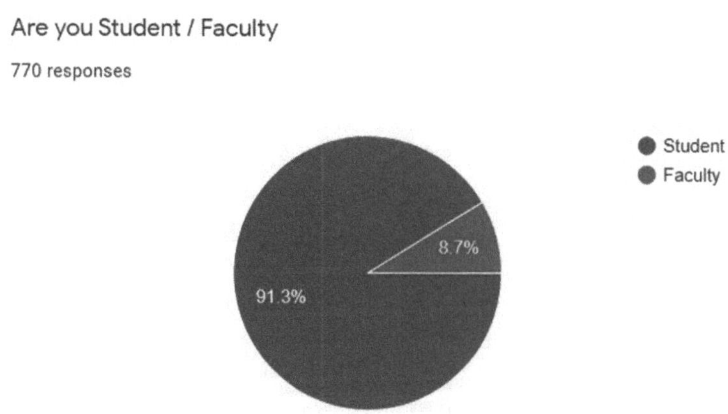

Figure 6.8 Google Forms responses (1).

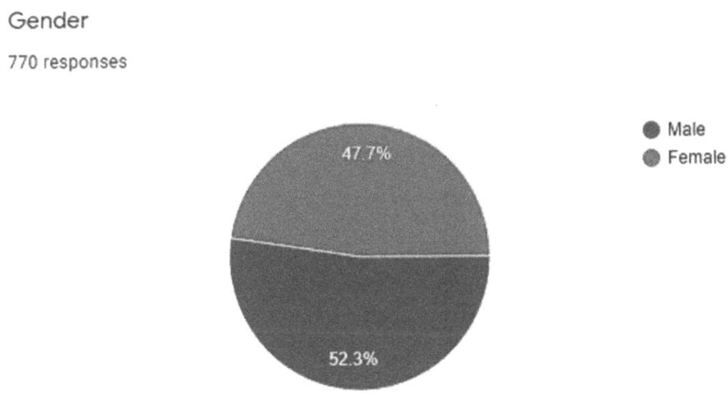

Figure 6.9 Google Forms responses (2).

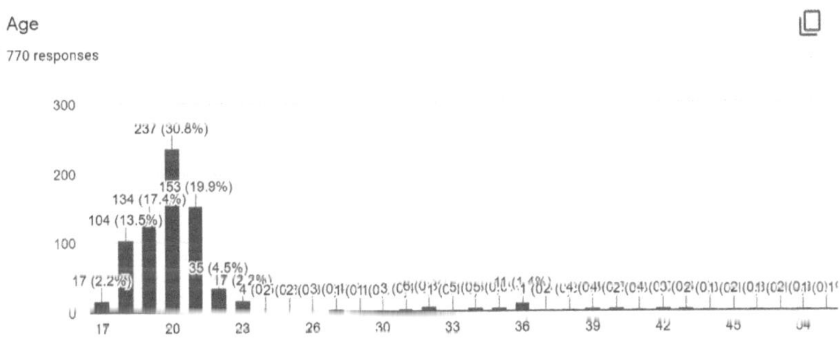

Figure 6.10 Google Forms responses (3).

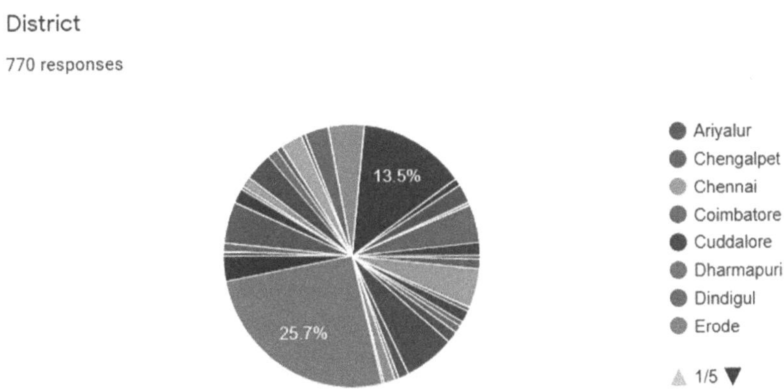

Figure 6.11 Google Forms responses (4).

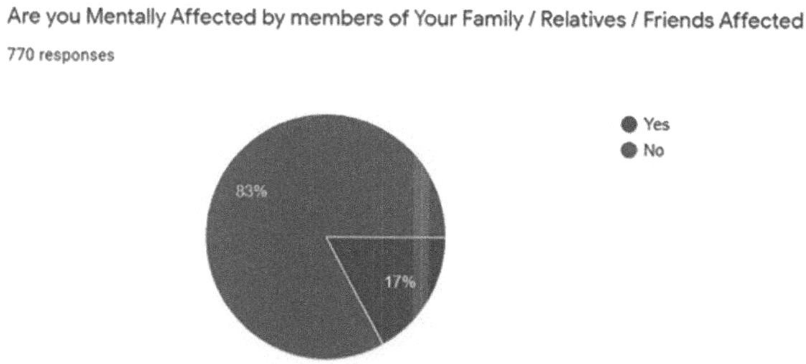

Figure 6.12 Google Forms responses (5).

The age category of students and staff is shown in the Fig. 6.10. Most responses belonged to the age group of 18—21 years. Students in the second year, pre-final year, and final year of engineering college responded. The faculty age group was scattered from in age from 23 to 55 years.

The questionnaire was circulated to students from all parts of the districts of Tamil Nadu. In response, 25.7% of State Headquarters of Tamilnadu (Chennai) has responded more and 13.5% contribution from Kancheepuram has responded and the Fig. 6.11 shows candidates from all over the Tamil Nadu state has contributed to a minimum extent.

In general query, the question posted to analyze the mental stress undergone by the students and staffs when their family members or close relatives and friends circle were affected by Covid -19 resulted in 83% respondent were able to withstand the situation and was not mentally depressed and 17% has acknowledged the stress and depression they inhaled during pandemic period.

Student section: A set of questions was posted to collect data for study and to analyze the mental status of students during the online course the students took. The questions were about overall satisfaction in the conduct of online mode of teaching. Comparison in terms of the offline versus online mode of teaching, the understandability of concepts, the difficulty faced during submitting assignments, satisfaction in attending internal and end of semester examinations, interaction, concentration, and appreciation experienced in online classes. Ratings with respect to eye-to-eye contact, one-to-one contact, effectiveness in conducting practical courses, and conducting group study were also requested. Parameters with respect to fear, anxiety, stress, loneliness, and frustration were collected to predict the mental health of students and staff during the pandemic.

Tables 6.1 and 6.2 provide the queries posted and the percentage of respondents as well as ratings.

Table 6.1 Students' responses to queries posted in terms of percentages, ratios, and ratings.

	Percentage	0%	20%	40%	80%	100%
1	Overall satisfaction in online mode of teaching	6.8%	10.7%	30%	38.5%	13.9%
Ratio		**0:100**	**20:80**	**50:50**	**80:20**	**100:0**
2	Comparison of offline and online modes of teaching	9.1%	14.2%	38.8%	30.7%	7.1%
3	Understandability of concepts: offline versus online	8.7%	12.1%	39%	33.6%	6.7%
4	Difficulty faced in submitting assignments offline versus online	14.2%	17.1%	42.8%	17.8%	8.1%
5	Satisfaction in attending internal/end of semester examination offline versus online	19.3%	16.9%	36.4%	17.1%	10.2%
6	Interaction in class offline versus online	9.4%	12.9%	38.5%	28%	11.1%
7	Concentration in attending class offline versus online	9.5%	12.1%	35.8%	31.6%	11
8	Recognition/applause/appreciation offline versus online	Satisfactory = 62.9%			Not satisfactory = 37.1%	
Ratings		**(1 = low; 5 = high)**				
9	Eye-to-eye contact in offline	9.7%	10%	29%	25.9%	25.5%
10	One-to-one contact in online	17.1%	18.1%	34.3%	18.1%	12.5%
11	Effectiveness on hands-on session	9.7%	12.2%	44.5%	23.3%	10.2%
12	Group study	20.6%	14.1%	29.9%	19.5%	15.9%
13	Fear owing to COVID	15.4%	9.5%	21.1%	17.4%	36.7%
14	Anxiety owing to COVID	14.1%	10.2%	28.9%	21.6%	25.2%
15	Loneliness owing to COVID	18.6%	10.2%	25%	18.5%	27.6%
16	Frustration owing to COVID	12.9%	10.8%	33.3%	17.9%	25%
17	Stress owing to COVID	14.1%	11.8%	22.6%	17.5%	34%

Table 6.2 Faculty responses to query posted in terms of percentages, ratios, and ratings.

1	Faculty vaccinated or not	Yes = 16.7%			No = 83.3%	
Percentage		**0%**	**20%**	**40%**	**80%**	**100%**
2	Overall satisfaction in online mode of teaching as faculty	2.4%	16.7%	46.4%	32.1%	2.4%
Ratio		**0:100**	**20:80**	**50:50**	**80:20**	**100:0**
3	Comparison of offline versus online mode of teaching	3.6%	16.7%	32.1%	44%	3.6%
4	Understandability of concepts by students: offline versus online	3.6%	16.7%	32.1%	42.9%	4.8%
5	Difficulty faced by students in submitting assignments offline versus online	8.3%	19%	42.9%	26.2%	3.6%
6	Satisfaction in conducting internal/end of semester examination: offline versus online	7.1%	16.7%	33.3%	35.7%	7.1%
7	Interaction with students in class offline versus online	3.6%	11.9%	25%	44%	15.5%
8	Concentration of students in attending class offline versus online	2.4%	10.7%	29.8%	46.4%	10.7%
9	Recognition/applause/ appreciation expressed to students online	Satisfactory = 44%			Not satisfactory = 56%	
Ratings		**(1 = low; 5 = high)**				
10	Eye-to-eye contact with students in class offline	16.7%	11.9%	9.5%	28.6%	33. 3%
11	One-to-one contact with students in class online	28.6%	31%	27.4%	6%	7.1%
12	Effectiveness on hands-on session	15.5%	14.3%	32.1%	28.6%	9.5%
13	Fear owing to COVID	8.3%	19%	32.1%	14.3%	26.2%
14	Anxiety owing to COVID	9.5%	10.7%	35.7%	25%	19%
15	Loneliness owing to COVID	19%	13.1%	29.8%	20.2%	17.9%
16	Frustration owing to COVID	16.7%	11.9%	27.4%	19%	25%
17	Stress owing to COVID	14.3%	10.7%	17.9%	28.6%	28.6%

9. Prediction of mental health in online mode of teaching using convolutional neural network

The main objective of this study using deep learning was to predict the mental health of higher education students during the pandemic. The prediction helps us to view the impact of online education in students and faculty and how to embed or take up online education in the future.

The objective is to predict the mental health of students and faculty in the offline versus online mode of teaching.

Data collection: Data are collected from students and staff in higher education institutions (engineering discipline) using social networks.

Prepare data: Preparing data is a crucial step that involves preprocessing works to clean, match, and blend the data. A survey is conducted and data are collected among 770 students and faculty. The distribution of responses to the queries is depicted in Fig. 6.13.

Select algorithm: Sixteen factors from the collected data are considered for input into the CNN model. Overall satisfaction in the online mode of teaching is set as the expected outcome. Input to the CNN model is a 4×4 matrix in which 16 places are filled by 16 factors collected from students. It is convoluted by 8 2×2 filters and then by 10 2×2 filters. This is then converted into fully connected layers of 40 neurons, and then a Softmax function is applied to it to predict the percentage of satisfaction in online learning. The designed CNN architecture is depicted in Fig. 6.14.

Training and testing: The collected dataset is split 70:30 for training and testing, respectively. Each data from the dataset is used to form the 4×4 matrix. Test model: During testing, the matrix is shuffled randomly for each part of the data to form different matrices for the same matrix (data augmentation).

Integrated model: Seventy percent of student data was given as input for training; 30% of student and staff data was fed as input for testing and the results were analyzed.

Results: The answers replied for the query of 16 questions was fed as input data and the answer of the overall satisfaction of the query was the expected outcome for training. The overall satisfaction of the students in online mode of teaching was analyzed and found that students satisfied above 80% is 13.9% and between 60 and 80% is 38.5% and between 40 and 60% is 30% and below 40% is 17.5%. Students below 40% were mentally disturbed by the conduct of online classes and students between 40 and 80 had less concentration online, which might have led to mental depression. When faculty data were analyzed, only 1.5% of staff was highly satisfied; 35.8% was satisfied above 60%, and 49.3% above 40% and 13.4% were not satisfied

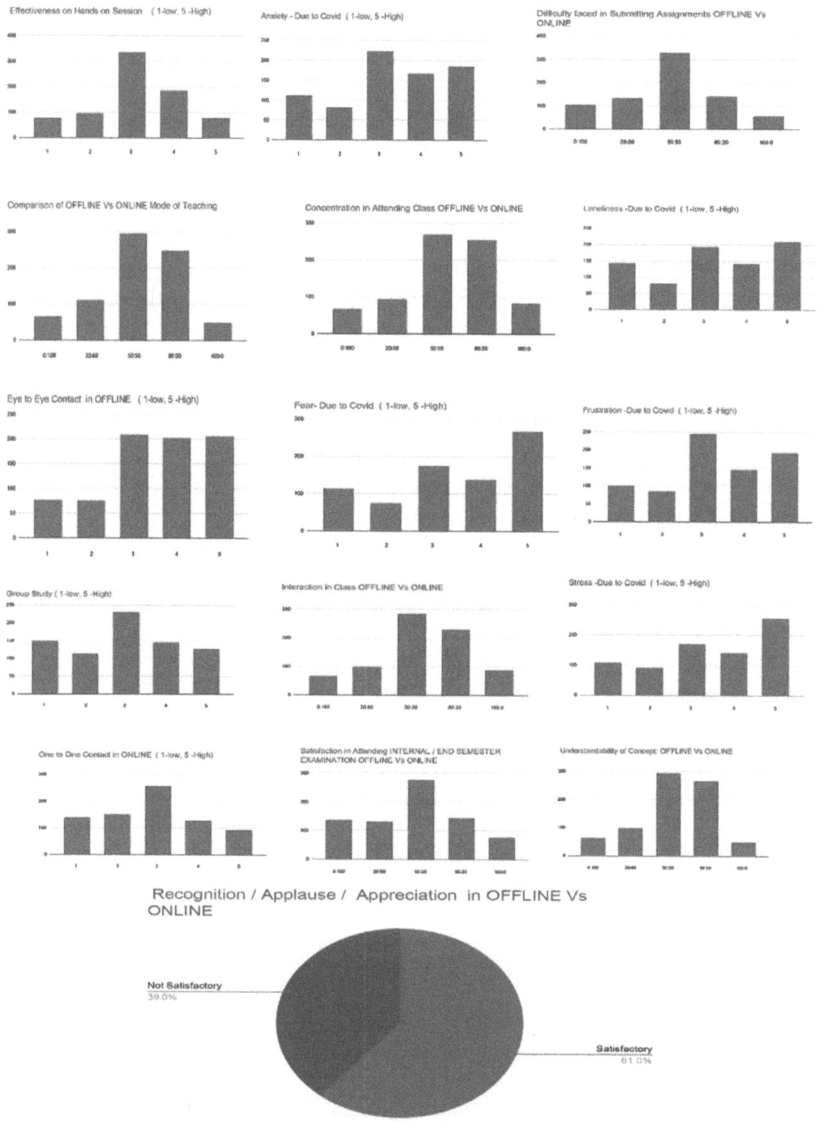

Figure 6.13 Distribution of students' queries considered for data preparation.

with the online mode of teaching. The overall satisfaction of students and staff in online mode of learning and teaching and an accuracy graph in terms of no of epoch are depicted in Fig. 6.15.

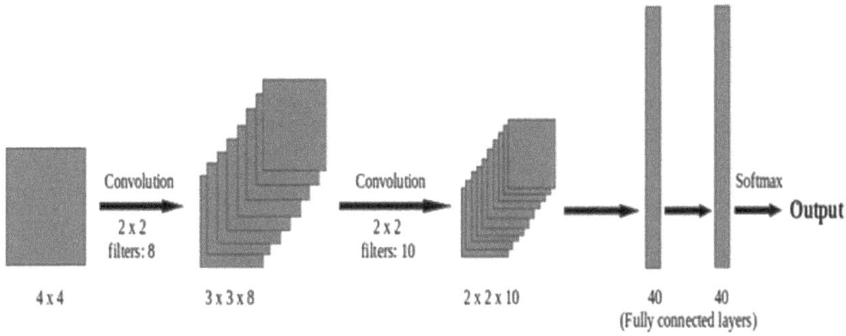

Figure 6.14 Designed convolutional neural network architecture.

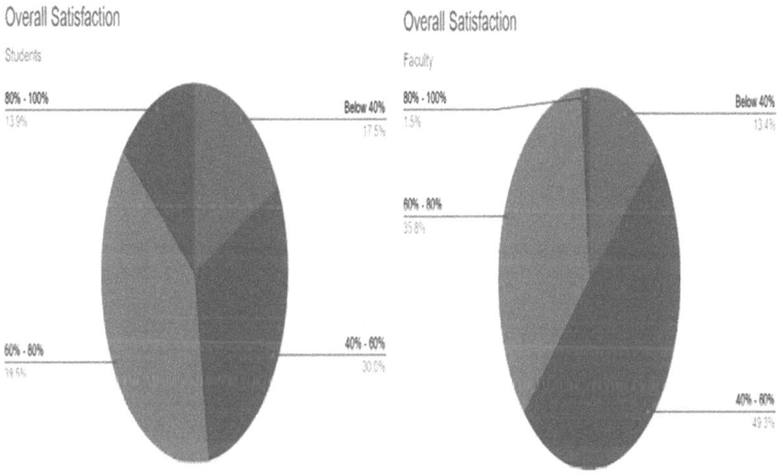

Figure 6.15 Overall satisfaction of students and staff.

Performance measure: The performance of the model was calculated by finding the true positive, true negative, false positive, and false negative. The sensitivity in Eq. 6.1, specificity in Eq. 6.2, and accuracy in Eq. 6.3 were calculated:

$$Sensitivity = \left[\frac{TP}{TP + FN}\right] \tag{6.1}$$

$$Specificity = \left[\frac{TN}{TN + FP}\right] \tag{6.2}$$

$$Accuracy = \frac{TP + TN}{TP + FP + FN + TN} \tag{6.3}$$

where TP = true positive, FN = false negative, FP = false positive, and TN= true negative. The accuracy of the prediction model was 92% (Fig. 6.16).

Tables 6.3 and 6.4 show the performance measure for students and faculty.

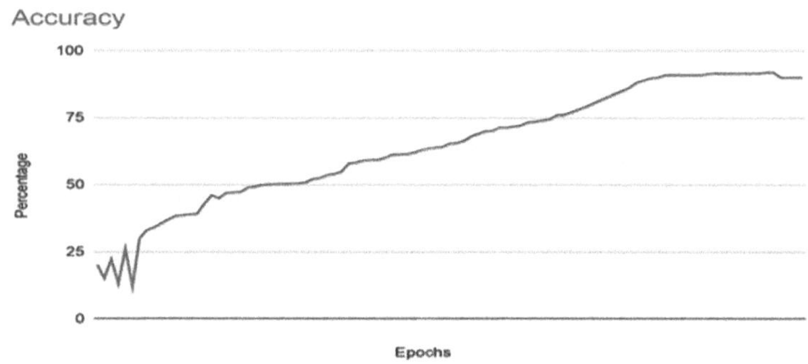

Figure 6.16 Accuracy of prediction model.

Table 6.3 Students' performance measure.

Performance measure	Values
True positive	83
True negative	69
False positive	8
False negative	4
Sensitivity	95%
Specificity	89%
Accuracy	93%
Prevalence	53%
Precision	91%

Table 6.4 Faculty performance measure.

Performance measure	Values
True positive	54
True negative	6
False positive	3
False negative	4
Sensitivity	93%
Specificity	67%
Accuracy	89%
Prevalence	86%
Precision	94%

9.1 Recommendations

Increasing screen time during the coronavirus pandemic was harmful to students' eyesight. Thus, time limitations each day need to be imposed in schools and colleges to avoid myopia. Research in Ireland concluded that 3 hours of screen time per day increases the odds of myopia in students. Research in Denmark concluded that the risk for myopia doubled in teenagers who had more than 6 hours of screen devices per day. It is recommended that outdoor activities be increased between screen times. China placed a recommendation of 40 min outdoor activity.

Some recommendations are:

1. Take a break from closeup work every 20 min.
2. Set a timer for reminders.
3. Digital media should be 18–20 inches from the face.

Government policy-makers must remember eye health strategies and protect students, faculty, and parents, and impose standard operating procedures for conducting online classes in schools and colleges.

The stress that developed during the entirely online mode of teaching that leads to depression in students and faculty can be avoided by imposing a blended mode of teaching.

Teacher-centric education does not help students to come up with innovative and creative ideas. A 70% teacher-centric method of imparting knowledge and 30% of student-centric activities can be designed in the curriculum to improve creative skills by combining teamwork in a student-centric mode with the online mode of teaching. Work assigned by the curriculum must not burden students; it may lead to stress and depression. The government is supposed to provide all technological stack like the device for online learning, internet connectivity, the standard operating procedure, etc., that is required for online mode of teaching.

10. Summary

AI has a vital role in the early detection of diseases. It helps doctors predict disease accurately and even enables diagnosis, decision-making, and treatment. Deep learning algorithms are deployed in the detection of pneumonia, skin cancer, and arrhythmia. Augmented reality microscopy helps in cancer detection. This chapter discussed COVID and its impact on the education sector, which led to an online mode of teaching. It reviewed how the online mode of teaching reached the students and faculty, and described a survey using deep learning analysis that predicted the impact of the online mode on education in students and staff. This analysis might provide insight to government policy-makers to come up with strategies in higher education for guidelines to frame a curriculum and syllabus in a blended mode of teaching to avoid stress and depression in students and maintain good health.

References

[1] The American Psychiatric Association – Anxiety Disorders – Article, What Are Anxiety Disorders, 2017. https://www.psychiatry.org/patients-families/anxiety-disorders/what-are-anxiety-disorders. (Accessed 6 May 2021).

[2] M. Behzadifar, M. Behzadifar, A. Sayehmiri, M. Behzadifar, M. Sarokhani, K. Sayehmiri, Economic factors influencing mental health using multiple regression model in Ilam province of Iran, Med. J. Islam. Repub. Iran 29 (292) (2015).

[3] World Health Organization – (Fact in Pictures), Mental Health, 2019. http://www.who.int/features/factfiles/mental_health/en/. (Accessed 6 May 2021).

[4] World Health Organization – (Fact Sheet), Mental Health: Strengthening Our Response, 2018. https://www.who.int/news-room/fact-sheets/detail/mental-health-strengthening-our-response. (Accessed 6 May 2021).

[5] The National Institute of Mental Health Information Resource Center – Health Topics – Article, US, Schizophrenia, 2020. https://www.nimh.nih.gov/health/topics/schizophrenia/index.shtml#part_145429. (Accessed 6 May 2021).

[6] The National Institute of Mental Health Information Resource Center – Statistics Article, US, Mental Illness, 2019. https://www.nimh.nih.gov/health/statistics/mental-illness.shtml. (Accessed 6 May 2021).

[7] Agarwal, S. Sharma, V. Kumar, M. Kaur, Effect of E-learning on public health and environment during COVID-19 lockdown, IEEE J. Big Data Mining Anal. 4 (2) (2021) 104–115.

[8] The National Institute of Mental Health Information Resource Center – Health Topics – Article, US, Bipolar Disorder, 2020. https://www.nimh.nih.gov/health/topics/bipolar-disorder/index.shtml. (Accessed 6 May 2021).

[9] The National Institute of Mental Health Information Resource Center – Brochures and Fact Sheets – Article, US, Looking at My Genes: What Can They Tell Me About My Mental Health?, 2020. https://www.nimh.nih.gov/health/publications/looking-at-my-genes/index.shtml#pub3. (Accessed 6 May 2021).

[10] T. Mitchell, Machine Learning, McGraw Hill, New York, 1997.

[11] Y. Bengio, Y. LeCun, G. Hinton, Deep learning, Nature 521 (7553) (2015) 436–444.

[12] A. Krizhevsky, I. Sutskever, G. Hinton, ImageNet classification with deep convolutional neural networks, in: Proceedings of the 25th International Conference on Neural Information Processing Systems - Volume 1, Curran Associates Inc., Red Hook, NY, USA, December 2012, pp. 1097–1105.

[13] J. Saha, B. Barman, P. Chouhan, Lockdown for COVID-19 and its impact on community mobility in India: an analysis of the COVID-19 Community Mobility Reports, 2020, Child. Youth Serv. Rev. 116 (2020). Article 105160.

[14] N. Kapasia, P. Paul, A. Roy, J. Saha, A. Zaveri, R. Mallick, B. Barman, P. Das, P. Chouhan, Impact of lockdown on learning status of undergraduate and postgraduate students during COVID-19 pandemic in West Bengal, India, Child. Youth Serv. Rev. 116 (2020). Article 105194.

[15] M. Adnan, K. Anwar, Online learning amid the COVID-19 pandemic: students' perspectives, J. Pedagog. Sociol. Psychol. 2 (2020) 2–8.
[16] E.M. Aucejo, J. French, M.P. Ugalde Araya, B. Zafar, The impact of COVID-19 on student experiences and expectations: evidence from a survey, J. Publ. Econ. 191 (2020). Article 104271.
[17] W. Bao, COVID-19 and online teaching in higher education: a case study of Peking University, Human Behav. Emerging Technol. 2 (2020) 113–115.
[18] N. Hasan, Y. Bao, Impact of "e-Learning crack-up" perception on psychological distress among college students during COVID-19 pandemic: a mediating role of "fear of academic year loss", Child. Youth Serv. Rev. 118 (2020). Article 105355.
[19] P. Odriozola-gonzalez, A. Planchuelo-gomez, M. Jesus, R. De Luis-garcía, Psychological effects of the COVID-19 outbreak and lockdown among students and workers of a Spanish university, Psychiatr. Res. 290 (2020). Article 113108.
[20] C. Son, S. Hegde, A. Smith, X. Wang, F. Sasangohar, Effects of COVID-19 on college students' mental health in the United States: interview survey study, J. Med. Internet Res. 22 (9) (2020) e21279.
[21] Khattar, P.R. Jain, S.M.K. Quadri, Effects of the disastrous pandemic COVID 19 on learning styles, activities and mental health of young Indian students - a machine learning approach, in: Proceeding of the 4th International Conference on Intelligent Computing and Control Systems (ICICCS), May 2020, pp. 1190–1195. Madurai, India.
[22] J. Lee, H.J. Jeong, S. Kim, Stress, Anxiety, and Depression Among Undergraduate Students during the COVID-19 Pandemic and Their Use of Mental Health Services, Innovative Higher Education, 2021.
[23] Anxiety & Depression Association of America – Article, USA, Facts & Statistics, 2020. https://adaa.org/about-adaa/press-room/facts-statistics. (Accessed 6 May 2021).

CHAPTER SEVEN

Machine learning based analysis and prediction of college students' mental health during COVID-19 in India

Aparajita Nanda, Sonal Tuteja and Sarishty Gupta
Department of Computer Science & Engineering and Information Technology, Jaypee Institute of Information Technology, Noida, Uttar Pradesh, India

1. Introduction

The COVID-19 pandemic has not only caused worldwide economic and social disruption but also drastically changed the lifestyle of people. The effects of this pandemic are also visible in the whole education system, starting from schools to universities. The traditional education system, which primarily focuses on peer-to-peer and interactive learning to engage students, has now changed to online learning [1]. In online learning, it is challenging for students to collaborate and interact with the faculty as well as peers. Other issues with online learning include social isolation, academic pressure, job insecurity, etc. Additionally, the change in the education system has led to mental-health-related problems for students, which needs to be addressed. The mental health of an individual provides essential clues in the behavioral pattern of a person, which vary according to different communities and the treatments. The broad category of communities includes high school students, college students, and working professionals, where mental stress and depressions are common. The rate of mental stress of college students differs with respect to their year, e.g., graduating-year students are more worried about getting a job than a first-year student. So the rate of the stress of a final-year student is much higher than the intermediate-year or fresher. Furthermore, the online education system complicates the scenarios for student communities and makes them grapple with social isolation, infrastructure issues, academic performance, depressive thoughts, etc., across the world. Hence, it is necessary to determine the stress level to address mental illness as a prevention.

Artificial Intelligence, Machine Learning, and Mental Health in Pandemics
ISBN: 978-0-323-91196-2
https://doi.org/10.1016/B978-0-323-91196-2.00001-6

Researchers have designed and analyzed parameters concerning the mental health of students from US universities [1,2]. Also, the analysis of parameters concerned with mental health of Chinese students has been discussed in Refs. [3,4]. Machine learning algorithms are employed to identify mental health issues in persons in terms of depression, anxiety, and stress scale [5,6]. Researchers have applied various machine learning algorithms to identify the stress level of patients [7]. However, the parameters concerning the mental health of Indian students have not been considered so far. The motivation for this work is to analyze the parameters of utmost concern to the students in Indian universities. The parameters of concern for Indian students can be different from other countries. We are interested in finding students with high mental stress who need attention. Therefore, the proposed framework thrusts upon:

- Analyzing the parameters that strongly impacted students' mental stress level due to COVID-19 through a survey.
- Designing classifier models to determine or predict the mental stress level of students from the abovementioned survey.

A module framework is designed to predict the students' mental stress level based on a set of benchmark questions, which is represented in Fig. 7.1. Firstly, we conduct a survey through an online questionnaire for students from Indian universities. The responses are collected into a dataset and preprocessed. Then, the dataset is used to categorize the students into two groups: high mental stress and low mental stress using k-means clustering. The labels identified by k-means are further validated by the students. Lastly, we apply different classification models such as naive Bayes (NB), Logistic regression (LR), Support Vector Machine (SVM), and Random Forest (RF) to predict the class label of students. Moreover, we also analyze students' responses to understand the parameters that are of more concern for the Indian students. Therefore, our proposed work can be used to find the mental stress level of students so that immediate action can be taken.

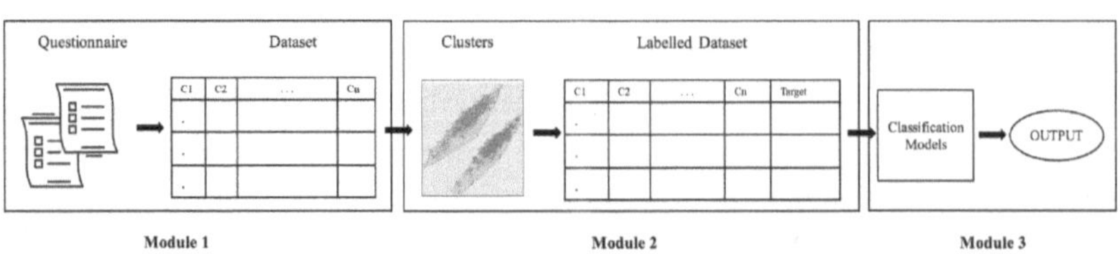

Figure 7.1 Overview of proposed modular framework.

The paper is organized as follows. Section 2 describes the related work. In Section 3, we discuss the proposed framework. The surveyed data is analyzed in Section 4. The experimentation and results analysis are presented in Section 5, which is followed by conclusion in Section 6.

2. Related work

We segregate the related work into two subsections. In Section 2.1, we describe the literature based on mental health analysis using machine learning. In Section 2.2, we discuss the related work based on COVID-19 analysis using machine learning.

2.1 Machine-learning-based mental health analysis

For many years, several countries have studied the relationships between mental health and total well-being of a person. Various researchers have used machine learning algorithms to predict mental health. Srividya et al. [6] identified a person's mental health by applying various machine learning algorithms such as NB classifier, decision tree, SVMs, LR, K- nearest neighbor. They applied clustering algorithms to discover the number of clusters. The cluster labels obtained from clustering were provided as input to build the classifiers. They performed analysis on different target groups. In the study [7], the authors used the Depression, Anxiety, and Stress Scale questionnaire (DASS 21) to collect data from different individuals. Five different machine learning algorithms were used in this study to assess five levels of stress, anxiety, and depression. Following the application of the various approaches, the confusion matrix revealed that classes were imbalanced. As a result, the F1 score was considered, which assisted in determining that the RF classifier had the best accuracy model. Sau et al. [8] applied different classification methods to identify anxiety and depression in elderly patients based on sociodemographic and health-related characteristics. With a dataset of 510 geriatric patients, 10 classifiers were examined and tested using the 10-fold cross-validation approach. With the RF approach, the highest prediction accuracy of 89% was achieved.

Kessler et al. [9] used World Mental Health (WMH) models to predict eventual major depressive disorder (MDD) severity and persistence. They compared the results of ML models' findings with more traditional LR models. Smets et al. [5] examined several machine learning algorithms to measure mental stress. The physiological responses were recorded, such as the electrocardiogram (ECG), galvanic skin response (GSR), respiration, and temperature. Their findings revealed that Bayesian networks and extended SVMs produced the best performance. Another study [10] used several machine learning algorithms such as CatBoost, NB, RF, etc., to detect mental health disorders among seafarers. They interviewed 470 seafarers and gathered their occupational, sociodemographic, and health information. The Hospital Anxiety and Depression Scale (HADS) [11] was then used to determine the existence of anxiety and depression. Consequently, the researchers discovered that CatBoost had the highest accuracy and precision of all the classifiers, at 82.6 and 84.1%, respectively.

2.2 COVID-19 analysis based on machine learning

The COVID-19 has raised attention to the mental health of those who have been impacted. Pandemics are known to increase or create new tensions, such as anxiety and worry for one's own or family members, restrictions on physical movement and social activities due to isolation, and abrupt lifestyle changes. Most of the existing material on COVID-19's psychological effects comes from the first hotspots in China and the United States. The study [3] examined the anxiety in university students in China amid the breakout of COVID-19. They investigated a total of 3611 college students from all around China aged 18−24. Anxiety was measured using the SAS (Self-Rating Anxiety Scale) [12]. According to their findings, undergraduate students in China were more anxious with COVID-19. A few more studies from China [4,13,14] concluded that college students' depression and anxiety levels grew dramatically during the COVID-19, which was linked to various causes such as economic pressures, effects on everyday living, and academic delays. The findings from these studies suggested that college students' mental health suffers greatly, and they require assistance and support from colleges, families, and society.

To further understand the impacts of the pandemic on students' mental well-being, the authors [1] conducted interviews with 195 students at a US university. Their findings implied that the COVID-19 pandemic has had a significant negative influence on various outcomes such as health, academic, and lifestyle. Wilson et al. [2] assessed US students through an online survey to look at the impact of the pandemic on stress, depression, and physical activity. They indicated that during COVID-19, there was a substantial decrease in physical activity and a substantial rise in depression symptoms in college students. In Ref. [15], the authors surveyed 2031 students of Texas University. The survey included two standardized depression and anxiety scales—the Patient Health Questionnaire-9 and the General Anxiety

Disorder-7. They found the number of people who report having anxiety, depression, or suicide thoughts is frightening. Respondents expressed concerns about the pandemic's impact on their academics, lifestyle, and health. They suggested that given the outbreak's unexpected length and intensity, these problems must be explored further and addressed.

Li et al. [16] obtained data from 640 foreign and local university students. The foundations for information about the COVID-19 pandemic and its impact on mental health and psychological well-being were developed using a cross-sectional technique. The snowball sampling strategy was used to collect data to reach the maximum number of participants in a short amount of time. The findings revealed significant negative consequences, including varying levels of stress, depression, and specific discomfort. The mental health of university students is most harmed by COVID-19, quarantine activities, and self-isolation. Mekonen et al. [17] conducted an institution-based cross-sectional survey at The University of Gondar in which 350 students were chosen using a basic random sampling procedure. A standardized questionnaire was used to collect data. The DASS-21 was used to assess depression, anxiety, and stress. They concluded that more than a third, a fifth, and over two-fifths of students, respectively, suffered anxiety, stress, and depression. In paper [18], an online survey was used to collect sociodemographic information from French students. Stress was measured using the existing perceived stress scale (PSS) [19], and social support was measured using the Multidimensional Scale of Perceived Social Support (MSPSS) [20]. To investigate the relationship between severe perceived stress and other parameters, LR models were used. The existing methods on mental health are classified into different states of mind for different communities with a specific observation. Similarly, COVID-19-based machine learning approaches mostly deal with the impact on the student community in different countries. From the abovementioned papers, it is required to design an approach to analyze and predict the students' mental health in Indian universities.

3. Proposed framework

The aim of the proposed framework is to identify the college student's mental stress during this COVID-19 pandemic. The overview of the module framework is described in Fig. 7.1, which comprises three modules: (i) Module 1: Preparing Questionnaire, Data Collection, and Preprocessing, (ii) Module 2: Clustering and Label Validation, and (iii) Module 3:

Classification Models. We prepared an online questionnaire to analyze the mental health of the students (Section 3.1). The responses to those questionnaires were collected into a dataset to categorize their stress levels (Section 3.2). The dataset was grouped into two different clusters, which were fed as input for the classification (Section 3.3). Further, the responses with their corresponding stress levels are fed into a classifier model to learn and predict future responses (Section 3.4). Hence, the proposed framework describes two objectives:

- To analyze the parameters that strongly impacted students' mental stress level due to COVID-19 through a survey.
- To design classifier models for determining the mental stress level of college students from the survey as mentioned above.

3.1 Preparing questionnaire

We have prepared a set of benchmark questions for analyzing students' mental health [1,2]. These questions have been designed and modified based on the Indian context. The details of the questionnaires and different possible responses are described in the following Table 7.1.

3.2 Data collection and preprocessing

We have collected data based on the above questionnaire from 600 students from different universities and different courses April 1–5, 2021. The data provided by each student consists of gender, academic year (fresher, intermediate, and graduating), and responses to the questionnaire. These responses were collected to form a dataset where each student was represented as a sample. Each question has multiple possible responses, which were chosen by the students.

The responses of the students were stored in a csv file having 600 records. The gender with two possible selected values (Male and Female) was converted into two numeric attributes using a one-hot encoding scheme [21]. Similarly, the academic year with three possible values (Fresher, Intermediate, Graduating) was converted into three numeric attributes. The question's value for a student is calculated as the number of selected options divided by the total number of possible options for that question. Therefore, the size of the dataset after preprocessing contains 600 rows and 17 columns.

3.3 Clustering and label validation

Clustering is the process of organizing similar objects into meaningful/useful groups such that the objects within a group are more similar than those in

Table 7.1 Questions and sets of responses.

Questions	Sets of responses
Have you been worried about health of?	Families and relatives with higher vulnerabilities, families with more interpersonal contact, families and relatives being infected
Have you faced difficulty in concentration due to?	Homely environment, lack of self-motivation and accountability, lack of self-motivation and accountability, lack of peer-learning, distractions due to usage of social media, phone, games etc.
Have you faced disruption in your sleeping patterns like?	Staying up or waking up late, irregularity in sleeping patterns, increased duration of sleep, difficulty in falling or staying asleep
Have you realized social isolation due to?	Reduced interactions with people, lack of in-person interactions, restricted outdoor activities
Have you felt worried about academic performance due to?	Change of teaching mode from offline to online, academic progress and future career prospects, marks/grades improvement, reduced motivation or procrastination
Have you been worried about job-related issues such as?	Difficulty in job searching, delay in job joining, not finding the desired role in job, not finding the desired packaged/salaried job
Have you faced any financial difficulties due to?	Financial situations of families, current or future employment
Have you faced any infrastructure issues at your home such as?	No proper internet connection, no hardware support for practical work
Have you faced any issues related to increased academic load such as?	Online courses and class projects, difficult assignments, coverage of the same coursework in less time period
Have you come across any depressive thoughts such as?	Loneliness, insecurity or uncertainty, powerlessness or hopelessness, concerns about academic performance, overthinking
Have you come across any suicidal thoughts due to?	Depressive thoughts, academic issues, problems with parents, insecurity

other groups. The aim of clustering in our work is to organize the students into clusters and analyze their behavior in terms of the parameters determining their mental health. As our dataset is unsupervised, we have applied k-means clustering algorithms [21] to label the dataset into two classes: high mental stress versus low mental stress. Additionally, other clustering methods such as hierarchical clustering and DBSCAN [22] have also been applied. However, the clusters generated using k-means clustering were better able to provide disjoint clusters due to the prefixed value of k as 2.

The class labels obtained from k-means are verified by the participated students to validate the exactness of the clustering. We gathered their views on resultant class labels (i.e., having low mental stress and high mental stress) and computed the percentage of students who agreed with the assigned label by the k-means algorithm. The percentage was calculated with a factor of the number of students agreed on the assigned label divided by the total number of students. After the validation process, the labels identified using clustering were taken as target output for the classification models. The features of data points with their corresponding class labels (target class) were employed to build the classifier models.

3.4 Classification models

Classifier models are considered a supervised machine learning technique used to determine the data points belonging to a specific class based on their set of features. We fed the collected data into a classification model for learning the responses parameter of students and predict the mental health of students. Classification models such as NB, LR, linear SVM, and ensemble-based RF are taken into consideration.

The NB classifier follows the Bayes theorem to predict a data point's class membership probability value, i.e., it provides a probability value for a sample belonging to a specific class. NB provides the presumption that for any given sample point with its class label, values of the features are conditionally independent of one another. Sentiment analysis was performed on a large dataset using an implemented NB classifier, and accuracy depends on the size of the dataset. As dataset size increases, accuracy also increases [23].

LR is a linear classification model, which predicts the classification based on the probability value. It follows the logit transform to estimate the probability values for given data points, which later on outputs two class labels as 0 or 1 for binary classifiers. It predicts the probability of occurrence of a sample by passing data to the logit function. A set of appropriate features helps to enhance the classification score [24,25].

SVM is a linear classifier used to classify the data points into different class labels by using hyperplanes. SVM can be used to classify both linear and nonlinear data. It segments the data by generating multiple separating hyperplanes in such a way that each segment represents data points from a particular class. SVM has been successfully employed for various applications such as classification of cancerous cells [26], handwritten digits [27], text categorization [28], etc. Hence, SVM is proven to perform well for categorical data.

RF is an ensemble-based technique that creates a forest of decision trees during its training. It works on the principle of bagging, which is known for minimizing the variation in predictions by combining the output of decision trees on samples of a dataset. It results in an output class in the same process as a class is assigned to an individual tree [29–31].

3.4.1 Performance measures for classifiers

The performance of the classifiers is measured through the confusion matrix, which is considered the foundation of computing the classifier accuracy on a test set for its known true label. The confusion matrix is used for the computation of optimal solutions during the training. The results are represented in a tabular form where predicted classes are described in the row and target classes are in the column. The true positive (TP), True Negative (TN), False Positive (FP), and False Negative (FN) are computed from the confusion matrix. TP and TN describe the number of sample points that are positively and negatively classified, respectively. Similarly, FP and FN are positively and negatively misclassified, respectively. Based on this, the performance measures for the classifier models are evaluated in terms of accuracy, precision, and recall. Table 7.2 defines the measures as mentioned above.

Classifier accuracy is defined as the percentage of correctly classified test data to the total number of data points in the test set. The average accuracy of different test sets for a dataset is considered to be the accuracy of the classifier. Precision measures the percentage of samples that are labeled as positive and are correctly classified as positive. It provides the exactness by identifying negative samples as negative. Similarly, recall provides the computation to find all positive samples, i.e., the percentage of positive samples also labeled as positive.

Table 7.2 Performance measures for classifiers.

Measures	Formula
Classification accuracy	$\frac{TP+TN}{P+N}$
Precision	$\frac{TP}{TP+FP}$
Recall	$\frac{TP}{TP+FN}$

4. Data analysis of students

In this section, we have analyzed the answers to understand the parameters of concern to the Indian students based on the responses collected from students for the questionnaire (Table 7.1). The study indicated that COVID-19 has negatively impacted (either low, medium, or high) college students' mental health, academics, and social environment. As shown in Fig. 7.2, out of 600 students, 467 (78%) were worried about own and their families' health, 487(81%) faced difficulty in concentration, 428 (71%) had disruption in their sleeping patterns, 590 (98%) comprehended increase in social isolation with 31% reported it as high, and 41% as moderate, 418 (70%) were concerned about their academic performance with 30% reporting as high, and 26% as moderate, 384 (64%) faced issues due to increased academic load with 39% stated it as high, 444 (74%) happened to have depressive thoughts with 11% recorded as high, and 38% as moderate, 366 (61%) came across some suicidal thoughts.

Worried about health: It is observed that 78% of students were worried about their own or their families' health due to COVID-19. As shown in Fig. 7.3, 45% of students were concerned about their families and relatives having high vulnerabilities like their grandparents or adults having some health issues. 39% of students showed their concern about family members having more interpersonal contact or exposure like doctors or other medical workers. 39% of students expressed their worries about family members being infected by the virus.

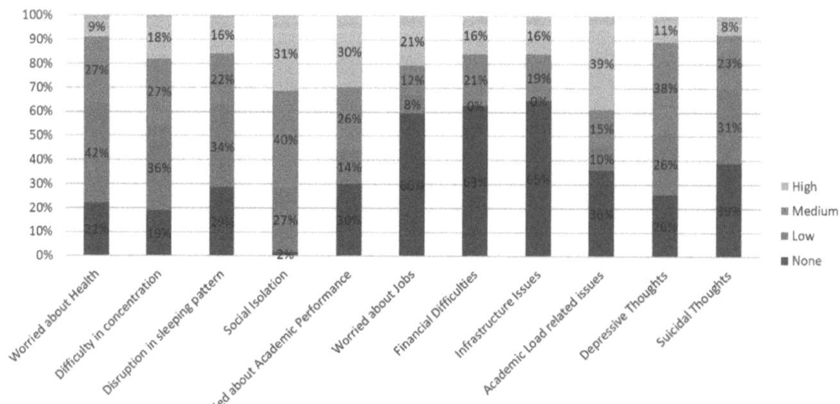

Figure 7.2 Concern level (none, low, medium, high) of students based on questionnaire.

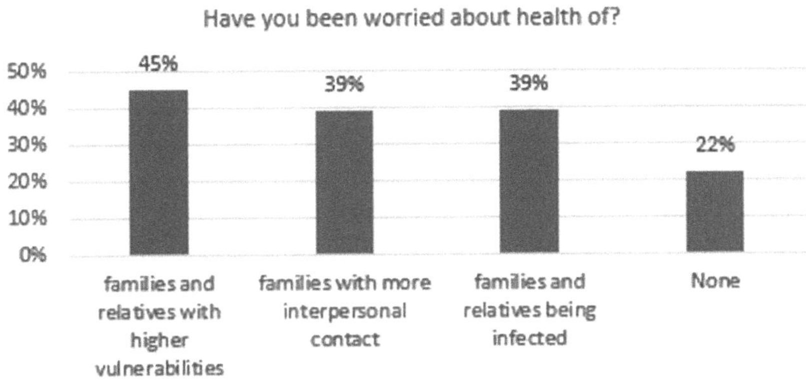

Figure 7.3 Percentage of students concerned about health parameters.

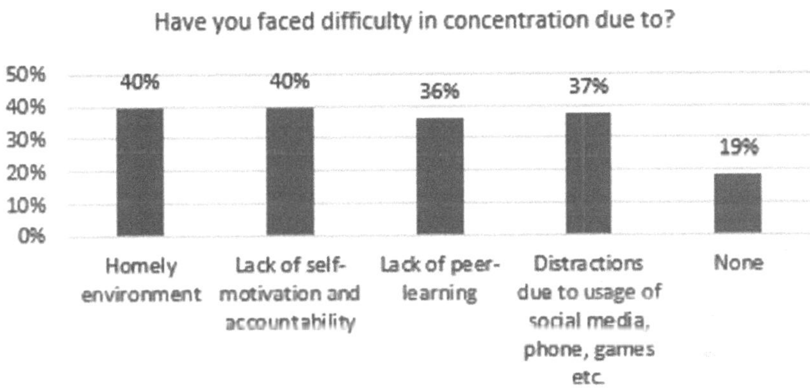

Figure 7.4 Percentage of students with issues in concentration.

Difficulty in concentration: A large number of students (81%) faced difficulty in concentration due to multiple reasons. As indicated in Fig. 7.4, 40% of students encountered distraction due to homely environment or lack of self-motivation. 36% of students faced difficulty due to lack of peer learning. 37% stated that they were distracted due to video games, mobile phones, or social media platforms.

Disruption in sleeping pattern: It is noticed that 71% of students faced disruption in their sleeping patterns. As shown in Fig. 7.5, 35% stated that they stayed up late or woke up late due to pandemic. 34% had irregularities in sleeping pattern, 32% mentioned increased duration of sleep. Some (28%) had difficulty in falling or staying asleep.

Social isolation: A vast number of students (98%) indicated that they had realized increased social isolation. As shown in Fig. 7.6, many students

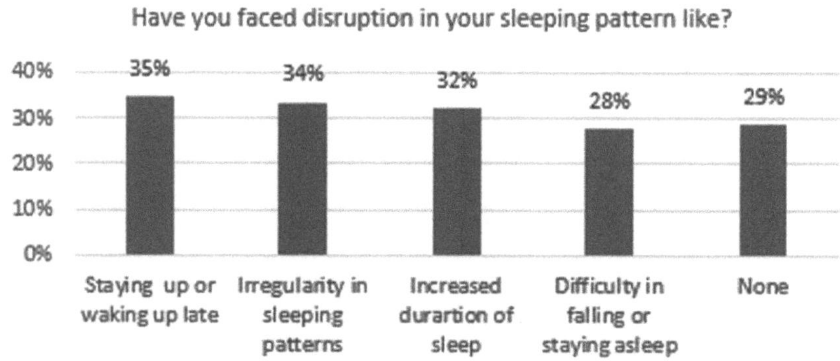

Figure 7.5 Percentage of students with disruptions in sleeping patterns.

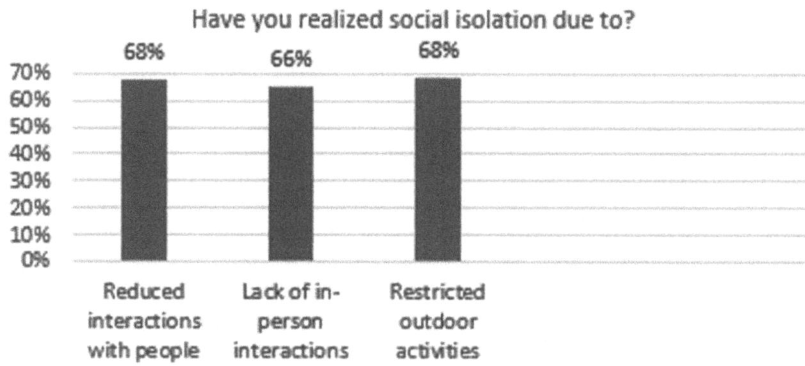

Figure 7.6 Percentage of students facing social isolation.

(68%) specified the reason as decreased interactions with people and restricted outdoor activities. Many (66%) mentioned the reason as lesser in-person interactions.

Worried about academic performance: A significant number of students (70%) mentioned that they were worried about their academic performance. As shown in Fig. 7.7, many students (46%) faced challenges due to the shift of teaching mode from offline to online. Many (48%) were worried about their progress in academics and other future aspects in their career. Some (39%) were concerned about improvement in their grades. Others (29%) reported the reduction in motivation and a habit of procrastination.

Academic load-related issues: Many (64%) students encountered problems of increased academic load as an impact of the pandemic. It can be seen from Fig. 7.8 that many (55%) were bothered by online classes and projects. Some (48%) found assignments challenging to be solved.

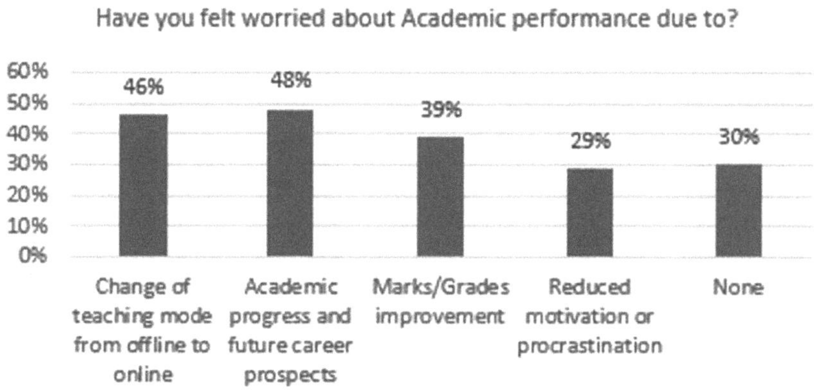

Figure 7.7 Percentage of students concerned about academic performance.

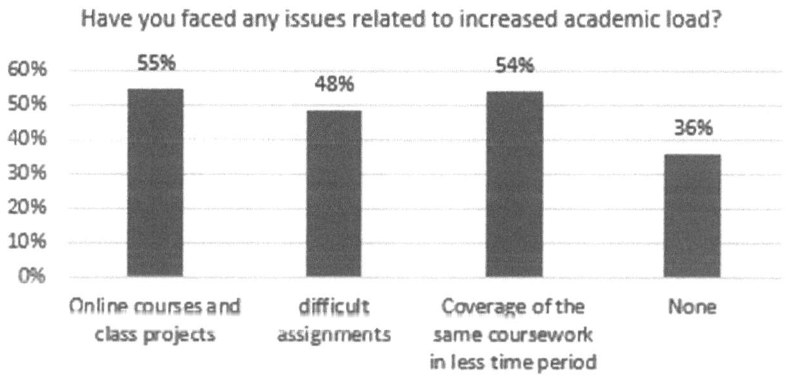

Figure 7.8 Percentage of students having issues with increased academic load.

Others (54%) experienced problems in covering the same coursework in reduced time duration.

Depressive thoughts: As an adverse effect of COVID-19, the majority of students (74%) reported that they encountered depressive thoughts. As described in Fig. 7.9, they came across many depressive thoughts such as loneliness (31%), uncertainty or insecurity (29%), hopelessness or powerlessness (28%), anxiety about performance of academics (34%), overthinking (38%).

Suicidal thoughts: Many students (64%) stated that they experienced suicidal thoughts due to pandemics. They had suicidal thoughts due to depressive thoughts (25%), academic issues (27%), problems with parents (24%), insecurity (28%), as depicted in Fig. 7.10.

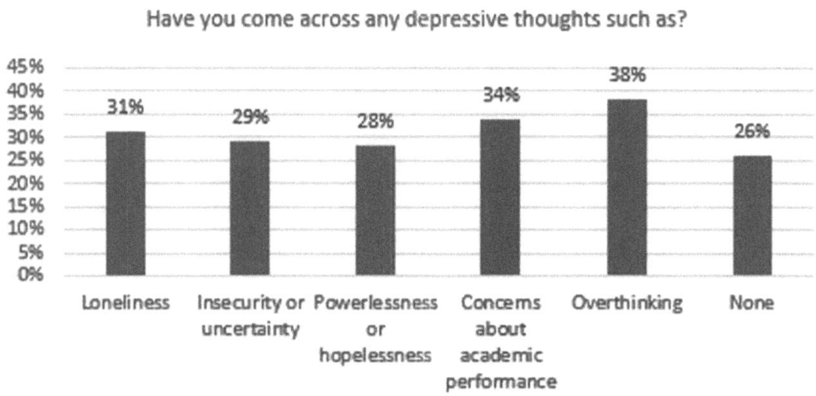

Figure 7.9 Percentage of students facing depressive thoughts.

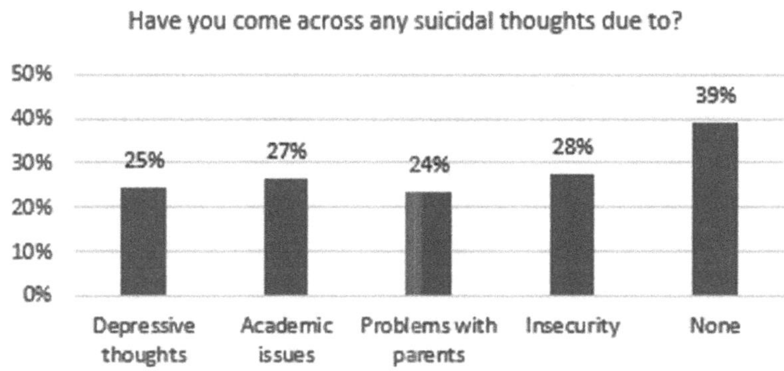

Figure 7.10 Percentage of students facing suicidal thoughts.

5. Experimentation and results

We surveyed data about the mental behavior of college students by preparing a questionnaire. It consisted of 11 questions and answers to these questions were responded to by 600 students (fresher, intermediate, graduating). Each of these questions is considered as a feature, and the responses collected are considered as data points. Each question had multiple options to choose from; the average value of these answers was computed to find the value of that parameter. Hence, in the dataset, we considered 17 features (gender, academic year, and 11 questions).

5.1 Clustering

The purpose of clustering in our work is to group the students into two different clusters representing students with high mental stress and low mental stress. As our data is unsupervised, we have used clustering techniques such as K-mean, K-medoids, and density-based clustering to group the data points into different clusters. As the number of clusters are fixed, and data points are numeric, k-means clustering has resulted in two disjoint clusters. One cluster represents the cases of low mental stress, whereas another cluster represents the cases of high mental stress.

5.1.1 Cluster analysis

We evaluated the clustering techniques on three different cases to determine the significant dependencies of features and their combination. Case 1 was defined by considering only the questionnaires and considered the questionnaires and the students' academic year in Case 2. All features, including gender, academic year, and questionnaires, were taken into consideration in case 3. The performance of K-mean subject to these cases is represented in Fig. 7.11.

Case 1: Considering only 11 questions as features for data points, the clusters were found to be overlapped as shown in Fig. 7.11A. In total, 370 students were in the overlapping regions of both clusters. The overlapping region represents the data points or students in both clusters, which signifies no meaning for classifying the mental stress of the students by only considering the questionnaire. However, the mental condition of a student definitely depends on the academic year. In this scenario, a more reasonable goal was to obtain disjoint subspaces where each subspace classifies the students' mental stress. Hence, we considered two more cases.

Case 2: In this, we have considered questions, as well as an academic year as features for 600 data points, the result of the K-mean clustering is shown

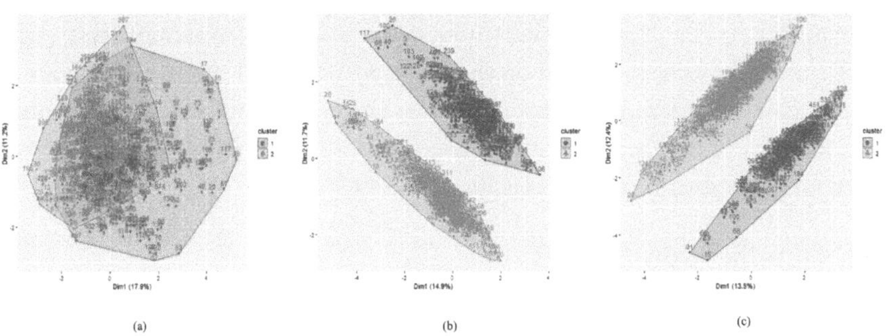

Figure 7.11 k-means clustering results using different parameters: (A) 11 questions only, (B) 11 questions and academic year, and (C) 11 questions, academic year and gender.

in Fig. 7.11B. The numbers of students in cluster 1 and cluster 2 are 313 and 287, respectively. In cluster 1, students are from the academic year as intermediate and graduating. However, the students in cluster 2 are primarily first-year students. As observed from the results, the students in cluster 1 are mostly concerned with job-related issues, academic load, and financial difficulty. However, the students in cluster 2 are more concerned about academic performance and social isolation. Also, features such as social isolation, infrastructure issues, and depressive thoughts are prevalent in both the clusters.

Case 3: In case 3, we have considered questions, academic year, and gender as features for all 600 data points. The motive here was to analyze mental stress with respect to gender. The clustering result for this case is shown in Fig. 7.11C. The numbers of students in cluster 1 and cluster 2 are 226 and 374, respectively. In the first cluster, most of the students have the value of gender as female. Whereas most of the students in cluster 2 have the value of gender as male. As observed from the results, the students in cluster 2 are more concerned with job-related issues, financial difficulty, and depressive thoughts.

From this result, we observed that the gender feature with all other features did not show a remarkable difference in clustering results when compared with the result of case 2. Hence, considering the gender feature with other features has a lesser impact on determining students' mental health. Based on this analysis, case 2 was considered only for designing classification models.

5.1.2 Validation of k-mean result

We communicate the class labels obtained from K-mean to the participated students to validate the exactness of the clustering. We gathered their views on class labels (i.e., having high mental stress and low mental stress), and 94.5% of students have agreed on the assigned class label. After the validation process, we considered the cluster labels as the class label for each data point. The features of data points with their corresponding class labels (target class) were employed to build the classifier models.

5.2 Classification models

5.2.1 Experimental setup

Our dataset for classification consists of 600 data points, 17 features, and two target classes. The dataset was partitioned into a training set and testing set in ratio as 70:30. The number of data points included in the training set and the testing set was 420 and 180. The testing was performed on the trained classification model with 10-fold cross-validation. The training and testing process is repeated 10 times, and the average prediction accuracy was reported for different classifiers. The training set was fed into multiple classifiers, and the models were built. With the above setup of training and test set, we employed four classification algorithms: NB, LR, SVM, and RF. We evaluated the performance of each classifier in terms of accuracy, precision, and recall. Although accuracy is hardly considered adequate for analyzing the results of a classifier, it provides a notion of the correctly classified samples in the testing dataset.

5.2.2 Results and analysis

The performance of the classifiers was represented through confusion matrices as shown in Fig. 7.12. Fig. 7.12A shows the performance of NB. Similarly, Fig. 7.12B–D describes the performance of LR, SVM, and RF, respectively. In the case of NB (Fig. 7.12A), 87 cases are high mental stress, out of which 78 cases are correctly detected. Also, from 89 cases of low mental stress, 80 have been detected correctly by the NB classifier. Similarly, in Fig. 7.12B, LR detects 82 cases correctly as high mental stress and 82 cases as low mental stress. In Fig. 7.12C, SVM classifier is able to detect 82 cases of high mental stress and 85 cases of low mental stress correctly. In contrast, RF classifier correctly detects 84 cases for high mental stress and 86 cases for low mental stress (Fig. 7.12D). It is observed that the six cases are incorrectly classified in both classes using RF, which is lesser as compared to other classifiers. Hence, from these metrics, it is observed that RF outperforms all other classifiers.

The performance in terms of accuracy is noted in Table 7.3. Though the performance of RF classifiers yields the best accuracy compared to others, it is still observed that the accuracies obtained from classifiers LR, SVM, and RF are nearly equal. Hence, to decide the correct classifier, we also calculated the precision and recall as performance measures.

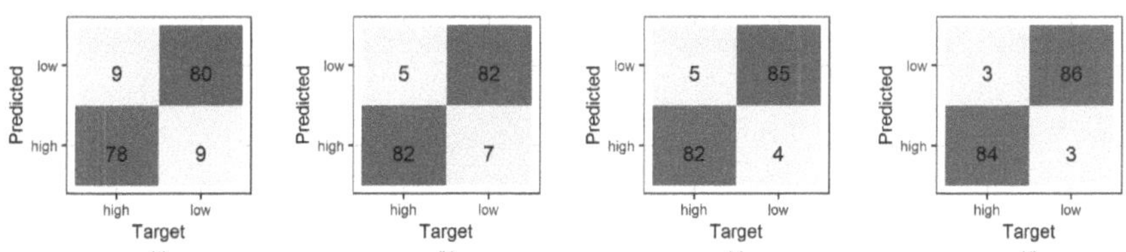

Figure 7.12 Confusion matrix for the test set using different classifiers: (A) NB (B) LR, (C) SVM, and (D) RF.

Table 7.3 Accuracy for different classifiers.

Model	NB	LR	SVM	RF
Accuracy	0.89	0.93	0.94	0.96

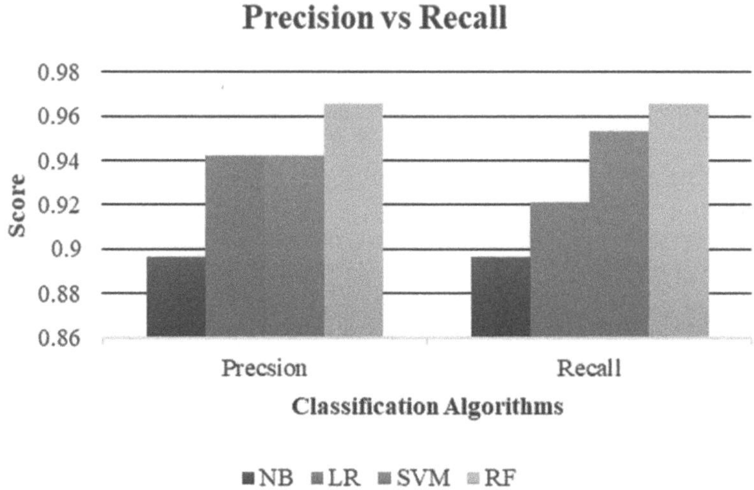

Figure 7.13 Precision vs recall for classifiers.

Fig. 7.13 depicts the values of precision and recall for all considered classifiers. Precision scores show the ratio of correctly identified students with high mental stress to all cases of high mental stress, which is the objective of our research. Fig. 7.13 shows the precision scores of classifiers as 0.89, 0.94, 0.94, and 0.96 for NB, LR, SVM, and RF, respectively. The value of precision score closer to 1 means the data points labeled high mental stress belong to that class in real. The precision values of LR, SVM show better performance than NB; however, the precision value of RF provides the best score among all.

Similarly, the recall values for all classifiers are shown in Fig. 7.13. Recall scores of the classifiers measure the effectiveness of the detected high mental stress cases. The score nearer to 1 represents the cases that are correctly classified as high mental stress. The recall scores for classifiers NB, LR, SVM, and RF are 0.89, 0.92, 0.95, and 0.96, respectively.

5.3 Discussion

For experimentation, initially, our dataset was clustered into two classes using the k-means algorithm considering the parameters: academic year and responses to 11 questions. These two classes represent students with high mental stress and low mental stress, respectively. These labels are further considered as target output for the classification models (NB, LR, SVM, RF). Based on the results generated, the RF model outperformed all other models for accuracy, precision, and recall. Following are the principal findings of our research work:

- From the surveyed data of university students, the parameters of concern for most of the students are: social isolation (98%), difficulty in concentration (80%), depressive thoughts (74%), disruption in sleeping pattern (71%), etc.
- By applying the k-means algorithm on the dataset, two clusters have been identified. The students in cluster 1, mostly intermediate and graduating academic year, are found to be concerned with job-related issues, academic load, and financial difficulty. However, the students in cluster 2, mostly first-year students, are concerned about academic performance and social isolation. Also, features such as social isolation, infrastructure issues, and depressive thoughts are prevalent in both the clusters.
- The performance of the NB classifier did not provide a commendable performance for our dataset, as the class label conditional assumption works better for large datasets. LR classifier, though it avoids overfitting and is robust to noise, still yields a fair performance. The SVM and RF have performed equally well; however, RF yielded a significant predictor of classes in determining the high mental stress and low mental stress cases in terms of accuracy, precision, and recall for our dataset.

It can be concluded from the above findings that COVID-19 has a negative impact on most of the students due to social isolation, difficulty in concentration, depressive thoughts, etc. However, the impact of gender parameters on finding mental stress of students is almost insignificant. Our classification model can help in predicting the mental health of the students. However, we need to test our model for larger datasets with more students.

6. Conclusion

The COVID-19 pandemic has shifted the focus from the traditional education system to online learning, which has affected students' mental health. We have proposed a framework that can be used to predict the mental stress of students. We collected the responses corresponding to the questionnaire and further designed to predict the mental stress. From the responses of the students, we found the parameters of concern for most of the students are: social isolation (98%), difficulty in concentration (80%), depressive thoughts (74%), disruption in sleeping pattern (71%), etc. Secondly, k-means clustering on the collected dataset yielded two clusters, one with students mostly concerned with job-related issues, academic load, and financial difficulty. However, the students in another cluster were more concerned about academic performance and social isolation. We also found that, considering the gender feature with other features has a lesser impact on determining the mental stress of students. These labels obtained from clustering were further considered as target outputs for the classification models (NB, LR, SVM, RF). Based on the experimental result and analysis, we found that the SVM and RF model performed better than other models in terms of accuracy, precision, and recall. The proposed framework is useful for analyzing and predicting the mental health of the students. In future, we will analyze our results on larger datasets by incorporating other parameters as well.

References

[1] C. Son, S. Hegde, A. Smith, X. Wang, F. Sasangohar, Effects of COVID-19 on college students' mental health in the United States: interview survey study, J. Med. Internet Res. 22 (9) (2020) e21279.

[2] O.W. Wilson, K.E. Holland, L.D. Elliott, M. Duffey, M. Bopp, The impact of the COVID-19 pandemic on US college students' physical activity and mental health, J. Phys. Activ. Health 18 (3) (2021) 272–278.

[3] C. Wang, H. Zhao, The impact of COVID-19 on anxiety in Chinese university students, Front. Psychol. 11 (2020) 1168.

[4] J. Guan, C. Wu, D. Wei, Q. Xu, J. Wang, H. Lin, C. Wang, Z. Mao, Prevalence and factors for anxiety during the COVID-19 pandemic among college students in China, Int. J. Environ. Res. Publ. Health 18 (9) (2021) 4974.

[5] E. Smets, P. Casale, U. Großekathöfer, B. Lamichhane, W. De Raedt, K. Bogaerts, I. Van Diest, C. Van Hoof, Comparison of machine learning techniques for psychophysiological stress detection, in: International Symposium on Pervasive Computing Paradigms for Mental Health, Springer, Cham, 2015, pp. 13–22.

[6] M. Srividya, S. Mohanavalli, N. Bhalaji, Behavioral modeling for mental health using machine learning algorithms, J. Med. Syst. 42 (5) (2018) 1–2.

[7] A. Priya, S. Garg, N.P. Tigga, Predicting anxiety, depression and stress in modern life using machine learning algorithms, Procedia Comput. Sci. 167 (2020) 1258–1267.

[8] A. Sau, I. Bhakta, Predicting anxiety and depression in elderly patients using machine learning technology, Healthc. Technol. Lett. 4 (6) (2017) 238–243.

[9] R.C. Kessler, H.M. van Loo, K.J. Wardenaar, R.M. Bossarte, L.A. Brenner, T. Cai, D.D. Ebert, I. Hwang, J. Li, P. de Jonge, A.A. Nierenberg, Testing a machine-learning algorithm to predict the persistence and severity of major depressive disorder from baseline self-reports, Mol. Psychiatr. 21 (10) (2016) 1366–1371.

[10] A. Sau, I. Bhakta, Screening of anxiety and depression among seafarers using machine learning technology, Inf. Med. Unlocked 16 (2019) 100228.

[11] I. Bjelland, A.A. Dahl, T.T. Haug, D. Neckelmann, The validity of the Hospital Anxiety and Depression Scale: an updated literature review, J. Psychosom. Res. 52 (2) (2002) 69–77.
[12] W.W. Zung, A rating instrument for anxiety disorders, Psychosomatics 12 (1971).
[13] X. Liu, J. Liu, X. Zhong, Psychological state of college students during COVID-19 epidemic, Lancet Global Health (2020). SSRN 3552814.
[14] W. Cao, Z. Fang, G. Hou, M. Han, X. Xu, J. Dong, J. Zheng, The psychological impact of the COVID-19 epidemic on college students in China, Psychiatr. Res. 287 (2020) 112934.
[15] X. Wang, S. Hegde, C. Son, B. Keller, A. Smith, F. Sasangohar, Investigating mental health of US college students during the COVID-19 pandemic: cross-sectional survey study, J. Med. Internet Res. 22 (9) (2020) e22817.
[16] H. Li, H. Hafeez, M.A. Zaheer, COVID-19 and pretentious psychological well-being of students: a threat to educational sustainability, Front. Psychol. 11 (2020) 4034.
[17] E.G. Mekonen, B.S. Workneh, M.S. Ali, N.Y. Muluneh, The psychological impact of COVID-19 pandemic on graduating class students at the University of Gondar, Northwest Ethiopia, Psychol. Res. Behav. Manag. 14 (2021) 109.
[18] S. Bourion-Bédès, C. Tarquinio, M. Batt, P. Tarquinio, R. Lebreuilly, C. Sorsana, K. Legrand, H. Rousseau, C. Baumann, Stress and associated factors among French university students under the COVID-19 lockdown: the results of the PIMS-CoV 19 study, J. Affect. Disord. 283 (2021) 108–114.
[19] S. Cohen, T. Kamarck, R. Mermelstein, A global measure of perceived stress, J. Health Soc. Behav. (1983) 385–396.
[20] G.D. Zimet, N.W. Dahlem, S.G. Zimet, G.K. Farley, The multidimensional scale of perceived social support, J. Pers. Assess. 52 (1) (1988) 30–41.
[21] Y.G. Jung, M.S. Kang, J. Heo, Clustering performance comparison using K-means and expectation maximization algorithms, Biotechnol. Biotechnol. Equip. 28 (Suppl. 1) (2014) S44–S48.
[22] G.W. Milligan, M.C. Cooper, Methodology review: clustering methods, Appl. Psychol. Meas. 11 (4) (1987) 329–354.
[23] B. Liu, et al., Scalable sentiment classification for big data analysis using naive bayes classifier, in: Big Data, 2013 I.E. International Conference on IEEE, 2013.
[24] S. Dreiseitl, L. Ohno-Machado, Logistic regression and artificial neural network classification models: a methodology review, J. Biomed. Inf. 35 (5) (2002) 352–359.
[25] M.T. Ribeiro, S. Singh, C. Guestrin, Why should i trust you?: explaining the predictions of any classifier, in: Proceedings of the 22nd ACMSIGKDD International Conference on Knowledge Discovery and Data Mining, ACM, 2016.
[26] A. Statnikov, L. Wang, C.F. Aliferis, A comprehensive comparison of random forests and support vector machines for microarray-based cancer classification, BMC Bioinf. 9 (1) (2008) 319.
[27] Y. Lee, Handwritten digit recognition using k nearest-neighbor, radial-basis function, and backpropagation neural networks, Neural Comput. 3 (3) (1991) 440–449.
[28] T. Joachims, Text categorization with support vector machines: learning with many relevant features, in: European Conference on Machine Learning, Springer, Berlin, Heidelberg, 1998, pp. 137–142.
[29] A. Vlahou, et al., Diagnosis of ovarian cancer using decision tree classification of mass spectral data, Biomed Res. Int. 2003 (5) (2003) 308–314.
[30] L. Breiman, Random forests, Mach. Learn. 45 (1) (2001) 5–32.
[31] P.O. Gislason, J.A. Benediktsson, J.R. Sveinsson, Random forests for land cover classification, Pattern Recogn. Lett. 27 (4) (2006) 294–300.

CHAPTER EIGHT

Modeling the impact of the COVID-19 pandemic and socioeconomic factors on global mobility and its effects on mental health

Shashank Uttrani[1], Bharti Nanta[1], Neha Sharma[2] and Varun Dutt[1]
[1]Applied Cognitive Science Lab, Indian Institute of Technology Mandi, Mandi, Himachal Pradesh, India
[2]Indian Institute of Information Technology Una, Una, Himachal Pradesh, India

1. Introduction

The outbreak of the coronavirus was declared a global health emergency by World Health Organization (WHO) in March 2020 [1]. COVID-19 pandemic was more than just a health crisis; its impact was widespread to all sectors, and overall, there was a massive impact on the economic sector [2]. Global lockdown stopped all the services and productions, causing economic instability [2,3]. During this phase, countries around the globe started imposing lockdown with varied stringency based on the severity of the condition in their area [4]. This was done to prevent the spread of infection and ensure social distancing everywhere to curb down the stretch as much as possible [5].

An immediate shutdown of worldwide air transport was implemented to control the spread of coronavirus across borders during the start of the pandemic [6]. This led to an exponential decline in the financial and economic sectors as manufacturing and trading of goods came to a sudden halt [2,3]. With the industrial sector suffering, millions of jobs were lost, and thousands of small to medium-scale businesses were shut down in India alone [7]. Eventually, this economic instability impacted the nation's GDP and per capita income [8]. The increasing death toll due to coronavirus also impacted the reproduction rate and human development index [9]. The imposed lockdown and social distancing protocols, however, had an adverse impact on people's mental health [10]. An alarming increase in

Artificial Intelligence, Machine Learning, and Mental Health in Pandemics
ISBN: 978-0-323-91196-2
https://doi.org/10.1016/B978-0-323-91196-2.00012-0

domestic violence and suicide cases was reported in India as well as other parts of the world during strict lockdown and quarantine rules [11]. The role of mobility, activity space, and the neighborhood is greatly discussed in the health geography literature [12]. Research has documented the association of limited activity space with a high risk of depression and anxiety as it reflects spatial and social confinement [12].

Prior research on COVID-19 lockdown explored the trend analysis of human mobility in both temporal and spatial dimensions [13]. However, these authors did not explore any correlation or association between COVID-19 and socioeconomic variables, which could have impacted human mobility. Similarly, research pertaining to COVID-19 has also examined the relationship between mobility and the COVID-19 variable, such as confirmed cases [14]. Specifically, using Community Mobility Report's data, researchers have looked at the association between COVID-19 confirmed cases and the mobility pattern levels [14]. However, the authors did not take any social or economic factors into consideration. Researchers have also investigated the incidence rate of COVID-19 and its relationship with the human development index [9]. This was an ecological study of COVID-19 basing upon the statistics of the reports sent to the WHO until April 30, 2020 [9]. However, the report did not present any implication of impact on mobility during the COVID-19 pandemic. Although researchers have proposed that people's ability to navigate through public places was dependent upon their decision-making strategies [15]. However, prior researchers did not consider the impact on mobility by the COVID-19, social and economic variables. Furthermore, little is known about how the COVID-19 pandemic and the imposed lockdown have impacted the mental health of people in India and around the world. Also, little is known about how computational models would predict global mobility under the influence of COVID-19 and socioeconomic variables. The primary objectives of this paper are to investigate the influence of the COVID-19 pandemic and socioeconomic variables on people's mobility worldwide and to develop a linear regression model to predict the future impact on mobility due to the COVID-19 pandemic.

In what follows, first, we recap the literature on the influence of the COVID-19 pandemic and socioeconomic variables on mobility. Next, we describe the mobility, COVID- 19 and socioeconomic datasets, and the linear regression model. Finally, we close the paper by discussing the implications of our results and highlighting the role of mobility on human mental health.

2. Background

Recent research in epidemiology has documented the impact of COVID-19 on social and economic factors along with the mobility of people around the world. Skórka et al. [16] showed that the number of COVID-19 cases, deaths, and rate of growth of infection were associated with global factors such as population density, gross domestic product, net migration rate, and the influx of tourists [16]. However, in their research, the authors did not perform a comprehensive analysis of factors other than the growth rate of COVID-19 cases. Spelta et al. [17] estimated the impact of lockdown on productive regional systems and economic consequences using the SIR model spread disease, focusing on virus spread and mobility restrictions in Italy [17]. However, their research was limited to only Italy in the geographic domain. They considered only the economic disruptions associated with the virus's spread with policy measures restricting mobility at a regional level.

Similarly, Roy et al. [18] studied the primary socioeconomic factors leading to the spread of infection and mortality [18]. However, this study used only the US dataset to identify the potential factors causing the virus's spread and did not include mobility patterns to see human interactions. Luo et al. [19] anatomized the cause of transmission of COVID-19 by taking the spring festival in China as a focal point [19]. However, this study included a minimal dataset of 2 months and only considered the crowd's mobility at the spring festival. Castex et al. [20] examined the effectiveness and compliance of lockdown policies using cross-country analysis of human mobility and behavioral response to risk perceptions to practice social distancing. However, the authors only discussed the voluntary practice of social distancing and behavioral traits to assess the effectiveness of policies.

Researchers have also investigated the impact of lockdown and the role of mobility on human mental health. Vallée et al. [12] investigated the influence of activity space and neighborhood on mental health and how limited activity space could develop severe depression symptoms among humans. Mittal and Singh [21] illustrated the increase in gender-based violence during imposed lockdown due to the COVID-19 pandemic [21]. Authors report economic insecurity and psychological instability as the major attributes contributing to the increase of such behavior among individuals. Similarly, Timms [22] investigated the relationship between social mobility and mental health. In this study, the author presented a strong association between mental health and occupational status among individuals [22].

Overall, we hypothesize that the COVID-19 and socioeconomic variables influenced human mobility in different categories, thereby adversely impacting the mental health of individuals around the world during the pandemic.

3. Methods

3.1 Data

The COVID-19 mobility dataset [23] used in the research was collected and provided by Google Inc. The COVID-19 and socioeconomic datasets [24] were provided by the Our World in Data repository. For our analyses, we considered 14-month time series data from both datasets in the period between April 1st, 2020, and May 31st, 2021. The start date was chosen to be April 1st, 2020, as most of the countries around the world started implementing nationwide lockdowns from the last week of March 2020 to take preventive measures against the COVID-19 pandemic. Thus, the start date allowed us to analyze the impact of lockdowns on mobility trends around the world. The end date was taken to be the latest date as much as possible. The mobility dataset contains movement trends in different regions around the world, across different categories of places. This time series dataset consists of six different variables, where each variable denotes the percentage change in mobility from baseline in six different categories in a region. These categories are retail and recreation, grocery and pharmacy, parks, transit stations, workplaces, and residential. The baseline was established as the median value of the movement in a region from January 3rd, 2020, to February 6th, 2020. For our analysis, we have considered the six most affected countries by COVID-19 around the world, namely, the United States, India, Brazil, Russia, France, and the United Kingdom. Fig. 8.1 shows time-series graphs of percentage change in mobility for different categories in India.

The COVID-19 and socioeconomic time series dataset comprises reported cases, deaths, testing, and vaccination in different countries during the COVID-19 pandemic. For our analyses, we have considered new cases, new cases per million, total cases per million, new deaths, new deaths per million, total deaths, new tests per 1000, total tests per 1000, tests per case, people fully vaccinated, people vaccinated per 100, positivity rate, reproduction rate, and stringency index.

3.2 Linear regression

The linear regression model assumes a linear relationship between single (or multiple) input variables (x) and an output variable (y). Specifically, "y" is

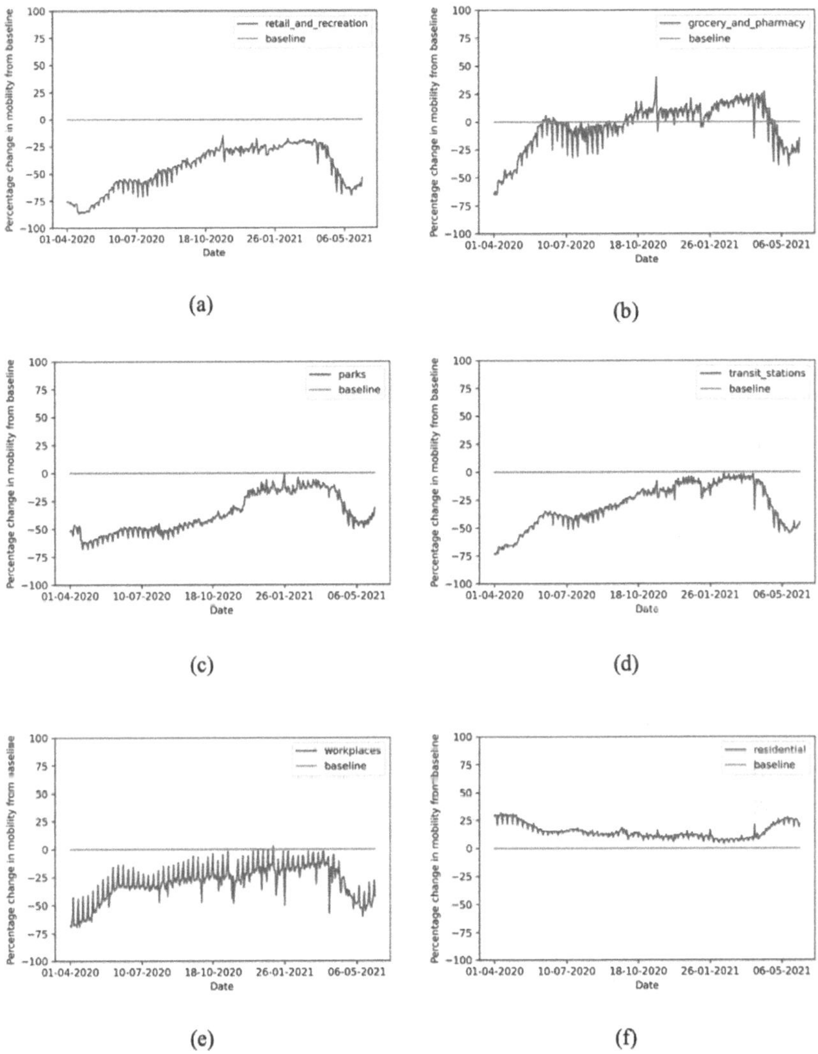

Figure 8.1 Percentage change in mobility in India during COVID-19 pandemic in (A) retail and recreation regions, (B) grocery and pharmacy regions, (C) parks, (D) transit stations, (E) workplaces, and (F) residential areas.

calculated using the linear combination of "x," i.e., the input variables. For a single input variable, the model is referred to as a simple linear regression model. However, for multiple input variables, it is referred to as a multiple linear regression model. In the simple regression model, the form of the equation would be:

$$y = B_0 + B_1 x$$

where B_0 is a constant, and B_1 is the slope of the regression line. For higher dimensions, i.e., when there are more than one input (x), the line is referred to as a plane or a hyperplane.

3.3 Data analyses

A multiple linear regression analysis was performed to predict the values of dependent variables, i.e., the percentage change in mobility from baseline in different regions of a country, using independent variables of COVID-19 and socioeconomic datasets. The "ENTER" method was used to select and enter the variables while performing the regression analyses. We tested our datasets for various assumptions of multiple linear regression analyses. All the assumptions of the multiple linear regression analysis were tested and met. First, a scatter plot was generated to test the assumption of the linear relationship between the dependent variable (mobility variables) and independent variables (COVID-19, social, and economic variables). The scatterplot produced a straight line suggesting a linear relationship between dependent and independent variables. Second, no multicollinearity was found among independent variables as the VIF score was below 10 and tolerance scores were greater than 0.2 for all the countries. Third, the assumption of independent residuals was met as the Dublin—Watson statistics test reported a value of 1.673. Fourth, the assumption of constant residual variance was also met as the residual plot did not appear to be funneled; instead, the points were randomly distributed. Fifth, the assumption of normal distribution of residuals was also met when tested by plotting the P-P plots for the model. All the Cook's distance values were under 1, implying that none of the individual cases influenced the model.

4. Results

The multiple linear regression was performed by taking mobility across retail and recreation, grocery and pharmacy, parks, transit stations, workplaces, and residential areas as the dependent variable. The standard beta (β) coefficients of the significant variables across different mobility regions for the developed multiple regression models are shown in Table 8.1 for India and Table 8.2 for the rest of the countries (global).

4.1 Impact of COVID-19 and socioeconomic factors on mobility in different regions in India

4.1.1 *Retail and recreation*

A significant regression model was found with an R^2 of 0.953 (F (14, 425) $= 589.24$, $p \leq .000$). For new deaths per million ($\beta = 0.426$,

Table 8.1 Standardized beta coefficients of the significant variables across different mobility regions in India.

Variables	Standardized β coefficients					
	Retail and recreation	**Grocery and Pharmacy**	**Parks**	**Transit stations**	**Workplaces**	**Residential**
Total deaths	—	—	—	-1.436^{a}	—	-3.065^{b}
Total cases per million	—	—	—	1.601^{a}	—	2.955^{b}
New deaths per million	0.426^{a}	0.393^{a}	—	0.484^{b}	0.774^{a}	-0.616^{b}
Reproduction Rate	0.479^{b}	-0.145^{a}	1.022^{b}	0.84^{a}	—	-0.224^{b}
Stringency index	-0.577^{b}	-0.762^{b}	0.675^{b}	-0.673^{b}	-0.648^{b}	0.713^{b}

$^{a}p \leq .05$.
$^{b}p \leq .01$.

Table 8.2 Standardized beta coefficients of the significant variables across different mobility regions around the globe.

Variables	Standardized β coefficients					
	Retail and recreation	Grocery and Pharmacy	Parks	Transit stations	Workplaces	Residential
Total cases	−0.52[b]	—	0.118[b]	−0.036[a]	—	0.130[b]
New cases	—	—	—	−0.87[a]	0.118[b]	—
Total deaths	0.73[b]	0.107[b]	0.110[b]	0.121[b]	0.089[b]	−0.152[b]
Total cases per million	0.176[b]	0.218[b]	0.060[b]	0.227[b]	0.193[b]	−0.209[b]
New cases per million	−0.36[a]	0.040[a]	0.050[b]	—	0.070[b]	0.028[a]
Total deaths per million	0.038[b]	−0.061[b]	—	—	−0.031[a]	—
New deaths per million	−0.280[b]	−0.157[b]	0.163[b]	−0.191[b]	−0.141[b]	0.190[b]
Reproduction Rate	−0.42[b]	−0.081[b]	0.025[b]	−0.022[b]	−0.037[b]	0.045[b]
New tests	0.096[b]	—	0.054[b]	0.044[b]	−0.045[a]	−0.081[b]
New tests per 1000	—	−0.045[b]	0.041[b]	−0.056[b]	−0.055[b]	0.059[b]
Positive rate	—	−0.049[b]	0.048[b]	−0.092[b]	−0.051[b]	0.029[b]
Stringency index	−0.649[b]	−0.531[b]	0.304[b]	−0.591[b]	−0.514[b]	0.594[b]
Population	−0.153[b]	—	0.042[b]	−0.068[b]	−0.096[b]	0.044[b]
Population Density	—	—	0.090[b]	0.103[b]	—	—
Median age	0.188[b]	—	0.273[b]	−0.049[a]	—	−0.183[b]
Aged 65 older	0.411[b]	—	0.828[b]	−0.249[b]	—	—
Aged 70 older	−0.388[b]	—	0.740[b]	—	—	—
Cardiovascular death rates	0.022[b]	0.033[b]	0.147[b]	0.175[b]	−0.075[b]	−0.187[b]
Diabetes prevalence	−0.093[b]	−0.152[b]	0.202[b]	−0.110[b]	—	0.084[b]

Female smoker	-0.092^{b}	-0.070^{b}	0.146^{b}	0.112^{b}	-0.032^{a}	-0.097^{b}
Male smoker	-0.030^{b}	0.110^{b}	0.059^{b}	—	0.032^{b}	—
Hospital beds per 1000	—	—	0.199^{b}	0.242^{b}	0.132^{b}	-0.080^{b}
Life expectancy	-0.277^{b}	-0.196^{b}	0.272^{b}	0.070^{b}		-0.040^{a}
Human Development index	-0.38^{a}	0.157^{b}	—	-0.285^{b}	-0.311^{b}	0.166^{b}

[a] $p \leq .05$.
[b] $p \leq .01$.

$p \leq .05$), reproduction rate ($\beta = 0.479, p \leq .01$), the standard coefficient (β) was positive, which articulates that there was an increase for every unit in the outcome of each predictor variable (see Table 8.1). For the stringency index ($\beta = -0.577, p \leq .01$), the standard coefficient (β) was negative, which articulates an increase for every unit in the outcome of each predictor variable (see Table 8.1).

4.1.2 Grocery and pharmacy

A significant regression model was found with an R^2 of 0.862 (F (10, 233) = 134.69, $p \leq .000$). For new deaths per million ($\beta = 0.393$, $p \leq .05$), the standard coefficient (β) was positive, which articulates that there was an increase for every unit in the outcome of each predictor variable (see Table 8.1). For reproduction rate ($\beta = -0.145, p \leq .01$) and stringency index ($\beta = -0.762$, $p \leq .01$), the standard coefficient (β) was negative, which articulates that there was an increase for every unit in the outcome of each predictor variable (see Table 8.1).

4.1.3 Parks

A significant regression model was found with an R^2 of 0.957 (F (10,233) = 108.90, $p \leq .000$). For reproduction rate ($\beta = 1.022, p \leq .01$), the standard coefficient (β) was positive, which articulates an increase for every unit in the outcome of each predictor variable (see Table 8.1). For stringency index ($\beta = -0.675$, $p \leq .01$), the standard coefficient (β) was negatively correlated, which articulates that there was a decrease for every unit in the outcome of each predictor variable (see Table 8.1).

4.1.4 Transit stations

A significant regression model was found with an R^2 of 0.950 (F (10,233) = 314.01, $p \leq .000$). For total cases per million ($\beta = 1.601$, $p \leq .05$), new deaths smoother per million ($\beta = 0.484$, $p \leq .01$) and reproduction rate ($\beta = 0.84, p \leq .05$), the standard coefficient (β) was positive, which articulates that there was an increase for every unit in the outcome of each predictor variable (see Table 8.1). For total deaths ($\beta = -1.436$, $p \leq .05$) and stringency index ($\beta = -0.673$, $p \leq .0$), the standard coefficient (β) was negatively correlated, which articulates that there was a decrease for every unit in the outcome of each predictor variable (see Table 8.1).

4.1.5 Workplaces

A significant regression model was found with an R^2 of 0.724 (F (10,233) = 44.10, $p \leq .000$). For new death per million ($\beta = 0.774$, $p \leq .01$), the standard coefficient (β) was positively correlated, which articulates that there was an increase for every unit in the outcome of the predictable variable (see Table 8.1). For the stringency index ($\beta = -0.648, p \leq .01$), the standard coefficient was negatively correlated, which articulates that there was a decrease to every unit in the outcome of the predictable variable (see Table 8.1).

4.1.6 Residential areas

A significant regression model was found with an R^2 of 0.869 (F (10,233) = 93.71, $p \leq .000$). For total cases per million ($\beta = 2.955$, $p \leq .01$) and stringency index ($\beta = 0.713$, $p \leq .01$), the standard coefficient (β) was positively correlated, which articulates that there was an increase for every unit in the outcome for each predictor variable (see Table 8.1). For total deaths ($\beta = -3.065, p \leq .01$), new deaths per million ($\beta = -0.616, p \leq .01$), reproduction rate ($\beta = -0.224, p \leq .01$), the standard coefficient (β) was negatively correlated, which articulates that there was a decrease for every unit in the outcome for each predictor variable (see Table 8.1).

4.2 Impact of COVID-19 and socioeconomic factors on mobility in different regions of the world

4.2.1 Retail and recreation

A significant regression model was found with an R^2 of 0.945 (F (29, 16,040) = 833.51, $p \leq .000$). For total deaths ($\beta = 0.73, p \leq .01$), total cases per million ($\beta = 0.176$, $p \leq .01$), total deaths per million ($\beta = 00.38$, $p \leq .01$), new tests ($\beta = 0.096$, $p \leq .01$), median age ($\beta = 0.188$, $p \leq .01$), aged 65 older ($\beta = 0.411$, $p \leq .01$), cardiovascular death rates ($\beta = 0.022$, $p \leq .01$), the standard coefficient (β) was positive, which articulates that there was an increase for every unit in the outcome of each predictor variable (see Table 8.2). For total cases ($\beta = -0.52$, $p \leq .01$), total cases per million ($\beta = -0.36, p \leq .05$), reproduction rate ($\beta = -0.42, p \leq .01$), stringency index ($\beta = -0.649$, $p \leq .01$), population ($\beta = -0.153$, $p \leq .01$), aged 70 older ($\beta = -0.388$, $p \leq .01$), diabetes prevalence ($\beta = -0.093$, $p \leq .01$), female smokers ($\beta = -0.092$, $p \leq .01$), male smokers ($\beta = -0.030$, $p \leq .01$), life expectancy ($\beta = -0.277$, $p \leq .01$), and human development index ($\beta = -0.38$, $p \leq .05$), the standard coefficient (β) was negative, which articulates that there was an increase for every unit in the outcome of each predictor variable (see Table 8.2).

4.2.2 Grocery and pharmacy

A significant regression model was found with an R^2 of 0.576 (F (29, 16,040) = 333.39, $p \leq .000$). For total deaths ($\beta = 0.107$, $p \leq .01$), total cases per million ($\beta = 0.281$, $p \leq .01$), new cases per million ($\beta = 0.040$, $p \leq .05$), cardiovascular death rate ($\beta = 0.033$, $p \leq .01$), male smokers ($\beta = 0.110$, $p \leq .01$), and human development index ($\beta = 0.157$, $p \leq .01$), the standard coefficient (β) was positive, which articulates that there was an increase for every unit in the outcome of each predictor variable (see Table 8.2). For total deaths per million ($\beta = -0.061, p \leq .01$), new deaths per million ($\beta = -0.157$, $p \leq .01$), reproduction rate ($\beta = -0.081$, $p \leq .01$), new tests per 1000 ($\beta = -0.045$, $p \leq .01$), positive rate ($\beta = -0.049$, $p \leq .01$), stringency index ($\beta = -0.531$, $p \leq .01$), diabetes prevalence ($\beta = -0.152$, $p \leq .01$), female smokers ($\beta = -0.070$, $p \leq .01$), and life expectancy ($\beta = -0.196$, $p \leq .01$), the standard coefficient (β) was negative, which articulates that there was an increase for every unit in the outcome of each predictor variable (see Table 8.2).

4.2.3 Parks

A significant regression model was found with an R^2 of 0.457 (F (29, 16,040) = 465.937, $p \leq .000$). For total deaths ($\beta = 0.110$, $p \leq .01$), total cases per million ($\beta = 0.060$, $p \leq .01$), new tests ($\beta = 0.054$, $p \leq .01$), population density ($\beta = 0.090$, $p \leq .01$), median age ($\beta = 0.273$, $p \leq .01$), aged 65 older ($\beta = 0.828$, $p \leq .01$), cardiovascular death rate ($\beta = 0.147$, $p \leq .01$), female smoker ($\beta = 0.146$, $p \leq .01$), the standard coefficient (β) was positive, which articulates that there was an increase for every unit in the outcome of each predictor variable (see Table 8.2). For total cases ($\beta = -0.118$, $p \leq .01$), new cases per million ($\beta = -0.050$, $p \leq .01$), new deaths per million ($\beta = -0.163$, $p \leq .01$), reproduction rate ($\beta = -0.025$, $p \leq .01$), new tests per 1000 ($\beta = -0.041$, $p \leq .01$), positive tests ($\beta = -0.048, p \leq .01$), stringency index ($\beta = -0.304, p \leq .01$), population ($\beta = -0.042, p \leq .01$), aged 70 older ($\beta = -0.740, p \leq .01$), diabetes prevalence ($\beta = -0.202$, $p \leq .01$), male smokers ($\beta = -0.059$, $p \leq .01$), hospital beds per 1000 ($\beta = -0.199$, $p \leq .01$), life expectancy ($\beta = -0.272$, $p \leq .01$), the standard coefficient (β) was negatively correlated, which articulates that there was decrease for every unit in the outcome of each predictor variable (see Table 8.2).

4.2.4 Transit stations

A significant regression model was found with an R^2 of 0.551 (F (29,16,040) = 679.78, $p \leq .000$). For total deaths ($\beta = 0.121$, $p \leq .01$), new deaths ($\beta = 0.066$, $p \leq .01$), total cases per million ($\beta = 0.227$, $p \leq .01$), new tests ($\beta = 0.044$, $p \leq .01$), population density ($\beta = 0.103$, $p \leq .01$), cardiovascular death rate ($\beta = 0.175$, $p \leq .01$), female smoker ($\beta = 0.112$, $p \leq .01$), hospital beds per 1000 ($\beta = 0.242$, $p \leq .01$), life expectancy rate ($\beta = 0.070$, $p \leq .01$), the standard coefficient (β) was positive, which articulates that there was an increase for every unit in the outcome of each predictor variable (see Table 8.2). For total cases ($\beta = -0.036$, $p \leq .05$), new cases ($\beta = -0.87$, $p \leq .05$), new deaths per million ($\beta = -0.191$, $p \leq .01$), reproduction rate ($\beta = -0.022$, $p \leq .05$), new tests per 1000 ($\beta = -0.056$, $p \leq .01$), positive rate ($\beta = -0.092$, $p \leq .01$), stringency index ($\beta = -0.591$, $p \leq .01$), population ($\beta = -0.068$, $p \leq .01$), median age ($\beta = -0.049$, $p \leq .05$), aged 65 older ($\beta = -0.249$, $p \leq .01$), diabetes prevalence ($\beta = -0.110$, $p \leq .01$), human development index ($\beta = -0.285$, $p \leq .01$), the standard coefficient (β) was negatively correlated, which articulates that there was a decrease for every unit in the outcome of each predictor variable (see Table 8.2).

4.2.5 Workplaces

A significant regression model was found with an R^2 of 0.343 (F (29,16,040) = 288.315, $p \leq .000$). For new cases ($\beta = 0.118$, $p \leq .01$), total deaths ($\beta = 0.089$, $p \leq .01$), new death ($\beta = 0.109$, $p \leq .01$), total cases per million ($\beta = 0.193$, $p \leq .01$), new cases per million ($\beta = 0.070$, $p \leq .01$), male smokers ($\beta = 0.032$, $p \leq .01$), and hospital beds per 1000 ($\beta = 0.132$, $p \leq .01$), the standard coefficient (β) was positive, which articulates that there was an increase for every unit in the outcome of each predictor variable (see Table 8.2). For new deaths ($\beta = -0.060$, $p \leq .05$), total deaths per million ($\beta = -0.031$, $p \leq .05$), total deaths per million ($\beta = -0.141$, $p \leq .01$), reproduction rate ($\beta = -0.037$, $p \leq .01$), new tests ($\beta = -0.045$, $p \leq .05$), new tests per 1000 ($\beta = -0.055$, $p \leq .01$), positive rate ($\beta = -0.051$, $p \leq .01$), stringency index ($\beta = -0.514$, $p \leq .01$), population ($\beta = 0.096$, $p \leq .01$), cardiovascular death rate ($\beta = -0.075$, $p \leq .01$), female smokers ($\beta = -0.032$, $p \leq .05$), human development index ($\beta = -0.311$, $p \leq .01$), the standard coefficient (β) was negatively correlated, which articulates that there was decrease for every unit in the outcome of each predictor variable (see Table 8.2).

4.2.6 Residential

A significant regression model was found with an R^2 of 0.568 (F (29,16,040) = 728.06, $p \leq .000$). For total cases ($\beta = 0.130$, $p \leq .01$), new cases per million ($\beta = 0.028$, $p \leq .05$), new deaths per million ($\beta = 0.190$, $p \leq .01$), reproduction rate ($\beta = 0.045$, $p \leq .01$), new tests per 1000 ($\beta = 0.059$, $p \leq .01$), positive rate ($\beta = 0.029$, $p \leq .01$), stringency index ($\beta = 0.594$, $p \leq .01$), population ($\beta = 0.044$, $p \leq .01$), diabetes prevalence ($\beta = 0.084$, $p \leq .01$), and human development index ($\beta = 0.166$, $p \leq .01$), the standard coefficient (β) was positively correlated, which articulates that there was an increase for every unit in the outcome of each predictor variable (see Table 8.2). For total deaths ($\beta = -0.152$, $p \leq .01$), new deaths ($\beta = -0.088$, $p \leq .01$), total cases per million ($\beta = -0.209$, $p \leq .01$), new tests ($\beta = -0.081$, $p \leq .01$), median age ($\beta = -0.183$, $p \leq .01$), cardiovascular death rate ($\beta = -0.187$, $p \leq .01$), female smokers ($\beta = -0.097$, $p \leq .01$), hospital beds per 1000 ($\beta = -0.080$, $p \leq .01$), and life expectancy ($\beta = -0.040$, $p \leq .05$), the standard coefficient (β) was negatively correlated, which articulates that there was decrease for every unit in the outcome of each predictor variable (see Table 8.2).

5. Discussion

Mobility is an important dimension of society, enabling people to access goods, services, and information, as well as jobs, markets, family, and friends [25]. Most of the research done in this regard inspects the impact of mobility on the communication of the virus [26]. However, the impact of socioeconomic and COVID-19 factors on the mobility of people has been less studied. Therefore, the aim of this research was to quantify the influence of socioeconomic factors and COVID-19 factors on human mobility during the pandemic across the world. The primary objective of this research was to study the mobility of various places, namely retail and recreation, grocery and pharmacy, parks, transit stations, workplaces, and residential areas. Furthermore, this research also studied the impact of COVID-19 and socioeconomic factors affecting mobility patterns.

In India, new deaths per million were positively related to mobility at retail and recreational centers. This shows that as more people were visiting such places, the average of people dying every day increased. Similarly, a positive correlation between reproduction rate and mobility was observed. This could be because even in this pandemic, people were celebrating the addition of a new member in their family. This shows that, even in a period of severe anxieties and panics, people did find some ways to be happy and positive. Meanwhile, because of a complete lockdown across the nation and specific other strict policies, mobility at recreational centers decreased with high stringency indexes. As a result, a negative correlation between the stringency index and mobility was observed. At the global level, the variables such as the total deaths, total cases per million, total deaths per million, and cardiovascular deaths rates were positively correlated to the mobility at retail and recreation. This shows that when more people visited the retail and recreational centers, the cases at the global level shot up. Furthermore, the median age and people older than 65 years also showed a positive correlation with mobility, as they were more susceptible to getting infected with the coronavirus. However, variables such as total cases, total cases per million, and total deaths per million were negatively correlated with the people's mobility at retail and recreation centers. This shows that due to fear and uncertainties, the average of people visiting these places decreased. The negative correlation of the stringency index shows that when more strict measures were taken to prevent mobility, mobility decreased. Moreover, a negative correlation among the people older than 70 years, diabetic prevalence, and female and male smokers were observed (as old people or people already having some chronic diseases are believed to have less immunity and hence were more vulnerable). This could be because such people were highly susceptible to coronavirus, which reduced their mobility. Also, when people showed high mobility, the chances of getting infected with coronavirus increased and hence, lower life expectancy rate.

New deaths per million were positively related to the mobility at the grocery and pharmacy in India. This could be because when the fatalities rates shoot up, anxiously more people rush toward grocery and pharmacy stores, probably to hoard the essential items at their homes. The reproduction rate was also negatively correlated with mobility. Most people prearrange medicines, pharmaceuticals, and other essential items at their homes if they have a pregnant lady at home. Hence, comparatively fewer people went to these places. Also, there was a higher chance for a pregnant lady or newborn to get infected with COVID-19 due to low immunity. The negative correlation between stringency index and mobility shows that people were restricted at their homes due to strict regulations in their homes and avoided going out of their homes unnecessarily. Similarly, total deaths, total cases per million, and new cases per million were positively correlated with the mobility at the grocery and pharmacy globally. This could be that when cases were increasing, people needed more medicines, food, and other essential household items, which increased their mobility. Similar reasons can also be associated with the positive correlation between mobility and cardiovascular death rate. Furthermore, with a sudden increase in demand for grocery items, medicines, and pharmaceutical products (probably because of hoarding behavior), this sector's economy increased. Hence, the Human Development Index was positively correlated with mobility. Total deaths per million were negatively correlated with mobility. This implies that when people availed more medicines, food, and other essential items, the death rate decreased despite getting infected with COVID-19. The negative correlation between new tests per 1000 and positive rate shows that when people took proper medicines and food and were taking good care of themselves, the rate of getting infected decreased. A negative correlation between diabetes prevalence and female smokers shows that their movement was restricted because of being highly susceptible to COVID-19 (due to health issues). Although, the mobility of male smokers was positively related. This could be associated with society's gender dimension, as males are supposed to be more responsible for the family outside duties than females. Furthermore, with the increased number of deaths and cases, the life expectancy was less, hence negatively correlated with mobility.

The stringency index was negatively related to the mobility trends across the parks in India. In the first scenario, this might have been due to the government's phases "unlock" series to lift mobility restrictions in several regions. With each passing phase of the series, the public's perception of the virus as a threat reduced, and it made them move around like before. It weakened the stringency measures as the public was getting less associated with the orders of the government. Lack of awareness might have even made them refrain from following their self-regulations and precautions. As these factors came into play, this also impacted the rise in the total number of cases infected and eventually led to an increase in deaths succumbed to the virus spread. At the same time, variables such as aged 65 older and cardiovascular death rate were positively correlated to the mobility trends in the parks in the rest of the world. It implies that increasing mobility in the parks increased the casualties of cardiovascular-related ailments as 65 years and above were moving around who were more susceptible. Male smokers and hospital beds per 1000 were negatively related to the mobility trends in the parks. This might be due to COVID-19 precautionary measures where there was a cut down in the tobacco supply, and few might have quit due to fear of respiratory issues in this scenario. It even implies that when mobility at parks was increased, it hampered the social distancing norms, likely causing virus spread. This led to a decrease in hospital beds available per 1000 as many infected people were admitted.

In India, the stringency index is negatively related to the mobility trends across the transit stations. Total deaths and a total of cases per million were positively related to the mobility across the transit stations. This might have been due to the reverse migration and lifting of the travel ban at all the interstate borders. It increased the number of commuters and the movement of the public at the transit stations. As the passengers had likely come into contact and mass gatherings, it contributed to the rise in the total number of cases infected and eventually led to an increase in deaths succumbed to the virus spread. However, the total number of deaths was positively related to the mobility trend across the transit stations around the world. It implies that the death rate was increasing as people were traveling and moving in the transit stations and likely encountered contact with the virus and infected people. Stringency index and aged 65 older were negatively related to the mobility trend across the transit stations. This implies that the preventive measures being less stringent might had facilitated passengers' physical contact at the transit stations and permitted the aged 65 older citizens to travel, which likely led to the spread of the virus. This increasing trend of mobility across the transit stations aligned with less stringent measures and increase in aged 65 older people articulates that group behavior had an impact on people's voluntary restrictions to avoid contact, i.e., as even the travel permit was granted, it implied that if everyone is traveling and complying to travel, it encouraged others to do the same.

The stringency index was negatively correlated with workplace mobility in India. This might be because people started going to workplaces because lockdown norms got less stringent. In the rest of the world, total cases per million, new cases, the total number of deaths, new deaths smoothed, and hospital beds per 1000 were positively correlated with mobility at the workplace. This implies that people at workplaces were violating social distancing norms. Therefore, there is an increase in the total number of cases, hence an increase in hospital beds per 1000 and consequently an increase in the total number of deaths as well. New tests per 1000, cardiovascular death rate, reproduction rate, stringency index, and Human development index were negatively correlated with workplace mobility. This implies that people were not turning up for COVID-19 tests because of the fear that they would be mistreated by society if they get positive. The cardiovascular death rate decreased as there was not much work stress, and the reproduction rate decreased during lockdown because, in the pandemic, mothers don't want to conceive. There was a reduction in the stringency index because the norms of lockdown became lenient. During the pandemic, there were school closures, GDP became low, and the health of people got affected; therefore, there was a reduction in the human development index as well.

The stringency index was positively correlated with the residential area's mobility in India. This implies that Indians were not following stringent norms of lockdown imposed to contain the virus. The reproduction rate was negatively correlated with the residential area's mobility. This implies that Indian mothers were refraining from conceiving during the pandemic because of the fear of the COVID-19 virus. Reproduction rate, Stringency index, population, and diabetes prevalence were positively correlated with the residential area's mobility in the rest of the world. This implies that there was an increase in diabetes prevalence, reproduction rate, and population because people during lockdown at their residences shifted to unhealthy dietary habits without any physical activity and violated family planning measures. Total deaths, new death smoothed, total cases per million, new tests, cardiovascular death rate, and hospital beds per 1000 were negatively correlated with the residential area's mobility. This implies that people were quarantined in their respective residences. Therefore, the spread of the virus was contained; hence total deaths, new death smoothed, total cases per million, and new tests were decreasing. The cardiovascular death rate was decreasing because people were spending more time with their families at their respective residences; therefore, there was a reduction in stress levels. Consequently, the cardiovascular death rate was also reduced. The hospital beds per 1000 decreased because there were infrastructural constraints in hospitals due to a sudden surge in COVID-19 cases.

6. Conclusion

The primary objectives of this research were to model the impact of the COVID-19 pandemic on Indian and global mobility using COVID-19 variables and socioeconomic variables and their effect on human mental health. In this research, various multiple regression models were developed to evaluate the impact of COVID-19 on global mobility trends and predict the future impact on global mobility. The R^2 value of linear regression models was used to evaluate the goodness of fit of the regression line. The models developed for India for different regions of mobility reported high accuracy in predicting future mobility.

This research has some implications for the research community. First, an implication from our result is that there is an inverse relationship between change in mobility and COVID- 19 variables. Second, it can be observed that the implementation of stringent policy measures on different forms of mobility helped in reducing the impact of the COVID-19 pandemic; however, with the increased stringency index, there was an adverse impact on people's mental health around the globe.

Certain ideas may be worthwhile investigating as part of future research. First, given the change in mobility over time, it might be interesting to develop machine learning and deep learning models that can predict future change in mobility due to the COVID-19 pandemic by encapsulating the essence of seasonality present within the data. Second, it might also be interesting to investigate and compare the effect of change in mobility on the mental health of people of different nationalities. We plan to continue experimenting with some ideas in our ongoing research on COVID-19.

References

[1] D. Cucinotta, M. Vanelli, WHO declares COVID-19 a pandemic? Acta Biomed. 91 (1) (2020) 157–160, https://doi.org/10.23750/abm.v91i1.9397.

[2] T. Laing, The economic impact of the Coronavirus 2019 (COVID-2019): implications for the mining industry, Extr. Ind. Soc. 7 (2) (2020) 580–582, https://doi.org/10.1016/j.exis.2020.04.003.

[3] M.I. Siddiquei, W. Khan, Economic implications of coronavirus, J. Publ. Aff. 20 (4) (2020) e2169, https://doi.org/10.1002/pa.2169.

[4] P. Pulla, COVID-19: India imposes lockdown for 21 days and cases rise, BMJ 368 (2020) m1251, https://doi.org/10.1136/bmj.m1251.

[5] B.K. Verma, M. Verma, V.K. Verma, R.B. Abdullah, D.C. Nath, H.T.A. Khan, A. Verma, R.K. Vishwakarma, V. Verma, Global lockdown: an effective safeguard in responding to the threat of COVID-19, J. Eval. Clin. Pract. 26 (6) (2020) 1592–1598, https://doi.org/10.1111/jep.13483.

[6] S. Nižetić, Impact of coronavirus (COVID-19) pandemic on air transport mobility, energy, and environment: a case study, Int. J. Energy Res. 44 (13) (2020) 10953–10961, https://doi.org/10.1002/er.5706.

[7] T. von Wachter, Lost generations: long-term effects of the COVID-19 crisis on job losers and labour market entrants, and options for policy, Fisc. Stud. 41 (3) (2020) 549–590, https://doi.org/10.1111/1475-5890.12247.

[8] A. Ghosh, S. Nundy, T.K. Mallick, How India is dealing with the COVID-19 pandemic, Sensors Int. 1 (2020) 100021, https://doi.org/10.1016/j.sintl.2020.100021.

[9] R. Gupta, R.K. Dhamija, K. Gaur, Epidemiological transition of COVID-19 in India from higher to lower HDI states and territories: implications for prevention and control, medRxiv (2020), https://doi.org/10.1101/2020.05.05.20092593.

[10] B. Pfefferbaum, C.S. North, Mental health and the COVID-19 pandemic, N. Engl. J. Med. 383 (6) (2020) 510–512, https://doi.org/10.1056/NEJMp2008017.

[11] A. Anurudran, L. Yared, C. Comrie, K. Harrison, T. Burke, Domestic violence amid COVID-19, Int. J. Gynecol. Obstet. 150 (2) (2020) 255–256, https://doi.org/10.1002/ijgo.13247.

[12] J. Vallée, E. Cadot, C. Roustit, I. Parizot, P. Chauvin, The role of daily mobility in mental health inequalities: the interactive influence of activity space and neighbourhood of residence on depression, Soc. Sci. Med. 73 (8) (2011) 1133–1144, https://doi.org/10.1016/j.socscimed.2011.08.009.

[13] F. Jiang, L. Deng, L. Zhang, Y. Cai, C.W. Cheung, Z. Xia, Review of the clinical characteristics of coronavirus disease 2019 (COVID-19), J. Gen. Intern. Med. 35 (5) (2020/05/01) 1545–1549, https://doi.org/10.1007/s11606-020-05762-w.

[14] M. Sulyok, T. Ferenci, M. Walker, Google trends data and COVID-19 in Europe: correlations and model enhancement are European wide, Transboundary Emerging Dis. 68 (4) (2021) 2610–2615, https://doi.org/10.1111/tbed.13887.

[15] H.F. Chan, A. Skali, D.A. Savage, D. Stadelmann, B. Torgler, Risk attitudes and human mobility during the COVID-19 pandemic, Sci. Rep. 10 (1) (2020) 19931, https://doi.org/10.1038/s41598-020-76763-2.

[16] P. Skórka, B. Grzywacz, D. Moroń, M. Lenda, The macroecology of the COVID-19 pandemic in the Anthropocene, PLoS One 15 (7) (2020) e0236856, https://doi.org/10.1371/journal.pone.0236856.

[17] A. Spelta, A. Flori, F. Pierri, G. Bonaccorsi, F. Pammolli, After the lockdown: simulating mobility, public health and economic recovery scenarios, Sci. Rep. 10 (1) (2020) 16950, https://doi.org/10.1038/s41598-020-73949-6.

[18] S. Roy, P. Ghosh, Factors affecting COVID-19 infected and death rates inform lockdown-related policymaking, PLoS One 15 (10) (2020) e0241165, https://doi.org/10.1371/journal.pone.0241165.

[19] G. Luo, M.L. McHenry, J.J. Letterio, Estimating the prevalence and risk of COVID-19 among international travelers and evacuees of Wuhan through modeling and case reports, PLoS One 15 (6) (2020), https://doi.org/10.1371/journal.pone.0234955 e0234955-e0234955.

[20] G. Castex, E. Dechter, M. Lorca, COVID-19: the impact of social distancing policies, cross-country analysis, Econ. Disaster Clim. Chang. 5 (1) (2021) 135–159, https://doi.org/10.1007/s41885-020-00076-x.

[21] S. Mittal, T. Singh, Gender-based violence during COVID- 19 pandemic: a mini-review, Front. Global Women Health 1 (4) (2020), https://doi.org/10.3389/fgwh.2020.00004.

[22] D.W. Timms, Social mobility and mental health in a Swedish cohort, Soc. Psychiatr. Psychiatr. Epidemiol. 31 (1) (1996) 38–48, https://doi.org/10.1007/bf00789121.

[23] Google, COVID-19 Community Mobility Reports, 2020. https://www.google.com/covid19/mobility/.

[24] OurWorldinData, COVID-19 Data, 2020. https://ourworldindata.org/coronavirus.

[25] L. Pappalardo, D. Pedreschi, Z. Smoreda, F. Giannotti, Using big data to study the link between human mobility and socioeconomic development, in: 2015 IEEE International Conference on Big Data (Big Data), 2015.

[26] C.-P. Kuo, J.S. Fu, Evaluating the impact of mobility on COVID-19 pandemic with machine learning hybrid predictions, Sci. Total Environ. 758 (2021) 144151, https://doi.org/10.1016/j.scitotenv.2020.144151.

CHAPTER NINE

Depression detection: approaches, challenges and future directions

Tara Rawat and Shikha Jain
Department of Computer Science & Engineering and Information Technology, Jaypee Institute of Information Technology, Noida, Uttar Pradesh, India

1. Introduction

In light of the emerging financial crisis and the multiple complexities surrounding the pandemic, individuals suffer from intense distress, panic, and rage, triggering suicidal attempts to happen and requiring immediate assessment or referral with a mental health facility for possible emergency. Social networks (SNs) have become an important part of our daily life because of its influence and attraction. Moreover, the exponential growth of new technologies is also promoting it to become an accepted part of our everyday lives. Nowadays people are becoming more and more comfortable with SN, they are habituated to share their emotions through their images, videos, recorded voice, daily schedule, and emotional phrases or words, etc., on social media. Nevertheless, the person who is stressed or depressed normally gets socially isolated and tends to be more active on these virtual media to share his emotions [1]. Hence, SN provides a vital platform to peep into their life while respecting their social isolation and extending help, if required.

According to the World Health Organization (WHO) [2], the number of people dealing with psychiatric illnesses is increasing gradually. The estimate of serious psychiatric illnesses reached 300 million, comprising 4.4% of the global population, which is quite a significant number. The reasons behind this increase in figure are lack of adequate mental health treatment and misunderstanding about common emotions and mental conditions. Mental disorder puts on a larger worldwide disability compared with physical disability and depression is ranked first (7.4%). Patients with mental illness have a burden death rate, which is 2.22 times higher than those of

Artificial Intelligence, Machine Learning, and Mental Health in Pandemics
ISBN: 978-0-323-91196-2
https://doi.org/10.1016/B978-0-323-91196-2.00002-8

stable patients. This is due to sufficiency in advance care intervention in case of accident and emergency [3].

This is a global trend, particularly in low-income countries where highly depressed people appear to have a higher prevalence of mental illness [4]. The causes of depressive illness may be deprivation, oppression, homelessness, fragility of life, alcohol and substance use, etc. [2]. Individuals with mental disorders are unable to deal with negative feelings, which are developed as a result of depression. It also results in a higher risk of suicide than with other nonphysical causes. A significant proportion of individuals who commit suicide are diagnosed with mental disorders according to western psychosocial studies [5,6]. Measures need to be taken to ensure that this sort of condition does not get worse. However, it is not possible to make a self-diagnosis based on the potential causes that induce depression. The mental illness manifestation that appears as early-stage signs should be observed and recorded to make a diagnosis in advance. The signs of illness, particularly in depression, often occur as a repetitive pattern, for instance, emotion changing or repeating one typical emotion within a period of time such as intense sadness for long. Nevertheless, people are not ready to accept that they are in depression. So, there arises a high need for a computational model that can detect mental disorders, especially depression, without interfering in someone's life. Symptoms can be obtained from the type of data a person is posting on SN. The data can be multimodal data. Each modality has its limitations and restrictions. To handle the complexities, increasing efforts are directed to design the psychological theory-based models.

Researchers are working toward depression detection either using questionnaire-based methods or using some computational model (automatic depression detection). Questionnaire-based method is based upon psychological evidence of symptoms. However, sometimes people are reluctant to talk about their true emotions. This leads to a major hindrance to come up with correct diagnosis using questionnaire-based methods. Hence, automatic detection of depression is required, in order to identify the signs that appear as early-stage signs that should be observed, considered, and recorded to make a diagnosis in advance. Long-term assessments of an individual's emotional state may be useful to better describe their emotions according to psychological aspects. We need to learn comprehensively how individuals communicate their true and daily experiences. We can choose social media to expand our corpus, which is more closely related to the daily lives of people. In the paper, we discuss the critical analysis of work done by researchers in this field.

The paper is organized as follows: Section 2 discusses the depression and need of detecting depression. Section 3 explains various datasets available for depression detection and existing challenges of the datasets. Section 4 mainly focuses on the various ways of depression detection such as questionnaire-based methods, psychological-theory-based methods, machine-learning (ML)-based methods, and microexpression (ME)-based methods. Also gaps and challenges with each method are listed there. Further, Section 5 discusses the role of personality in depression detection. Section 6 presents the summary of work done by various researchers to give an insight to the state of the art of the field followed by discussion in Section 7, which highlights the findings of our study. Finally, the paper concludes with future directions in Section 8.

2. Depression

Depression can be defined as "a psychiatric illness marked by extreme feelings of hopelessness and inadequacy usually followed by loss of motivation and interest in life." [2]. It is described in many various forms in the medical and social sciences [7,8]. It has a profound effect on a wide variety of practitioners including psychologists, sociologists, biologists, statisticians, and medical providers and has resulted in the publication of comprehensive diagnostic guidelines for mental illness.

People with depression are often isolated from their family and society and deprived of the necessities of life or healthful environmental influences. It has become the major cause of several nontreatable diseases such as cancer, heart diseases, diabetes, alcoholic and metabolic disorders [9]. With the prevalence of depression and suicide risk, it is becoming increasingly critical to find new diagnosis and therapeutic techniques at the early stage (Fig. 9.1) of depression to avoid any unfortunate happening.

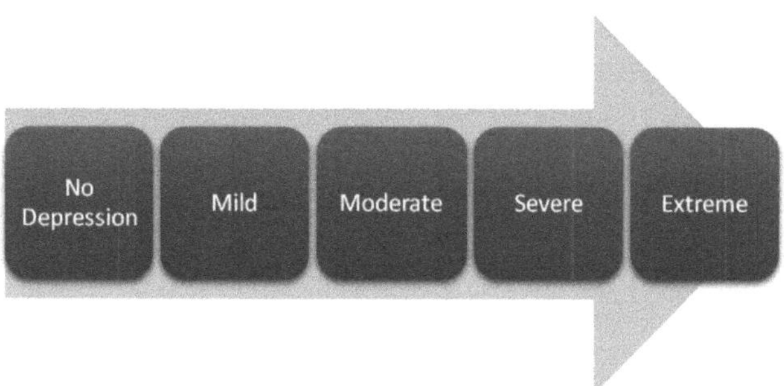

Figure 9.1 Stages of depression.

2.1 Need of automatic depression detection

Depressed people should consciously reach out to mental health practitioners in order to get a diagnosis. In reality, because of limitations on mobility, flexibility, costs, and encouragement, it can be difficult for them to get professional attention. However, with the increase of smart mobile devices, possible types of healthcare approaches have begun to change in creating innovations to mental health well-being.

Current diagnostic standards are subjective [10] and interview-based [11], which lead to conflicting and vague diagnosis. Such measures are useful to some extent. However, they are not systematic or effective means of integrating behavioral findings that indicate the presence and severity of depression. Therefore, more than 80% of people are hesitant to seek any consultation with a doctor, in their early stages of depression, which leads to further worsening of their conditions [9].

There are various reasons for the high rate of under treatment. Some of them are mentioned as below:

- Failure to obtain assistance, since the issue is not known.
- Fear of inadequate medication.
- Believe the problem is not serious and want to fix it without external support.
- Lack of awareness about mental illness.
- Accessibility issues: Minimal or lack of resources available in certain areas or for other populations.
- Financial factors.
- Other than that, the need for both pharmacological and psychological care remains largely unmet.

Hence, to tackle these limitations and strengthen the depression diagnosis process, the automatic monitoring of human communication, daily activities, and behavior contributes a lot.

3. Depression datasets

The process of depression detection is highly interdisciplinary (psychology, biology, science, computer science, etc.), which brings an important set of skills and understanding to the problem. Nevertheless, it is not always possible to work with people from every field in a particular idea to implement. Therefore, cooperation can be promoted by arranging competitions and making data and code publicly available. The National Comorbidity

Survey-Revised (NCS-R) has shared their data in the public domain. This is an epidemiological study of DSM, including depression. The Audio/Visual Emotion Recognition (AVEC) depression subchallenge [12–17] is an example of depression detection system challenges that pushed interest, encouraged research, and created connections across the research community.

Behavioral signs such as prosodic features of speech [18] and facial expression have proven to be outstanding components for predicting depression [19]. Commonly used datasets such as DementiaBank Database, BlackDog, Pitt, AVEC 13–17, D3-HDS, and other datasets used by researchers are listed in Table 9.1.

A challenge for automatic measurement of depression severity is basically the lack of available datasets that have clinically relevant depression. As most of the data is gathered in the controlled environment, it is based on the patient's activity under observation. The current clinical assessment does not represent psychological symptoms of mental disorders.

Some of the data collection challenges in controlled environment are as follows:

1. The participant may not be pleased with detailed video-recording interviews or use.
2. Participants may be nontalkative individuals or uneducated.
3. Participant may be disinterested in commenting on disease or speaking in detail about disturbing subjects
4. Conveniently ignoring and frustrating scheduled meetings to gather info.
5. Memory deficiencies about illness, treatments undergone.
6. Lethargy and disconnection leading to ignorance or misunderstanding.

Often people with emotional or dissociative disorders have trouble communicating or learning. During data collection, mood disorder may trigger anxiety, inattentiveness, and perseverance on a limited spectrum of topics. Any people with attitude and environmental problems put off forever or disagreed with follow-up appointments. However, it is also difficult to follow the most reliable source(s) of information due to the time taken to go through and analyze the vast volume of evidence in real time. There are numerous functional and assessment considerations such as psychometric questionnaires or measuring changes in values over time [47,48]. Besides these problems, data analysis and use of recorded results for patients have a range of difficulties to implement [49]. Therefore, it is necessary to evaluate depressive people in their natural environment in order to better understand a patient's well-being or behavior.

Table 9.1 Literature survey summarization.

Ref.	Dataset used	Modality	Depression scale used/approach	Techniques used	Procedure	Limitation
[20]	DementiaBank database	Audio + Video + Text	HAMD	Bidirectional hierarchical recurrent neural network combined with an attention mechanism (BHANN)	Interview	- Limited number of respondents - Lack of personality assessment - Issue in generalization among different languages as most of the dataset are available in English language.
[21]	BlackDog	Audio + Video	DSM-IV	SVM	Interview	- Dataset size is too small - Personality traits assessment is missing
[22]	Pitt	Audio + Facial images	DSM-IV and HRSD	Logistic Regression + SVM	Interview	- Lack of personality assessment - Issue in generalization
[23]	AVEC 13-17	Audio + Video	BDI scores	CNN + RNN	Spatio-temporal information from videos	- Imbalanced dataset that reduces depressive state identification efficiency and induces overfitting
[24]	D3-HDS	Text	Facebook post + CES-D Score+	RNN	By collecting facebook post and CES-D questionnaire	- Away from psychological aspect - Nonstandardized text format

[25]	SemEval-2014 task (ShARe-corpus)	Text	Manual annotation for depression	MaxEnt, SVM, CRF	Identification and normalization of commonly arising illnesses and conditions In clinical reports.	- Manual label annotation - Very less information - Generalization issue
[26,27]	OXYGEN	Audio + Video	Virtual human interaction	Neural network	Family interaction	- Limited features - Limited information
[28]	ORI	Audio + Video	DSM-IV	GMM + SVM	Family interaction	- Limited number of respondents - Lack of personality assessment
[29]	PDBH	Audio	DSM-IV	QDA	Reading story	- Dataset size is very small
[30]	WCGS	Audio	CESD	SVM	Interview	- Limited number of respondents - Lack of personality assessment - Controlled environment
[31]	DAIC	Audio + Video	PHQ-9(Self report)	SVM + Naive Bayes	Virtual human interaction	- Brief nature of the assessment - Carried out at different moments, the psychological symptoms may be the state-dependent effect of the person i.e., a short-term emotional impact triggered by an immediate occurrence rather than long-term depression-related affective characteristics

(Continued)

Table 9.1 Literature survey summarization.—cont'd

Ref.	Dataset used	Modality	Depression scale used/approach	Techniques used	Procedure	Limitation
[32]	eRisk 2017 shared task	Text	Writing features (WFs)	SVM + Random forest	Post from social media platform	- Away from psychological aspect - Nonstandardized text format
[33]	mPower voice	Audio	PDQ-8+ MDS-UPDRS	SVM + Randomforest + DNN	Voice recording on the mobile app	- Less accuracy due to the controlled environment.
[34]	Danish depression dataset	Text	HAM-D17	Conventional technique	Interview	- Personality traits are missing
[35]	Facebook user comments	Text	LIWC2015	Decision tree classifier + SVM + KNN + Ensemble	Analyzing the mental, spatial, linguistic characteristics of the facebook message	- Limited emotional features
[36]	Tweets	Text	Emotion artificial intelligence	Naive Bayes + SVM	Applying NLP on tweets	- Less accuracy due to the nonstandardize text format
[37]	Sensor data and self-reports	Sensing data	DSM-5 + PHQ-9	SVM + Random forest	Mobile devices	- Small dataset due to the time constraint imposed on patients. - Model overfitting
[24]	Heterogeneous data sources (D3-HDS	Text	CES-D	RNN	Analyzing the living situation, actions and sharing of material on social media	- Problem may occur if any of the key features are missing in the facebook profile.

[38]	Textual and multimodal depression dataset	Text + images	Multi-agent reinforcement learning method	Markov decision processes (MDPs)	Collecting text and photographs shared on social media by people.	The findings of identification could not be properly clarified with regard to the related field theories, which makes it impossible to perform a more thorough study of certain processes such as emotional state, mood etc.
[39]	College student videos	Images	FACS coding	SVM	GUI is built to capture photos	- Nonintrusive - Limited number of participants
[40]	DAIC	Audio	PHQ-8	CNNs	Virtual human interaction	- Nonintrusive - Controlled environment
[41]	SEMAINE	Video	Local binary pattern texture	SVM + RBF + PCA	Virtual human interaction	- Nonintrusive - Controlled environment - Weak image segmentation method
[42]	DAIC-WOZ	Audio + Video + Text	PHQ-8	Attention-based fusion network and deep neural network (DNN)	Interview	- Limited number of respondents - Lack of personality assessment

(Continued)

Table 9.1 Literature survey summarization.—cont'd

Ref.	Dataset used	Modality	Depression scale used/approach	Techniques used	Procedure	Limitation
[43]	AVEC 2019 (DAIC-WOZ)	Audio + Video	PHQ-8	BERT + CNN	Interview	- Limited samples - Nonintrusive
[44]	Tweets	Text + images	Ekman's model discrete emotion	Random Forest + SVM + CNN + Logistic regression	Collecting phrases, demographic details and photographs shared on social media by people.	- The scarcity of demographic factors (e.g., age, class, race) inside the data is a significant constraint to in-depth analysis.
[45]	Wizard of Oz (DAICWOZ)	Audio + Video + Text	PHQ-8	LSTM	Interview	- Lack of personality assessment - Required more rational means of recording gesture/ movement data
[46]	CHI-MEI	Audio	DSM-IV	Multivariate feature and discriminant analyses	Interview	- Use of nonstandardized recording procedures.

4. Depression detection

Researchers are working toward depression detection either using questionnaire-based methods or using some computational model (ML-based depression detection) in various domains as shown in Fig. 9.2. The next section provides overview of various techniques or approaches and discusses the pros and cons of various depression techniques.

4.1 Questionnaire-based depression detection

Clinicians and mental health professionals use questionnaires to analyze patient's behavior and also look into their e-health records if available. Patient's mood and responses are assessed, as per the predefined depression criteria. Some of the traditional tools are discussed below, which are commonly used for assessing depression:

1. The clinicians often use the standard method for the treatment and assessment of depression is the Patient Health Questionnaire (PHQ) and Hospital Anxiety and Depression Scale (HADS). This questionnaire contains the criteria for DSM-IV depression in a brief self-report tool, which asks if people are happy, bored, poor appetite, whether having trouble in focus, unable to sleep, etc. [50].
2. For face-to-face interviews, professionals use the commonly used Diagnostic and Statistical Manual of Mental Disorders criteria. It is the summary of mental disorders, a catalog of criteria to be used for their diagnosis, and a systematic method for description, organization, and

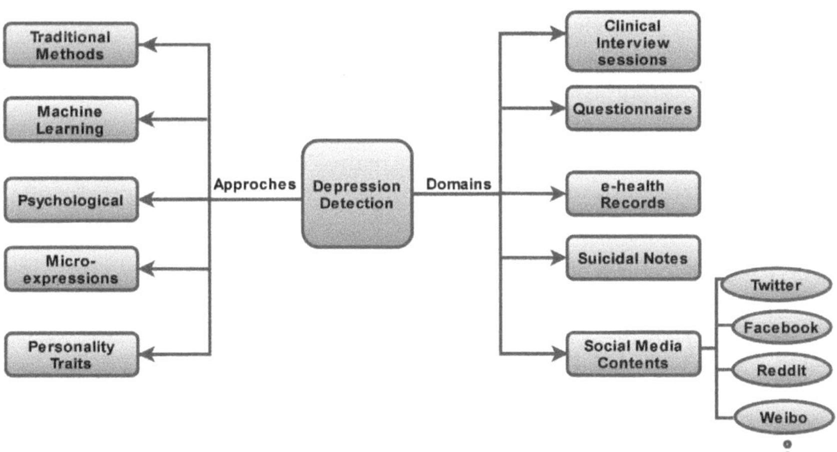

Figure 9.2 The categorization of depression detection domains and approaches.

classification. The guidelines identify the characteristic patterns of daily life and include nine types of symptoms of depression [51]. The Beck Depression Inventory (BDI) is a questionnaire of 21 sets of statements and is graded by intensity and rated from 0 to 3 in each set. The statements reflect rising feelings in depression (e.g., remorse, low self-esteem, and suicidal ideation). Every collection includes 10 positive and 10 negative statements, which is often confusing to patients [52].

3. Center for Epidemiological Studies Depression Scale (CES-D) consists of 20 items that the patient notes on the level of encounters over the past week. The index covers perceptual, affective, and somatic objects [53].
4. Hamilton Depression Scale consists of 17 elements evaluated by the analyst, instead of the individual [54].

To date, most of the work [55,56] has been undertaken using traditional psychological questionnaires, such as the abovementioned scales and many others. It is not unusual today that many different measures exist for evaluating the same psychological symptoms. For example, the clinician can choose between scales such as the BDI, the CES-D, the Hamilton Depression Rating Scale (HAM-D), and so on, for an analysis of depressive symptoms. Though such scales are rooted measures used in psychology and psychiatry studies, it is difficult to know which measure has the best sensitivity for an individual while conducting a test. This could be the issue when used in various age groups. Hence, there is a need to create and incorporate new, sophisticated measures that can be modified to measure possible behavioral disorders.

The questionnaire-based methods take time and are difficult to obtain adequate data to ensure the robustness of the results. Moreover, depression symptoms cannot be covered in already defined depression criteria as for every patient, symptoms can vary widely. Sometimes patients are ashamed or unaware of their condition that they would not consult with doctors. Moreover, the detection cost could be higher due to the need for health professionals to conduct questionnaires orally to communities with low literacy rates.

The healthcare practitioners are trained to monitor patient outcomes but may be less familiar with measuring psychiatric outcomes and commitment to diagnosis. There is a need for more practical tools and strategies intended to help both clinicians and patients to monitor their experiences with depression. Approaches are needed to reduce the cost of time and human capital and improve the efficiency of diagnosis in depression and other low-resource settings.

4.2 Psychological-theory-based depression detection

Psychological theories explain the long-term consequences of human behavior and provide robust evidence-based clarifications as to why people believe, behave, and react how they do. These theories discuss factors of personality, early experiences, and interpersonal relations. Such an evaluation process allows for strong clinical insights that may be helpful in identifying the patient's mental state. Peterson [57] discusses various psychological paradigms of abnormality, the identification and management of psychiatric disorders and strengths as well as weaknesses of each psychological model.

Ekman's [58], psychological assumption proposed a categorical emotion model, defines six basic emotions (anger, fear, disgust, excitement, sorrow, and surprise) or a variant of these. Therefore, according to this psychological hypothesis, all humans possess a common set of basic emotions, and each individual's emotional state can be categorized as one of these emotional sets. To the contrary, the dimension model proposed by Russell and Mehrabian [59], a valence—arousal—dominance (VAD) model, where emotional states can be assessed in terms of three emotional dimensions. These values cover a wide range of real-valued numbers representing the intensity and orientation on each dimension [59].

Mehrabian [60] extended and introduced a model where individual mood characteristics contain three key components—pleasure, arousal, and dominance (PAD). These three characteristics are almost distinct and form a three-dimensional space of mood. Axes ranging from −1.0 to 1.0 for each dimension are used for applying the PAD mood space. An individual mood is defined in each of the three mood space axes with the following understanding: + P and −P for friendly and negative, + A and −A for aroused and calm, and + D and −D for dominant and compliant. The Pleasure—Arousal—Dominance paradigm (1995) of Mehrabian presented a 3Dmodel that provides a set of emotional responses. For instance, if the value of the trait happiness is negative, the value of the trait arousal is negative, and the value of the trait dominance is also negative, a person's distinct mood profile is depressed or intensely sad or anxious. In Ref. [61], the author has shown the mapping for various emotions into the PAD 3D model that can be used for identifying human mental state.

Other theories/hypotheses regarding the psychological and social causes of depression and their theory-related, evidence-based treatments are discussed in Refs. [62—64]. Riskind et al., [65] presented an existing and very promising psychological model of cognitive vulnerability to anxiety disorders, which is becoming a fast approachable vulnerability model of anxiety. Their focus is on self-identification of anxiety disorders and also emphasized on the link with social, personality, and general psychological theories. The study emphasizes the role of future-oriented cognition in the psyche. In Ref. [66], the author has surveyed the association of cognitive vulnerability with adverse events and has been shown to be a specific risk factor for potential depression. Two cognitive hopelessness theories (HT; Abramson, Metalsky, & Alloy) [67] and Beck's cognitive theory (BT; Beck) [68] have been specifically tested in the report. The role of cognitive bias in depression and its correlation with evaluation bias was discussed by Mehu and Scherer [69]. The negative behavior relies on emotional reactions across evaluation processes, interconnecting with negative impact in the form of irregular behavior, which leads to an extreme state of sadness and anxiety, known as depression.

In [70], authors have proposed a dynamic computational mood model, which is based on psychological theories: OCC theory [71], Aaron Beck depression theory [67], and Thayer theory (2-D model) [68]. With two criteria, the author analyzes stress events: coping and resilience. Islam et al., [72], presented an emotion analysis method called DEVA for text information engineering. With the help of the 2-D model, they also capture the emotional state of the user. Rottehberg [73] has presented the study on people with mood disorders to figure out how mood affects their thought process. According to research results conducted by the author, poorer emotional reactivity to sad circumstances is linked with severe depression.

4.3 Automatic (machine learning) depression detection

ML is generally defined as a computing approach that automatically assesses methods and parameters to achieve an appropriate solution to a problem [74]. ML intends to deliver new ways for improving health risk factor identification, forecasting disease advancement, and designing customized health strategies. Fig. 9.3 shows the general framework of depression detection using ML technique. To date, research has begun to investigate the detection of depression via inferences of people's activities on social media, internet searches, or uses of cell phone apps, as well as various methods for evaluating or constantly tracking a person's mental well-being and associated symptoms through measuring sleep, mood, stress, or physical activity through audio, visual, or biological stimulus processing. Particularly in mental health, evidence and judgments influenced by ML can have far-reaching psychological, social, and economic effects. Hence, we need to be very careful of what reasonable inferences can be drawn from relevant data. Moreover,

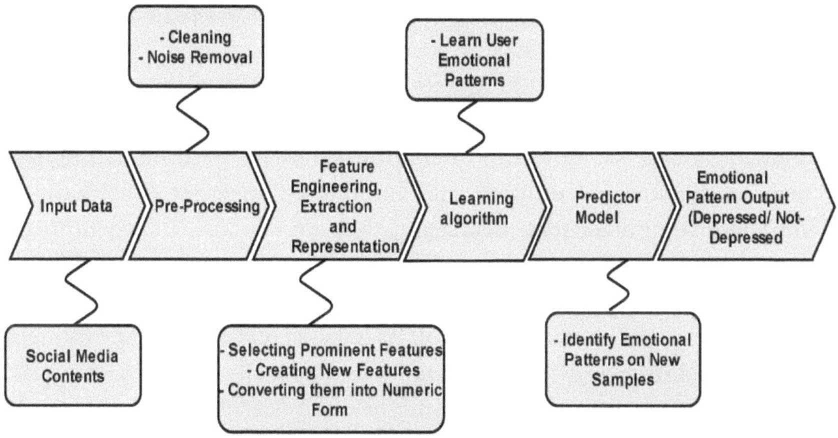

Figure 9.3 General framework of depression detection.

we should construct interfaces that help people understand machine inferences appropriately and ensure that finally, people stay in charge of, and responsible for, critical ML-informed decisions.

Some of the challenges in automatic depression detection are as follows:

1. There are no large-scale public comparison repositories available for depression studies.
2. There are several dimensions of the actions of people on social media. Characterizing people from selective viewpoints is challenging, and understanding the interaction through various modalities.
3. While the activities of people are extensive and varied, only handfuls are signs of depression, and the depressive-oriented elements on social media are scarce and difficult to catch.
4. These approaches are away from the psychological aspect.
5. The reliability of statistical methods is inadequate to classify depression, as the dynamic signs are continuously revealed as different expressions of emotions.

Previous studies [75,76] have confirmed that depression appears to occur as a set of emotions or exists continuously as a single emotion. Hence, the research based on the current statistical method can be done more on the emotional level, which can be better understood by psychological perspective. Therefore, emotions with gradual changing as a linear sequence will help describe depressed people's symptoms.

A multimodal approach, which is a combination of text, audio, visuals, posture, hand gestures, facial expressions, etc., provides a thorough understanding of an individual's mind. Much of the work [77,78] to date on mental illness has focused on unimodality and a number of datasets have been created for predicting the outcome measure. A single modality is less insightful because it only offers one-sided knowledge and might miss the inherent parameter. Due to the multidimensional nature of mental illness, if multimodal data is evaluated and interpreted together, it provides a comprehensive and accurate depression detection modal. In recent years, depression detection using multimodal assessments has developed an interest in the advantages that this technique may offer in providing useful insights into challenging circumstances [79,80]. As social media is evolving exponentially, information is available in multiple formats such as audio, video, text, behavioral pattern, etc. Although some research has addressed multimodal structures [81] and demonstrated significant improvement in assessing the disease. Several studies have established connections between depression and a variety of factors, including psychological, physiological, verbal—nonverbal, textual, daily routine patterns, etc. [82—84].

Following are the challenges with multimodal depression detection:

1. Depression is a subject of various disconnected fields that makes it difficult to assess.
2. Variations in behavior and lack of labeled behavioral datasets.
3. Lack of research in integrating various modalities.
4. Need tools to encourage greater collaboration and cooperation, especially across the different modalities, since large amounts of data and balanced data are highly challenging.

4.4 Microexpressions-based depression detection

MEs are hidden, brief facial gestures that show true emotions and hold useful knowledge for varying situations. They appear in different parts of the face and last just a fraction of a second, i.e., 1/25th to 1/3rd of a second. Since MEs may show emotions that individuals can seek to conceal, understanding MEs can benefit therapists or psychiatrists by offering information for detecting and intercepting depression and other problematic circumstances.

In 1969, Ekman had noticed MEs when he reviewed a video interview of a depressed patient [85]. A lot of work in MEs has been done by Ekman, Frank and O'Sulliva [86] and Portets [87]. These MEs have been established as an important behavioral basis for the identification of depression and vulnerabilities of behavior. Such facial micromovements are short and occur unconsciously, which is displayed by the human face as they attempt to conceal or manipulate emotions. In Ref. [88], the authors proposed two types of MEs tagging schemes, emotion groups and the Facial Action Coding System (FACS). FACS tags facial expressions with Units of Action (AU). A particular AU describes a facial expression variable; hence an expression is represented through a set of AU.

Unlike traditional facial expressions, MEs are immediate and spontaneous human emotional impressions. Researchers have recently been researching MEs, which can represent true emotions [89,90]. MEs act as a crucial guideline for the acute treatment of depression by emotional state monitoring and lies detection.

5. Importance of personality in depression detection

Psychological aspects that cause depression include critical thought and decision biases and a lack of interpersonal skills. The characteristics of people's personalities can affect them in such a manner that they are more or less likely to behave in ways that can lead to depression.

Several clinical works [91,92] have focused on recognizing the personality characteristics associated with major depression and the consequences of these correlations for the interpretation and treatment of major depression. As per [93], various personality factors increase mental disorder risk. A recent analysis [94] shows that low extraversion, high neuroticism, and poor sensitivity are the predicted depressive symptoms. A number of models have been suggested for the relationship between personality and mood disorders [95–98]. These possible relations include:

(a) The prevalent causes of personality and depressive disorders;
(b) A continuous continuum is created by personality and depressive disorders;
(c) The precursor to depressive conditions is personality;
(d) The predisposition of personality to having depressive disorders;
(e) There are known to be involved effects of personality on depression;
(f) Personality traits are state-dependent cooccurrence of depressive episodes; and
(g) Traits of personality are implications of depressive episodes.

Several researchers [99–101] have attempted to link personality measures to the result of depression in early trials during the 1980–90s. Such findings show that personality disorders in people who experience depression are widespread. In studying this relationship, some significant methodological difficulties were identified by researchers; resultant study on personality disorder characteristics in people with depression is limited.

Also latest findings show a close link between emotional behavior in social networks and mental illnesses [102–104]. Such findings use the techniques of ML to construct diagnostic models [32,105]. Psychological explanations of depression, however, reveal more than just predictive analytics in mental health according to the WHO Action Plan [106]. Moreover, only the ML algorithms-based examination of mental disorders such as depression can result in a broad boundary between various types of mental disorders and reduce the precision of the diagnosis. Hence, there is a need to incorporate psychological theories, personality aspects along with other attributes to detect depression using ML methods. The American Psychological Association (APA) believes that sentiments play a significant part in the treatment of psychological disorders [107], because people with psychological problems are often strongly associated with negative emotions.

6. State of the art

A number of papers are studied and reviewed in the field of depression detection using different modalities such as text, images, audio, and videos. Table 9.1 presents a summary of some important research. The table gives an insight to various dataset, modalities, depression scales, and different approaches used to detect depression through different procedures. Moreover, it discusses existing gaps and the limitations of those approaches.

7. Discussion

This systematic review discusses the various approaches and available datasets for depression detection and also identified the pros and cons of each approach. This review found that the traditional techniques of treatment are comparatively ineffective because psychiatrists are unable to identify a patient's regular feelings while doing a manual diagnosis of depression. They can learn about the patient's medical history by using a few standard questionnaires and may enquire about patient's behavior from family members or friends.

This study represents an overview of how social media network can be useful in detecting depressive state of the social media users. There is a vast amount of data on social media in various formats such as images, text, audio, and video. People share their everyday activities, sentiments, emotions, and thoughts, as well as offer feedback and evaluations based on their preferences.

Although the study has discussed various pros and cons of each depression detection techniques in the above sections, this study has also suggested a robust predictive model using a correlation between psychological aspect and ML techniques. As there is so much data available, the ML techniques can now be able to compile data for mental health professionals to help them in doing their job better. However, one patient's behavior might differ from that of another. Therefore, the standard questionnaire-based database or traditional treatment may not assist in predicting the correct output despite of using ML techniques. Several research studies identified that a depressive state can be described using psychological or cognition-based emotion mining theories. Cognitive approaches talk about human belief and behavior. These approaches are the core of psychological aspect in defining human behavior. Therefore, psychological aspect provides evidence-based clarifications of human mental state, which aid in developing robust predictive models.

Other important findings of this review suggest that mental illness is multidimensional and unimodal (say only audio modality) may miss the important aspect as finding balanced information in a single modality will be highly challenging. ME identification is one of the important aspects on the symptoms of depression. Few studies have suggested that severely depressed people fake their expressions socially. Therefore, to prevent suicidal attempts, further study is needed in identifying deception in depressed people.

This thorough investigation also sheds light on the link between personality and depression. Several models have been developed in this area, to understand the link between personality and depressive illnesses as personality changes over time with emotional experiences. As a result, studying the link between personality and depression might provide helpful information for creating depression detection predictors.

8. Conclusion and future directions

There are disturbing effects of the Covid-19 pandemic for individual, public safety, mental and social functioning. Depressive state tends to generate negative emotions. Psychological perspectives can help an individual to identify his optimal emotional level. In this paper, we present a review of the various approaches for understanding and working with depression, covering questionnaire, psychological, ML and ME-based approaches. The outcome of each approach draws a robust and structured formulation of concepts to understand mental health in a clear way. We also discussed the challenges and consequences of mental health if not detected in an early stage and handled appropriately. In terms of clinical relevance, this study highlights the need for automatic early-stage depression detection and use of psychological aspects for strong clinical insights.

Concern about mental health has grown rapidly in recent years. The following research directions need to addressed in providing efficient and evidence-based depression detection approaches:

1. Research on depression detection using psychological approaches and on ML techniques has developed quite independently. Yet both can be integrated in building a robust system. Efforts to combine these fields conceptually and empirically seem to be necessary.
2. Identifying useful noninvasive methods, which provide a natural environment. Then only, it will be possible to come up with more logical and diverse explanations for various elements of depression.
3. Due to the complex and multidimensional nature of mental illness, a considerable amount of time and effort may be required in analyzing the trustworthiness of user-generated content (social media) as a means of collecting real-time feedback on ground-level emotions. Therefore, preprocessing and feature engineering must be one of the important aspects while studying mental health from social media.
4. Consideration of psychological aspects in long-term assessments of an individual's emotional state describes emotions and mood of an individual. Therefore, we need to learn comprehensively how individuals communicate their true and daily experiences.
5. Research studies on building Individual-centric prediction algorithms that scan a person's social media feeds and give early warning/intervention if there are any out of the ordinary behavioral problems.

References

[1] F. Trefflich, S. Kalckreuth, R. Mergl, C. Rummel-Kluge, Psychiatric patients' internet use corresponds to the internet use of the general public, Psychiatr. Res. 226 (1) (2015), https://doi.org/10.1016/j.psychres.2014.12.037.

[2] Geneva: World Health Organization, Depression and Other Common Mental Disorders: Global Health Estimates, 2017.

[3] E.R. Walker, R.E. McGee, B.G. Druss, Mortality in mental disorders and global disease burden implications a systematic review and meta-analysis, JAMA Psychiatr. (2015), https://doi.org/10.1001/jamapsychiatry.2014.2502.

[4] N. Hoertel, et al., Mental disorders and risk of suicide attempt: a national prospective study, Mol. Psychiatr. (2015), https://doi.org/10.1038/mp.2015.19.

[5] E.C. Harris, B. Barraclough, Suicide as an outcome for mental disorders. A meta-analysis, Br. J. Psychiatry 170 (3) (1997) 205–228.

[6] L. Brådvik, Suicide risk and mental disorders, Int. J. Environ. Res. Publ. Health (2018), https://doi.org/10.3390/ijerph15092028.

[7] F. Draft, Depression in adults (update) depression: the treatment and management of depression in adults, Depression 12 (2009).

[8] M. Marcus, M.T. Yasamy, M. van Ommeren, D. Chisholm, Depression, a Global Public Health Concern, 2012. WHO Department of Mental Health and Substance Abuse.

[9] B.H. Hidaka, Depression as a disease of modernity: explanations for increasing prevalence, J. Affect. Disord. 140 (3) (2012), https://doi.org/10.1016/j.jad.2011.12.036.

[10] J.A. Bilello, Seeking an objective diagnosis of depression, Biomarkers Med. 10 (8) (2016), https://doi.org/10.2217/bmm-2016-0076.

[11] K.M. Smith, P.F. Renshaw, J. Bilello, The diagnosis of depression: current and emerging methods, Compr. Psychiatr. 54 (1) (2013), https://doi.org/10.1016/j.comppsych.2012.06.006.

[12] M. Valstar, et al., AVEC 2013 - the Continuous Audio/Visual Emotion and Depression Recognition Challenge, 2013, https://doi.org/10.1145/2512530.2512533.

[13] M. Valstar, et al., AVEC 2014 - 3D dimensional affect and depression recognition challenge, in: AVEC 2014 - Proc. 4th Int. Work. Audio/Visual Emot. Challenge, Work. MM 2014, 2014, pp. 3–10, https://doi.org/10.1145/2661806.2661807.

[14] M. Valstar, et al., AVEC 2016 - Depression, Mood, and Emotion Recognition Workshop and Challenge, 2016, https://doi.org/10.1145/2988257.2988258.

[15] F. Ringeval, et al., AVEC 2017 - Real-Life Depression, and Affect Recognition Workshop and Challenge, 2017, https://doi.org/10.1145/3133944.3133953.

[16] F. Ringeval, et al., AVEC 2018 Workshop and Challenge: Bipolar Disorder and Cross-Cultural Affect Recognition, 2018, https://doi.org/10.1145/3266302.3266316.

[17] F. Ringeval, et al., AVEC 2019 Workshop and Challenge: State-of-Mind, Detecting Depression with AI, and Cross-Cultural Affect Recognition, 2019, https://doi.org/10.1145/3347320.3357688.

[18] Z. Yang, H. Li, L. Li, K. Zhang, C. Xiong, Y. Liu, Speech-based automatic recognition technology for major depression disorder, in: Lecture Notes in Computer Science (Including Subseries Lecture Notes in Artificial Intelligence and Lecture Notes in Bioinformatics), vol. 11956, LNCS, 2019, https://doi.org/10.1007/978-3-030-37429-7_55.

[19] A. Jan, H. Meng, Y.F.A. Gaus, F. Zhang, S. Turabzadeh, Automatic depression scale prediction using facial expression dynamics and regression, in: AVEC '14: Proceedings of the 4th International Workshop on Audio/Visual Emotion Challenge, 2014, https://doi.org/10.1145/2661806.2661812.

[20] Y. Pan, B. Mirheidari, M. Reuber, A. Venneri, D. Blackburn, H. Christensen, Automatic hierarchical attention neural network for detecting AD, in: Proceedings of the Annual Conference of the International Speech Communication Association, INTERSPEECH, 2019, https://doi.org/10.21437/Interspeech.2019-1799.

[21] J. Joshi, et al., Multimodal assistive technologies for depression diagnosis and monitoring, J. Multimodal User Interfaces 7 (3) (2013), https://doi.org/10.1007/s12193-013-0123-2.

[22] J.F. Cohn, et al., Detecting depression from facial actions and vocal prosody, in: Affective Computing and Intelligent Interaction and Workshops, 2009. ACII 2009. 3rd International Conference on, 2009, https://doi.org/10.1109/ACII.2009.5349358.

[23] W.C. De Melo, E. Granger, A. Hadid, Combining global and local convolutional 3D networks for detecting depression from facial expressions, in: 14th IEEE International Conference on Automatic Face and Gesture Recognition, 2019, https://doi.org/10.1109/FG.2019.8756568.

[24] M.Y. Wu, C.Y. Shen, E.T. Wang, A.L.P. Chen, A deep architecture for depression detection using posting, behavior, and living environment data, J. Intell. Inf. Syst. 54 (2) (2020), https://doi.org/10.1007/s10844-018-0533-4.

[25] S. Pradhan, N. Elhadad, W. Chapman, S. Manandhar, G. Savova, SemEval-2014 Task 7: Analysis of Clinical Text, 2015, https://doi.org/10.3115/v1/s14-2007.

[26] K.E.B. Ooi, M. Lech, N.B. Allen, Multichannel weighted speech classification system for prediction of major depression in adolescents, IEEE Trans. Biomed. Eng. 60 (2) (2013), https://doi.org/10.1109/TBME.2012.2228646.

[27] K.E.B. Ooi, L.S.A. Low, M. Lech, N. Allen, Prediction of Clinical Depression in Adolescents Using Facial Image Analysis, 2011.

[28] N.C. Maddage, R. Senaratne, L.S.A. Low, M. Lech, N. Allen, Video-based detection of the clinical depression in adolescents, in: Annu. Int. Conf. IEEE Eng. Med. Biol. Soc., 2009, https://doi.org/10.1109/IEMBS.2009.5334815.

[29] E. Moore, M.A. Clements, J.W. Peifer, L. Weisser, Critical analysis of the impact of glottal features in the classification of clinical depression in speech, IEEE Trans. Biomed. Eng. 55 (1) (2008) 96–107, https://doi.org/10.1109/TBME.2007.900562.

[30] M.H. Sanchez, et al., Using Prosodic and Spectral Features in Detecting Depression in Elderly Males, 2011.

[31] S. Scherer, et al., Automatic audiovisual behavior descriptors for psychological disorder analysis, Image Vis. Comput. 32 (10) (2014), https://doi.org/10.1016/j.imavis.2014.06.001.

[32] F. Cacheda, D. Fernandez, F.J. Novoa, V. Carneiro, Early detection of depression: social network analysis and random forest techniques, J. Med. Internet Res. (2019), https://doi.org/10.2196/12554.

[33] Y. Ozkanca, M. Göksu Öztürk, M.N. Ekmekci, D.C. Atkins, C. Demiroglu, R. Hosseini Ghomi, Depression screening from voice samples of patients affected by Parkinson's disease, Digit. Biomarkers 3 (2) (2019), https://doi.org/10.1159/000500354.

[34] P. Videbech, A. Deleuran, The Danish depression database, Clin. Epidemiol. 8 (2016), https://doi.org/10.2147/CLEP.S100298.

[35] M.R. Islam, M.A. Kabir, A. Ahmed, A.R.M. Kamal, H. Wang, A. Ulhaq, Depression detection from social network data using machine learning techniques, Health Inf. Sci. Syst. 6 (1) (2018), https://doi.org/10.1007/s13755-018-0046-0.

[36] M. Deshpande, V. Rao, Depression detection using emotion artificial intelligence, in: 2017 International Conference on Intelligent Sustainable Systems (ICISS), 2018, https://doi.org/10.1109/ISS1.2017.8389299.

[37] N. Narziev, H. Goh, K. Toshnazarov, S.A. Lee, K.M. Chung, Y. Noh, STDD: short-term depression detection with passive sensing, Sensors 20 (5) (2020), https://doi.org/10.3390/s20051396.

[38] T. Gui, et al., Cooperative multimodal approach to depression detection in twitter, Proc. AAAI Conf. Artif. Intell. 33 (Jul. 2019) 110–117, https://doi.org/10.1609/aaai.v33i01.3301110.

[39] N.S. Parameswaran, D. Venkataraman, A computer vision based image processing system for depression detection among students for counseling, Indones. J. Electr. Eng. Comput. Sci. 14 (1) (2019) 503–512, https://doi.org/10.11591/ijeecs.-v14.i1.pp503-512.

[40] K. Chlasta, K. Wołk, I. Krejtz, Automated speech-based screening of depression using deep convolutional neural networks,, Procedia Comput. Sci. 164 (2019) 618–628, https://doi.org/10.1016/j.procs.2019.12.228.

[41] B.G. Dadiz, C.R. Ruiz, Detecting depression in videos using uniformed local binary pattern on facial features,, Lect. Notes Electr. Eng. 481 (2019) 413–422, https://doi.org/10.1007/978-981-13-2622-6_40.

[42] S.A. Qureshi, S. Saha, M. Hasanuzzaman, G. Dias, E. Cambria, Multitask representation learning for multimodal estimation of depression level, IEEE Intell. Syst. 34 (5) (2019) 45–52, https://doi.org/10.1109/MIS.2019.2925204.

[43] W. Fan, Z. He, X. Xing, B. Cai, W. Lu, Multi-modality depression detection via multi-scale temporal dilated CNNs, in: AVEC '19: Proceedings of the 9th International on Audio/Visual Emotion Challenge and Workshop, 2019, https://doi.org/10.1145/3347320.3357695.

[44] A.H. Yazdavar, et al., Multimodal mental health analysis in social media, PLoS One 15 (4) (Apr. 2020), https://doi.org/10.1371/journal.pone.0226248.

[45] M. Rohanian, J. Hough, M. Purver, Detecting depression with word-level multimodal fusion, in: Proceedings of the Annual Conference of the International Speech Communication Association, INTERSPEECH, 2019, https://doi.org/10.21437/Interspeech.2019-2283.

[46] D.J. France, R.G. Shiavi, Acoustical properties of speech as indicators of depression and suicidal risk, IEEE Trans. Biomed. Eng. 47 (7) (2000) 829–837, https://doi.org/10.1109/10.846676.

[47] D. Revicki, R.D. Hays, D. Cella, J. Sloan, Recommended methods for determining responsiveness and minimally important differences for patient-reported outcomes, J. Clin. Epidemiol. (2008), https://doi.org/10.1016/j.jclinepi.2007.03.012.

[48] P.M. Fayers, D. Machin, Quality of Life: The Assessment, Analysis and Interpretation of Patient-Reported Outcomes, second ed., 2007.

[49] N.H.I. Hjollund, L.P. Larsen, K. Biering, S.P. Johnsen, E. Riiskjær, L.M. Schougaard, Use of patient-reported outcome (PRO) measures at group and patient levels: experiences from the generic integrated PRO system, WestChronic, J. Med. Internet Res. (2014), https://doi.org/10.2196/ijmr.2885.

[50] M.J.B. Wilkinson, P. Barczak, Psychiatric screening in general practice: comparison of the general health questionnaire and the hospital anxiety depression scale, J. Roy. Coll. Gen. Pract. 38 (312) (1988) 311–313.

[51] T.A. Widiger, W.L. Gore, Mental disorders as discrete clinical conditions: dimensional versus categorical classification, in: Adult Psychopathol. Diagnosis, seventh ed., 2014.

[52] A.T. Beck, C.H. Ward, M. Mendelson, J. Mock, J. Erbaugh, An inventory for measuring depression, Arch. Gen. Psychiatr. (1961), https://doi.org/10.1001/archpsyc.1961.01710120031004.

[53] S.T. Cheng, A.C.M. Chan, The center for epidemiologic studies depression scale in older Chinese: thresholds for long and short forms, Int. J. Geriatr. Psychiatr. (2005), https://doi.org/10.1002/gps.1314.

[54] M. HAMILTON, A rating scale for depression, J. Neurol. Neurosurg. Psychiatry (1960), https://doi.org/10.1136/jnnp.23.1.56.

[55] F. Serra, A. Spoto, M. Ghisi, G. Vidotto, Formal psychological assessment in evaluating depression: a new methodology to build exhaustive and irredundant adaptive questionnaires, PLoS One 10 (4) (2015), https://doi.org/10.1371/journal.pone.0122131.

[56] K. Kroenke, R.L. Spitzer, J.B.W. Williams, The PHQ-9: validity of a brief depression severity measure, J. Gen. Intern. Med. 16 (9) (2001), https://doi.org/10.1046/j.1525-1497.2001.016009606.x.

[57] C. Peterson, Psychological approaches to mental illness, in: A Handbook for the Study of Mental Health, 2012.

[58] P. Ekman, An argument for basic emotions, Cognit. Emot. (1992), https://doi.org/10.1080/02699939208411068.

[59] J.A. Russell, A. Mehrabian, Evidence for a three-factor theory of emotions, J. Res. Pers. (1977), https://doi.org/10.1016/0092-6566(77)90037-X.

[60] A. Mehrabian, Pleasure-Arousal-Dominance: a general framework for describing and measuring individual differences in temperament, Curr. Psychol. (1996), https://doi.org/10.1007/bf02686918.
[61] A. Mehrabian, Analysis of the big-five personality factors in terms of the PAD temperament model, Aust. J. Psychol. 48 (2) (1996) 86−92.
[62] A.T. Beck, Cognitive therapy: past, present, and future, J. Consult. Clin. Psychol. 61 (2) (1993), https://doi.org/10.1037/0022-006X.61.2.194.
[63] R. Law, Interpersonal psychotherapy for depression, Adv. Psychiatr. Treat. 17 (1) (2011), https://doi.org/10.1192/apt.bp.109.007641.
[64] P. Cuijpers, A psychoeducational approach to the treatment of depression: a meta-analysis of Lewinsohn's 'Coping with Depression' course, Behav. Ther. 29 (3) (1998), https://doi.org/10.1016/S0005-7894(98)80047-6.
[65] J.H. Riskind, E. Calvete, Anxiety and the dynamic self as defined by the prospection and mental simulation of looming future threats, J. Pers. 88 (1) (2020), https://doi.org/10.1111/jopy.12465.
[66] B.L. Hankin, L.Y. Abramson, N. Miller, G.J. Haeffel, Cognitive vulnerability-stress theories of depression: examining affective specificity in the prediction of depression versus anxiety in three prospective studies, Cognit. Ther. Res. (2004), https://doi.org/10.1023/B:COTR.0000031805.60529.0d.
[67] A.T. Beck, B.A. Alford, Depression: Causes and Treatment, second ed., 2009.
[68] R.E. Thayer, Mood regulation and general arousal systems, Psychol. Inq. 11 (3) (2000) 202−204.
[69] M. Mehu, K.R. Scherer, The appraisal bias model of cognitive vulnerability to depression, Emotion Rev. 7 (3) (2015) 272−279, https://doi.org/10.1177/1754073915575406.
[70] H.H. Son, ScienceDirect toward a computational model of mood, Procedia Comput. Sci. 110 (2017) 199−206, https://doi.org/10.1016/j.procs.2017.06.085.
[71] N. Ahmadpour, OCC model: application and comparison to the dimensional model of emotion, in: KEER2014. Proc. 5th Kanesi Eng. Emot. Res. Int. Conf. Link{ö}ping; Sweden; June 11−13, no. 100, 2014, pp. 607−617.
[72] R. Islam, M.F. Zibran, DEVA : Sensing Emotions in the Valence Arousal Space in Software Engineering Text, 2018, pp. 1536−1543.
[73] J. Rottenberg, Mood and emotion in major depression, Curr. Dir. Psychol. Sci. 14 (3) (2005) 167−170, https://doi.org/10.1111/j.0963-7214.2005.00354.x.
[74] A. Husseini Orabi, P. Buddhitha, M. Husseini Orabi, D. Inkpen, Deep learning for depression detection of twitter users, in: Proceedings of the Fifth Workshop on Computational Linguistics and Clinical Psychology: From Keyboard to Clinic, May 2018, pp. 88−97, https://doi.org/10.18653/v1/w18-0609.
[75] X. Cheng, X. Wang, T. Ouyang, Z. Feng, Advances in emotion recognition: link to depressive disorder, in: Mental Disorders, 2020.
[76] S. Alghowinem, Multimodal analysis of verbal and nonverbal behaviour on the example of clinical depression, Diss. Abstr. Int. Sect. B Sci. Eng. 77 (2-B(E)) (2016).
[77] S. Poria, E. Cambria, R. Bajpai, A. Hussain, A review of affective computing: from unimodal analysis to multimodal fusion, Inf. Fusion 37 (2017), https://doi.org/10.1016/j.inffus.2017.02.003.
[78] C. Su, Z. Xu, J. Pathak, F. Wang, Deep learning in mental health outcome research: a scoping review, Transl. Psychiatr. 10 (1) (2020), https://doi.org/10.1038/s41398-020-0780-3.
[79] E. Garcia-Ceja, M. Riegler, T. Nordgreen, P. Jakobsen, K.J. Oedegaard, J. Tørresen, Mental health monitoring with multimodal sensing and machine learning: a survey, Pervasive Mob. Comput. (2018), https://doi.org/10.1016/j.pmcj.2018.09.003.

[80] T. Baltrusaitis, C. Ahuja, L.P. Morency, Multimodal machine learning: a survey and taxonomy, IEEE Trans. Pattern Anal. Mach. Intell. (2019), https://doi.org/10.1109/TPAMI.2018.2798607.
[81] S. Alghowinem, et al., Multimodal depression detection: fusion analysis of paralinguistic, head pose and eye gaze behaviors, IEEE Trans. Affect. Comput. 9 (4) (2018), https://doi.org/10.1109/TAFFC.2016.2634527.
[82] N. Cummins, V. Sethu, J. Epps, S. Schnieder, J. Krajewski, Analysis of acoustic space variability in speech affected by depression, Speech Commun. (2015), https://doi.org/10.1016/j.specom.2015.09.003.
[83] J.K. Darby, H. Hollien, Vocal and speech patterns of depressive patients, Folia Phoniatrica Logop. (1977), https://doi.org/10.1159/000264098.
[84] M. De Choudhury, S. Counts, E.J. Horvitz, A. Hoff, Characterizing and predicting postpartum depression from shared facebook data, in: CSCW'14: Proceedings of the 17th ACM conference on Computer supported cooperative work & social computing, 2014, https://doi.org/10.1145/2531602.2531675.
[85] P. Ekman, W.V. Friesen, Nonverbal leakage and clues to deception, Psychiatry (1969), https://doi.org/10.1080/00332747.1969.11023575.
[86] P. Ekman, Telling Lies: Clues to Deceit in the Marketplace, Politics, and Marriage, 1985.
[87] S. Porter, L. Ten Brinke, Reading between the lies: identifying concealed and falsified emotions in universal facial expressions, Psychol. Sci. (2008), https://doi.org/10.1111/j.1467-9280.2008.02116.x.
[88] P. Ekman, W.V. Friesen, Facial action coding system: a technique for the measurement of facial movement, J. Pers. Soc. Psychol. (1971), https://doi.org/10.1037/h0030377.
[89] D. Borza, R. Itu, R. Danescu, Micro expression detection and recognition from high speed cameras using convolutional neural networks, in: 13th International Joint Conference on Computer Vision, Imaging and Computer Graphics Theory and Applications at: Madeira, Portuga, 2018, https://doi.org/10.5220/0006548802010208.
[90] M. Verma, S.K. Vipparthi, G. Singh, S. Murala, LEARNet: dynamic imaging network for micro expression recognition, IEEE Trans. Image Process. (2020), https://doi.org/10.1109/TIP.2019.2912358.
[91] W.S. Chow, J. Schmidtke, A. Loerbroks, T. Muth, P. Angerer, The relationship between personality traits with depressive symptoms and suicidal ideation among med ical students: a cross-sectional study at one medical school in Germany, Int. J. Environ. Res. Publ. Health 15 (7) (2018), https://doi.org/10.3390/ijerph15071462.
[92] D.N. Klein, R. Kotov, S.J. Bufferd, Personality and depression: explanatory models and review of the evidence, Annu. Rev. Clin. Psychol. 7 (2011), https://doi.org/10.1146/annurev-clinpsy-032210-104540.
[93] C. Hakulinen, M. Elovainio, L. Pulkki-Råback, M. Virtanen, M. Kivimäki, M. Jokela, Personality and depressive symptoms: individual participant meta-analysis of 10 cohort studies, Depress. Anxiety 32 (7) (2015), https://doi.org/10.1002/da.22376.
[94] Y. Li, et al., Linking personality types to depressive symptoms: a prospective typology based on neuroticism, extraversion and conscientiousness, Neuropsychologia 136 (2020), https://doi.org/10.1016/j.neuropsychologia.2019.107289.
[95] H.S. Akiskal, R.M.A. Hirschfeld, B.I. Yerevanian, The relationship of personality to affective disorders: a critical review, Arch. Gen. Psychiatr. 40 (7) (1983), https://doi.org/10.1001/archpsyc.1983.01790060099013.
[96] M.H. Klein, S. Wonderlich, M.T. Shea, Models of relationships between personality and depression: toward a framework for theory and research, in: Personality and Depression, 1993.

[97] S. Stuart, Personality and depression: a current view, Psychiatr. Serv. 46 (4) (1995), https://doi.org/10.1176/ps.46.4.415.
[98] R.F. Krueger, J.L. Tackett, Personality and psychopathology: working toward the bigger picture, J. Pers. Disord. 17 (2) (2003), https://doi.org/10.1521/pedi.17.2.109.23986.
[99] C.F. Duggan, A.S. Lee, R.M. Murray, Does personality predict long-term outcome in depression? Br. J. Psychiatry 157 (1990) https://doi.org/10.1192/bjp.157.1.19.
[100] D.S. Charney, J.C. Nelson, D.M. Quinlan, Personality traits and disorder in depression, Am. J. Psychiatr. 138 (12) (1981), https://doi.org/10.1176/ajp.138.12.1601.
[101] L.A. Clark, D. Watson, S. Mineka, Temperament, personality, and the mood and anxiety disorders, J. Abnorm. Psychol. 103 (1) (1994) 103–116, https://doi.org/10.1037/0021-843X.103.1.103.
[102] S. Tsugawa, Y. Kikuchi, F. Kishino, K. Nakajima, Y. Itoh, H. Ohsaki, Recognizing depression from twitter activity, in: The 33rd Annual ACM Conference, 2015, https://doi.org/10.1145/2702123.2702280.
[103] J.D. Henry, W. Von Hippel, P. Molenberghs, T. Lee, P.S. Sachdev, Clinical assessment of social cognitive function in neurological disorders, Nat. Rev. Neurol. (2016), https://doi.org/10.1038/nrneurol.2015.229.
[104] X. Wang, C. Zhang, Y. Ji, L. Sun, L. Wu, Z. Bao, A depression detection model based on sentiment analysis in micro-blog social network, in: Pacific-Asia Conference on Knowledge Discovery and Data Mining, 2013, https://doi.org/10.1007/978-3-642-40319-4_18.
[105] X. Wang, C. Zhang, L. Sun, An improved model for depression detection in micro-blog social network, in: Proceedings of the 2013 IEEE 13th International Conference on Data Mining Workshops, 2013, https://doi.org/10.1109/ICDMW.2013.132.
[106] S. Saxena, M. Funk, D. Chisholm, WHO's Mental Health Action Plan 2013–2020: what can psychiatrists do to facilitate its implementation? World Psychiatr. (2014) https://doi.org/10.1002/wps.20141.
[107] V. Del Barrio, Diagnostic and statistical manual of mental disorders, in: The Curated Reference Collection in Neuroscience and Biobehavioral Psychology, 2016.

CHAPTER TEN

Improving mental health surveillance over Twitter text classification using word embedding techniques

Reno Ardian Syaputra and Rashid Ali
Department of Computer Engineering, Aligarh Muslim University, Aligarh, Uttar Pradesh, India

1. Introduction

As the web quickly develops, web users are also evolving. People are progressively connecting, sharing, and working together using social media. The size of social web growing exponentially is caused by the huge amount of collective information. This condition leads to the difficulties of refining knowledge from data, especially to monitor a person mental development through comments they leave on social media such as twitter. Twitter has been growing very fast as one of the most popular social networking websites. It reaches up to 284 million monthly active users and sends over 500 million tweets per day [1]. Moreover, content on the web is only suitable for human consumption and hard to be processed by machine [2]. This is where Natural Language Processing (NLP) methods have a contribution in text analysis.

The main benefit of the NLP methods is direct application in text mining. Text mining or intelligent text analysis can obtain important information and knowledge from those unstructured textual data. Choosing proper NLP techniques reduces time to find patterns and decision-making. This is relevant since most of the information from the web is more than 80% stored as text [3]. However, text cannot be fed for machine learning algorithms right away. Text should be encoded as numbers either as input or output of neural network models [4].

Word embedding or word vector is one of the possible ways for representing words into numbers. This model is often referred to as semantic distribution in computational linguistics [5]. Importantly, word embeddings

Artificial Intelligence, Machine Learning, and Mental Health in Pandemics
ISBN: 978-0-323-91196-2
https://doi.org/10.1016/B978-0-323-91196-2.00014-4

allow us to maintain usable meaning and similarity relationships while having it on numerical type data. The idea behind this concept is to look at the word context. A word, which appears in a paragraph, has a context represented by the set of words that appear nearby within a fixed-size window [6].

One of the profound word embedding algorithms is called Word2Vec [7]. The algorithm consists of two models developed over neural networks, namely Skip-gram and Continuous-Bag-of-Word. Despite these advances, most of the word embedding techniques have the same problem, where each word must be encoded all its potential meanings into one vector [8]. For polysemy words [9], regardless of a sentence where a word appears, its number representation is always the same. For example, the word "Jaguar" will always have the same matrix either as an animal or a brand. Thus, this method is called static word embedding [10].

Many new methods have been proposed since the milestone of word embedding. More recent works that are occupying deep neural language models such as ELMo [11] and BERT [12] have succeeded in developing contextual word representations. These models are sensitive word vectors toward the context in which it appears. Replacing static word embeddings with contextual representations has resulted in significant improvements for many NLP tasks [13]. ELMo and BERT differ from their predecessors. They can capture different latent syntactic-semantic information of the same word based on a contextual use [14].

Given the number of choices of word embedding models, it raises the question of their performance in text classification. Previous experiments on analyzing Twitter data showed that word embedding can be used as a complement to a clustering algorithm for topic classification [1]. Measurement in similarity, which formulated as the sum of semantic combinations and syntactic metrics, is the main feature of detecting topics. Using the similarity score of the clustered words, tweets can be classified.

The objective of this project is to analyze the tweets by performing text classification-based clustering using different word representation methods (Word2Vec, ELMo, and BERT). Then, these clusters are evaluated for their quality in which the representation gets the best quality of clusters. Performance evaluation is done through confusion matrix observation.

2. Related work

The use of word embedding is gaining popularity interest because of the usefulness in variety problems domains. With word embeddings, deep-learning-based techniques have recently gotten a lot of interest. Word2Vec is a word embedding framework that encodes multiple aspects of words using dense, low-dimensional, and real-valued vectors [7]. Since then, deep-learning-based word representation models provide contextualized embeddings, which have progressively developed, namely ELMo in 2018 [11] and BERT in 2016 [12].

Many text classification tasks showing improvement by incorporating word embedding models with clustering [1] have performed word embedding based on clustering method, which has ever been conducted for health issue by classifying tweets. In the research done over Twitter data, the context of words in tweets is represented by the vectors of word embeddings. Using cosine similarity, words in tweets can be split into clusters whether it is related or not to the health issue. The tweets are classified based on the similarity measure of the clusters of words. If the similarity score is toward 1, then it is most likely related to the topic. The proposed method shows a better result compared to standard Naive Bayes method.

Word embedding can also be used for feature reduction [15]. Combining Word2Vec with several classifiers showed that feature reduction achieved along with improvement in classification accuracy. Especially for K-means clustering with word embedding method, a research has shown a result where word embedding techniques are successfully applicable for a large variety of disciplines or a given problem domain, according to a study that sought to extract subject from bibliometric data [16].

3. Methodology

The framework of this project is shown in Fig. 10.1 and can be illustrated as follows.

3.1 Dataset

In Twitter, an original text that is posted directly by the user is called as a tweet. An original tweet can be shared to other platform or retweeted by any other users. In this experiment, we are interested in collecting tweets that are not a reshared or retweeted but the original tweet by streaming them. The tweet was streamed with the topics "corona virus" "covid-19" and "covid pandemic." We streamed from Twitter API to collect the datasets. The result of this process is a JSON file format, which is the standard format used by Twitter for information exchange.

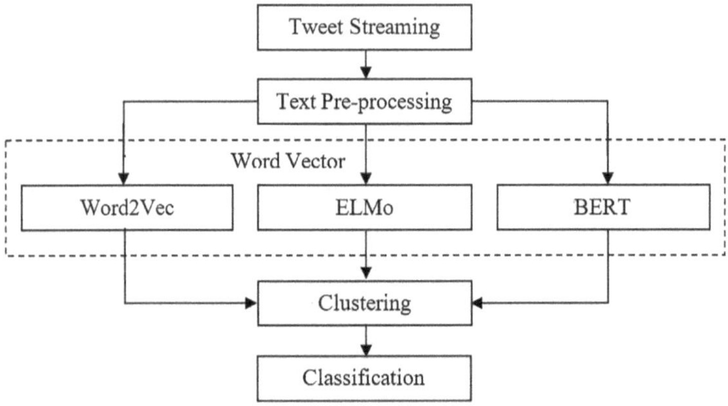

Figure 10.1 Workflow of the tweets classification.

3.2 Text-preprocessing

Tweets collected through Twitter Streaming API are real-time broadcasted. Random tweets that have shared publicly about certain topics are unclean. Text preprocessing is the method of tokenizing or normalizing tweets that include diverse noise text including such hash tags, slangs, abbreviations, or URLs. In this process, JSON file needed to be filtered out of noise and meaningless symbols that have no contribution in the text analysis framework. The steps to clean text in this process are shown in Fig. 10.2.

3.3 Word vector conversion

Words in tweet are converted because machine learning model is not able to process the raw text directly. The fundamental objective of word conversion is to provide the classifier a collection of training datasets that have been sorted into one or more preset classes in numeric data format. The machine learning model then trains using the word vector dataset to automatically classify fresh incoming inputs that have never been seen before.

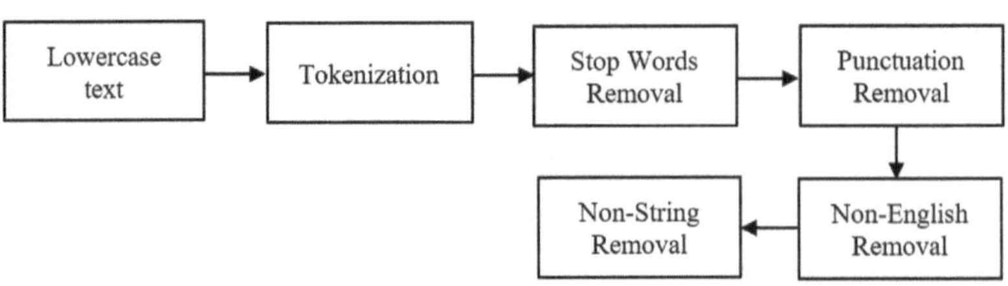

Figure 10.2 Text-preprocessing steps.

Many real-world applications have investigated the difficulties of the implementation of text classification. Furthermore, many researchers have tried in building applications that use text classification algorithms by combining the word embedding on the neural network-based model. The initial step of text classification is always done by processing the raw text dataset. Textual datasets, in general, contain text sequences from documents, which is denoted as $D = \{X1, X2, X3, \ldots, XN\}$ where Xi is a data point with s number of sentences, each of which includes w_s words with l_w letters. A class value is assigned to each point from a collection of k as different discrete value indices [17].

The primary four steps of the text classification framework can be deconstructed into feature extraction, dimension reductions, classifier selection, and model evaluation. Text is an unstructured data collection in general. However, because it is utilized in mathematical modeling as part of the classification, this unstructured text sequence needs to be transformed into a structured feature [3]. Data must be cleaned to remove superfluous letters and words, thus preprocessing must be completed before feature extraction methods can be used.

Weighted word techniques and word embedding are two well-known methods for feature extraction. But, this project is primarily concerned with the usage of word embedding because of its high accuracy rate for evaluating semantic similarity between two words with low computing cost [15]. Word embedding is a characteristic of the learning approach in which each sentence is assigned to a real number N random space from the lexicon. To convert unigrams into numbers for machine learning algorithms, many approaches of word embedding have been utilized.

Because text datasets frequently contain a large number of unique words, the processes of the text preprocessing might take a long time and require a lot of memory. The use of dimensionality reduction techniques is a popular solution to this problem. However, these methods do not have a good performance when applied in some datasets [17]. Many researchers choose to utilize dimensionality reduction to lower the memory usage burden of their systems in order to prevent performance degradation.

The classifier algorithm is the most critical stage in the text classification process. The algorithms such as Random Forest, Naive Bayes, and K-Nearest neighbor are still widely employed, but in this work we implemented K-Means++ clustering [18]. Support vector machines (SVMs), particularly kernel SVM, are another popular classification approach. For document categorization, tree-based classification algorithms such as decision trees and random forests are also quick and accurate. These popular classification algorithms will be used as the baseline models for the comparison with our word embedding-based clustering model.

Evaluation is the final step in the text classification pipeline. Performance evaluation is done to examine different parts of the performance tweet classification tasks. In practice, model evaluation is used to estimate the performance of the model through cross-validation [17]. The parameters used for measuring performance in this work are using confusion matrix. This metrix gives an understanding that reflects information about the true positive, true negative, false positive, and false negative (TP, TN, FP, and FN respectively) class from classification. From the metrix, we calculate the measurement parameters such as recall, precision, F1-measure, and accuracy.

3.3.1 Word embedding

NLP is a subfield of computer science, which combines artificial intelligence and linguistics. NLP appears to facilitate human in the sense that machine can communicate through natural language [19]. Using intelligence techniques, NLP enables computer to learn the meaning behind words. Meaning can be defined as the idea that is represented by a word, phrase, or any other particular conceptual relation behind the physical appearance. Common linguistic way to think about meaning is called denotational semantics. Using this idea, thus the word "chair" is the semantic representation, which comes from the actual chair in the real world.

Syntactic and semantic are the two primary terms to understand human language. Syntax refers to the sentence structure and grammatical arrangement. Even though people can do what they want with language, syntax helps general users of a language as well as machine to understand words organization. Semantics, on the other hand, refers to the meaning of a sentence it self. For example, the sentence "a rabbit is chasing dog" might make sense on the syntactic level, but it is odd when it comes to semantics. That is why intelligence techniques are needed in processing natural language, because textual data does not appear just like numbers.

There are a lot of NLP preprocessing techniques known to clean text datasets from noise. Because, unnecessary noise and features can degrade system performance in many statistical and probabilistic learning methods. So, before moving on to the feature extraction section, the text must be cleaned. Lowercasing, lemmatizing, stemming, stop word removal, tokenization, and non-English word removal are the main preprocessing techniques used in NLP. Despite being simple, tokenization works better than more complex preprocessing techniques such as lemmatization or many word groupings, except for certain domains where data set performing poorly [20].

Conventional NLP regards words as discretes symbols where words are represented in a vectors consisting of 0 and 1. This method is called one-hot word vectors representation [9]. Using this way, a vector may end up with a very high dimension, because the length of the vector is derived from the number of words in the model. For example, if a model consists of 30 millions words, then it has 30 million dimensions just for representing a word in one-hot vector, and the rest are zero. The problem with one-hot vector representation is that it is orthogonal, meaning there is no similarity relationship among the words in the model.

A binary vector is used to represent a category variable in one-hot encoding. Each word's value is represented as a binary vector with all zero values except for the word's index, which is 1. Table 10.1 is the illustration of one-hot encoding matrix. It is easy to implement and work fast, but during the process, the meaning of the word in the sentence is lost. Thus, hot encoding is not widely used in NLP applications.

Common solution for having usable word meaning representation in a machine is using WordNet. WordNet is a large lexical English database, which divides lexicons into five categories, nouns, verbs, adjectives, adverbs, and function word. Nouns, verbs, and adjectives are organized into a set of synonyms, each representing one underlying lexical concept. Additionally, this model also covers list of hypernyms. Hypernyms are words that have general meanings as opposed to hyponyms.

Problem with WordNet and any other resource in the same types are lacks of nuance. For example, the word "proficient" is listed as a synonym for "good." This may be true, but it is only correct in some context. The word "proficient" can also have a synonym of "expert." Furthermore, developing WordNet requires human labor, and it is impossible to keep up-to-date. Thus it is not scalable.

Table 10.1 The illustration of one-hot encoding matrix.

Word	One-hot vector					
Man	1	0	0	0	0	0
Woman	0	1	0	0	0	0
Person	0	0	1	0	0	0
People	0	0	0	1	0	0
Horse	0	0	0	0	1	0
Elephant	0	0	0	0	0	1

Distributional semantic is the most successful idea in the modern statistical NLP. The idea of this method is developing word vectors model by looking at the words context. A word, which appears in a paragraph, has a context represented by the set of words that appear nearby within a fixed-size window. For example, consider the sentences below:

1. As happened in 2009, government debt concerns morphed into *banking* crises.
2. Claiming that Europe requires a unified *banking* regulatory framework to replace the patchwork.
3. India's *banking* system has just received a boost.

The word "banking" might have several meanings. Those words surrounding the "banking" word are the contexts that support the meaning of banking. Words and context are what need to be represented in numerical form so that they can be processed by machines.

Word embedding as a numerical representation of words is also known as word vector. The concept is discussed as semantic distribution in the linguistic field [4]. Word embeddings have emerged as a research topic in NLP because of its usefulness in the downstream tasks. The model can encode syntactic and semantic word relationship, thus making the representation carry information about the meaning of words.

Table 10.2 shows the simplified version of word embeddings, which each dimension captures meaning shown in numbers. For example, the word "Man" has the vector [0.4, 0.4, 0.09, −0.01, 0.14], which represents how close it relates each other. Several studies have shown that word embedding is a valuable tool for enhancing NLP tasks including part-of-speech tagging, chunking, syntactic parsing, named entity identification, and semantic role labeling [5].

Table 10.2 The illustration of the word embedding concept.

		Dimensions				
Vectors	**Word**	**Animal**	**Domesticated**	**King**	**Woman**	**Pet**
	Man	0.4	0.4	0.09	−0.01	0.14
	Woman	0.15	0.02	0.07	−0.2	0.08
	Person	0.19	−0.5	0.4	0.54	−0.68
	People	0.08	−0.14	0.34	0.7	−0.02
	Horse	0.7	0.41	−0.44	−0.02	0.03
	Elephant	0.27	0.1	−0.01	0.02	0.04

Word embedding represents the word as a multidimensional continuous number where similar words are mapped to the nearest point in geometric space. This means that words such as "proficient" and "good" must have a vector similar to the word "expert" due to the similar meaning. In simplified terms, each dimension in word vector represents a meaning and the numerical weight of the word on that dimension captures the closeness of its relationship [6]. Thus, the semantics of the word are embedded in all dimensions of the vector.

The correlation between "Man" and "King" may be derived from Table 3.2 by calculating the vector distance between them. For the purpose of illustration, a two-dimensional word vector is presented in Fig. 10.3. In the real practice, the vector is on high dimensional. Because a high-dimensional vector cannot be read easily, dimensionality reduction should be applied for the visualization purpose. As addition, the distance is expressed in Cosine, which is the distance between two points in vector space (Fig. 10.3).

Suppose we have the following word vectors "King" "Man" and "Woman" to predict the word vector of the "Queen" based on the word embedding model in Fig. 10.3. This can be explained as if what is the closest vector relationship to the result of the equation:

$$\text{vec(King)} - \text{vec(Man)} + \text{vec(Woman)} = \text{vec(queen)}$$

This indicates that the vector distance between linked words is less than the vector distance between unrelated words from a mathematical standpoint.

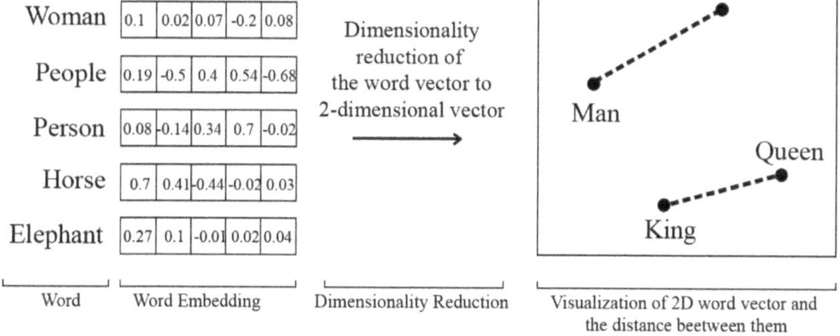

Figure 10.3 Word vector visualization.

3.3.2 Word2Vec

Different approaches have been proposed for developing word embedding over neural networks. Mikolov [7] presented the improvement architecture of word embedding called word-to-vector or Word2Vec through two hidden layer neural network. With Word2Vec we are able to predict word based on its neighboring words in a fixed-size window. By grouping related words together, the distributed representation of words in the vector space aids the learning algorithm in achieving higher performance for NLP tasks. Word2Vecs has two architectures: Continuous Bag-of-Words (CBOW) and Skip-Gram.

The core model of Word2Vecs is quite similar in algorithm. The CBOW model learns to predict target words by using of all the words in its environment. On the other hand, the Skip-Gram model does inverse learning to predict words based on the neighboring words. As a result, if we put a word, the model will learn to predict words in its context [5]. Finding word representation that is useful for prediction process of the context words in a sentence is the objective of the Skip-Gram model. In detail, consider this sequence of training words $w1,\ w2,\ w3,\ \ldots,\ w_T$. The goal of the Skip-gram model, as stated in the equation below, is to maximize the average probability.

$$\frac{1}{T}\sum_{t=1}^{T}\sum_{-c\leq j\leq c,\, j\neq 0} log\, p\left(w_{t+j}\mid w_t\right)$$

Where c is a metric for the learning process, which can be a function of the center word wt. When c is resulting greater, it will generate more training instances and hence greater accuracy, but as the cost of increased training time [7]. The basic Skip-Gram probability formula is defined using the softmax function shown in the formula below.

$$p(w_O\mid w_I) = \frac{\exp\left(v'_{wo}\, T_{v_{wI}}\right)}{\sum_{w=1}^{W}\exp\left(v'_{wo}\, T_{v_{wI}}\right)}$$

In the formula above, v_w and v'_w are the "input" and "output" vector representations of w, and W is the amount of words in the data set. The way neural network trained into Skip-Gram model uses tricks called fake task, which can be seen in other machine learning algorithm. A hidden layer neural network is utilized to perform a specific job; however, the model will not be used for the purpose for which it was trained. Instead, the goal is to figure out what the concealed layer weights are. The "word vector" is made up of these weights.

The neural network's fictitious goal in the Skip-Gram model is to examine neighboring words. The input word is a specific word that appears in the midst of a sentence. The algorithm then selects one word at random from the adjacent words in the fixed-size window. The network then tells the probability of each word in the vocabulary of being "closest word" that was chosen. When compared to Skip-gram, the fake job in CBOW is slightly different. The model still takes a pair of words and teaches the model the likelihood of words occurring together. The distinction is that the algorithm adds input words for the same target word instead of errors.

A typical window size of the Skip-Gram model is 5, which means five words behind and five words ahead and 10 in total. The likelihood of the output is proportional to the chance of each vocabulary term being found near the input word. For example, given a trained network the word "Man" as the input, the probability of the output will be higher for words "Woman" and "King" than for unrelated words "Cat" and "Horse" The word pairings discovered in the training text are used to train the neural network.

The examples in Fig. 10.4 show the training examples of word pairs taken from the sentence "The brown fox is quick to jump over a lazy dog" For the purpose of illustration, the small window size of 2 is used. Words highlighted in gray are the input words. By using word pairs in fixed-size window, the neural network will learn the probability of how much times each pair appears. For example, the network will get more training samples ("Lazy", "Dog") than ("Smart", "Dog"). After the training

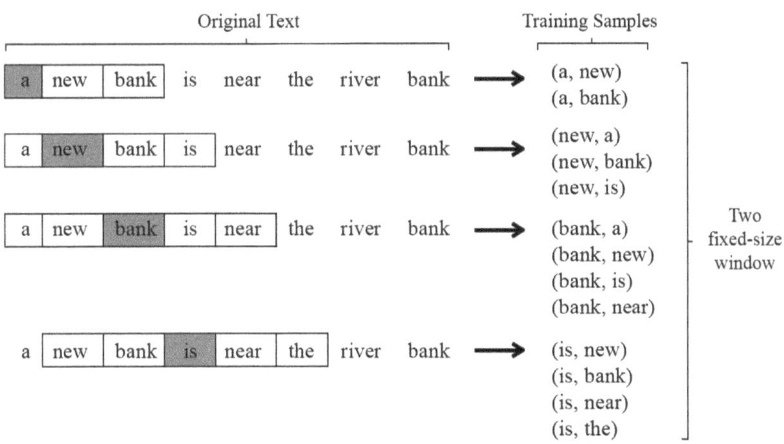

Figure 10.4 Word pairs illustration in two fixed-size windows.

is over, if the word "Lazy" is used as test input, the result will show the probability higher for the word "Dog" rather than "Fox."

Textual data set cannot be implemented in neural network directly. So, word needs a way to be represented as number for the network. One way to do this is by building a vocabulary word from our training set, for example, a vocabulary that consists of 10000 words. One-hot vector will be used to represent the words as input. Each word in the lexicon will have 10,000 dimensions in this vector. The one-hot vector model will have a value of "1" in the location corresponding to a specific word and 0 in the remaining places. For the record, the network's output for each word in the vocabulary is a single vector with 10,000 dimensions. Fig. 10.5 is the neural network architecture of the Skip-Gram model for the text "a new bank is near the river bank" as the input.

In Fig. 10.5, the input is shown to be a single-hot vector encoding the input word "bank." The output word is also represented by the training output, which is a one-hot vector. The output vector of a trained network assessed on an input word, however, is a probability distribution rather than a one-hot vector. In addition to this, in Fig. 10.5, the hidden layer neurons have no activation function, while the output layer employs softmax, as explained in the formula above.

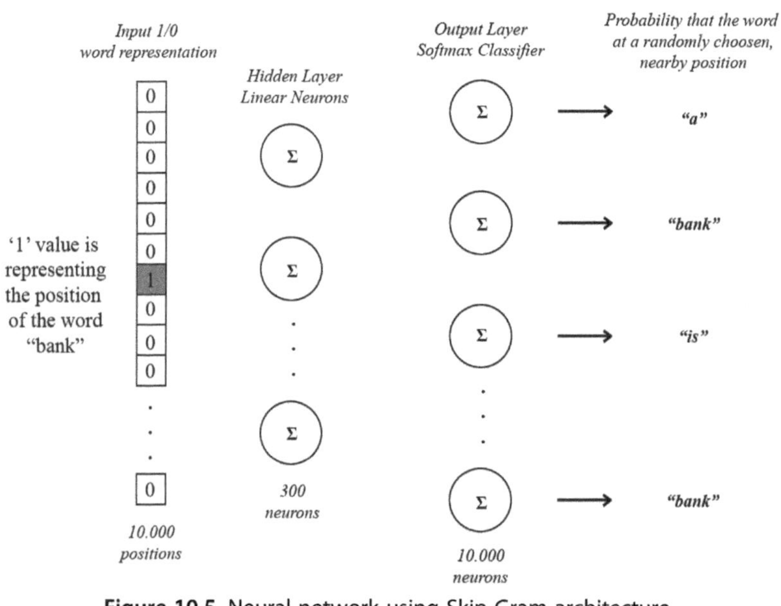

Figure 10.5 Neural network using Skip-Gram architecture.

3.3.3 ELMo

Word2Vec has achieved great success in solving most of NLP task, even though it still suffers a problem of polysemic words. This happens because the words in the model are represented by static word embeddings. This means that each word is represented by a vector that remains constant in its environment. Under this situation, for a polysemous word [9], regardless of a sentence where a word appears, its number representation is always the same. An alternative way to overcome the polysemic problem is to use contextual embeddings, where vector representations change according to words context.

Embedding from Language Model (ELMo) is a word representation that provides deep contextual embeddings for both syntactics and semantics. This model is able to handle various linguistic contexts, particularly for polysemy words. The ability comes from the bidirectional LSTM (bi-LSTM), which is pretrained on a large unlabeled text corpus. ELMo word vector is built on a two-layered two-way language model (bi-LM) with character convolutions. This bi-LM model has two layers stacked up together, which each layer then has two passes called feed forward and backward.

The ELMo architecture creates word representations based on character embeddings using a character convolutional neural network (Char-CNN). This approach reduces the number of parameters while also minimizing out-of-vocabulary (OOV) issues. The ELMo architecture uses a character convolutional neural network to construct word representations based on character embeddings (Char-CNN). This method minimizes out-of-vocabulary (OOV) problems while reducing the amount of parameters.

The motivation of using ELMo is that word embeddings should understand word level characteristics as well as contextual semantics. Previously, word embeddings are not context-specific, meaning that they study based on word concurrence, so they do not know about sequential context. For example, in these two sentences, "I slice apples" and "I bought an Apple phone," the word "apples" refers to very different meanings but they have the same word vector representation. The answer is based on a product of all of the bi-internal LSTM's layers. To obtain the final embeddings, ELMo generates vectors for each of the internal functions of each layer and merges them in a weight.

ELMo learns to predict the next word in a word sequence and therefore gains language comprehension. This is the task of Language Modeling. Instead of assigning each word a fixed word vector, ELMo examines the full phrase before assigning each word a number, resulting in slightly varied embeddings for each occurrence. For instance, consider this sentence "The broadway play was premiered yesterday" The word "play" in the above example will be assigned to one static vector representation if standard word embeddings such as Glove, Fast Text, or Word2Vec are implemented. Despite that the word "Play" has several meanings such as the verb to play or in this case, a theater house.

The bi-LM concept is clearly stated in the ELMo original paper [11]. Given a sequence of N words, ($w1$, $w2$, ..., wN), a forward language model will compute the probability of the given sequence by modeling the probability of word wk given the previous words ($w1$, $w2$, ..., wk-1), the backward model; on the other hand, moves in the opposite directionA backward LM are identical to a forward LM, except it predicts the previous word based on the future context in reverse ($wk + 1$, ..., wN). The biLM model combines both a forward and backward concept. The forward and backward functions' log probabilities are simultaneously maximized in this approach:

$$L = \sum_{t=1}^{N} (\log P(w_t|w_1, w_2, \ldots, w_{t-1}) + (\log P(w_t|w_{t+1}, w_{t+2}, \ldots, w_N)$$

ELMo is a special task combination of intermediate layer representations in biLM. For each context, the biLM has L-layer LSTMs, which produces $2L + 1$ representations for word w_t:

$$R_t = \left\{ x_t, \overrightarrow{h_{t \cdot j}}; \overrightarrow{h_{t \cdot j}} \middle| j = 1, \ldots, L \right\} = \left\{ \overrightarrow{h_{t \cdot j}} \middle| j = 1, \ldots, L \right\}$$

Where $h_{t,0} = x_t$ is the output of the character CNN, and $h_{t.j}$ is the concatenation of the j-th-layer hidden representations of forward and backward LSTMs. When applying the ELMo to downstream tasks, the simplest way is to select the top layer $h_{t,L}$. Generally, task-specific weighting of all biLM layers is calculated as:

$$\text{ELMo}_t = \lambda \sum_{j=0}^{L} S_j h_{t \cdot j}$$

ELMo successfully learns an unlimited unlabeled data collection to dynamically represent words. It improves NLP tasks such as question answering, semantic labeling, textual entailment, entity extraction, and sentiment analysis significantly. Much of the work on this model has focused on transfers linguistic information drawn from large text without labels for downstream task. ELMo does this by pretraining a language model on unlabeled data before fine-tuning it for a specific purpose. As a result, this sort of study is known as pretraining language modeling, and contextual representation is usually regarded a by-product.

3.3.4 BERT

Previous models, such as ELMo, have effectively learnt information from vast amounts of unlabeled data in order to do better downstream tasks by fine-tuning language modeling on target tasks. The use of LSTM networks has hampered their models' capacity to capture long-range relationships [9]. To deal with this problem, Generative Pre-Training (GPT) model is proposed by Ref. [21]. To learn a longer-range language structure, GPT employs transformer networks. Despite the advance model, GPT and other language model-based methods are limited by the language model's unidirectional aim, which restricts the model's perspective to just left or right context during pretraining.

Bidirectional Encoder Representations from Transformers (BERT) was proposed to maximize the potential of the pretrained contextualized representation. The two pretraining objectives allow the model to be used on any single sequence and sequence-pair tasks without substantial specific modifications. Pretraining and fine-tuning are the two phases in the BERT system. The model is trained on unlabeled data across several pretraining tasks during pretraining. The BERT model is fine-tuned by initializing it with the pretrained parameters and then fine-tuning all of the parameters using labeled data from the downstream tasks.

Based on the original implementation detailed in the Transformer paper, BERT's model architecture is a multilayer bidirectional Transformer Encoder [22]. The designs are utilized in both pretraining and fine-tuning, in addition to the output layers. For various downstream jobs, the same pretrained model parameters are utilized to initialize models. All settings are fine-tuned during fine-tuning. [CLS] is a special symbol added in front of every input example, and [SEP] is a special separator token (e.g., separating questions and answers). Transformer uses a layered self-attention and pointwise architecture with fully linked layers for the encoder and decoder.

BERT pretrained consists of two unsupervised tasks, the Masked Language Model (MLM) and Next Sentence Prediction (NSP). MLM's goal is to forecast the words in a context that is randomly masked, allowing the model to capture both left and right. NSP, on the other hand, is used to predict if a sentence A follows a sentence B, with the training data coming from any monolingual corpus. NSP has been proven to be beneficial in tasks such as Question Answering and Natural Language Inference.

With its large number of parameters, BERT is essentially a neural network design. The number of people in the range might be anywhere from 100 million to over 300 million. As a result, starting from scratch with a short dataset and training a BERT model would result in overfitting. Thus for task-specific model, for example, text classification, fine-tuning BERT model is preferable. There are several benefits to doing this rather than training a specialized deep learning model, such as CNN, BiLSTM, or others.

BERT may be fine-tuned in three different ways. First, we can easily create a model. A lot of information about words is already contained in the pretrained BERT model weights. As a result, training our fine-tuned model takes less time than creating a specific neural network. Second, for fine-tuning, use a smaller data set. We can fine-tune our job on a lot smaller dataset using pretrained weights than we could with a model created from scratch. Third, it relatively produces a better result. Adding one fully connected layer on top of a pretrained BERT model and then training the tweaked model for a few epochs is what fine-tuning is all about. For a wide range of tasks, including as text categorization, semantic similarity, language inference, and question-answering, this technique has demonstrated to accomplish minimum task-specific modifications.

3.4 K-means clustering

Clustering is a widely used unsupervised learning approach for evaluating the context of natural language text data [23]. It is a method for gathering and segmenting related material into clusters using mathematics. It reduces the amount of unstructured language in a document and makes the material easier to grasp and arrange. The clustering algorithm K-means finds a user-specified number of clusters represented by their centroids. Based on the provided features, the method allocates each point to one of the *k* groups repeatedly, and the points are clustered based on feature similarity [16].

This project adopts the K-means clustering algorithm to classify words that have been converted into word vectors. This converted word has a weighted value that occupies the euclidian space. K-means clustering algorithm is described in the following sequence.

1. Let $X = \{x_1, x_2, x_3, \ldots, x_n\}$ be the set of data points and $V = \{v_1, v_2, \ldots, v_c\}$ be the set of centers;
2. Randomly select "c" cluster centers using the formula below;

$$J(V) = \sum_{i=1}^{c} \sum_{j=1}^{c_i} (||x_i - v_i||)^2$$

Where:

"$||x_i - v_j||$" is the Euclidean distance between x_i and v_j.
"c_i" is the number of data points in ith cluster.
"c" is the number of cluster centers

3. Calculate the distance between each data point and cluster centers.
4. Assign the data point to the cluster center with the shortest distance between it and all other cluster centers.
5. Recalculate the new cluster center using the formula below:

$$v_i = \left(\frac{1}{c_i}\right) \sum_{j=1}^{c_i} x_i$$

Where:

"c_i" is the number of data points in ith cluster.

6. Recalculate the distance between each data point and new obtained cluster centers.
7. If no data point was reassigned then stop, otherwise repeat from step 3.

3.5 Classification

Tweets can be categorized as a binary option (related or unrelated) to a defined subject vector based on similarity metrics across all clusters. The cosine similarity metric was employed in this experiment to determine if the clusters of words were connected to "mental health" or not. The aggregation vector of a cluster is indicated by C (Cluster Vector). Then the average number of the clustered vector is calculated to aggregate the text vectors representation. The full equation is shown below.

$$similarity(x, y) = \frac{\sum_{i=1}^{n} (x_i y_i)}{\sqrt{\sum_{i=1}^{n} x_i^2 \sum_{i=1}^{n} y_i^2}}$$

In the similarity formula above, x and y are vectors of length n according to this formula. C may be determined by averaging all of the cluster's vectors. Then, the averaging number is compared in terms of cosine similarity with the word vector of the "mental health." Using cosine similarity, one may compute a similarity score from the subject vector T and the cluster vector C by designating T as the vector of the topic word. For example, we use the vector of the "mental health" as the topic vector T_{topic}. We then compute the similarity score s between T_{topic} and each cluster C. The cosine equation is a measure of how similar two nonzero vectors in the inner product space are by measuring the cosine from their corner. If the cosine similarity value is near to 1, the two vectors are highly similar.

4. Evaluation and results

4.1 Datasets

The number of tweets obtained are 3.778 tweets. After text-preprocessing or text cleaning, there are 3.645 tweets that could be used as a training set. Among them, there are no retweeted text and duplicate data included. It is structured as token separated words in English language only. There are 2.535 tweets (69%, 54%) labeled as related to "mental health" and the remaining 1.110 (30%, 45%) tweets are labeled as nonrelated to "mental health."

4.2 Word embedding-based clustering

The three word embedding techniques compared have different characteristics. As mentioned in the original paper, ELMo and BERT capture word context better than Word2Vec. When comparing words that have several different contexts, ELMo and BERT give the output of two different vectors, while Word2Vec returns the output of only one vector value. Word2-Vec has a one-dimensional vector with the length of 300 digits each word. ELMo has a number of three-dimensional tensor data types with a length of 1.024 digits for each word. Whereas BERT has a one-dimensional vector with the length of each word being 4.864 digits.

All words that have been converted to vector can be grouped into several clusters. This is done to classify the words in each tweet based on the closest context. Each word that has a close context is grouped into one cluster. In practice, the three clusters are determined using the K-means algorithm. The three clusters were chosen because the more the number of clusters, the words in the

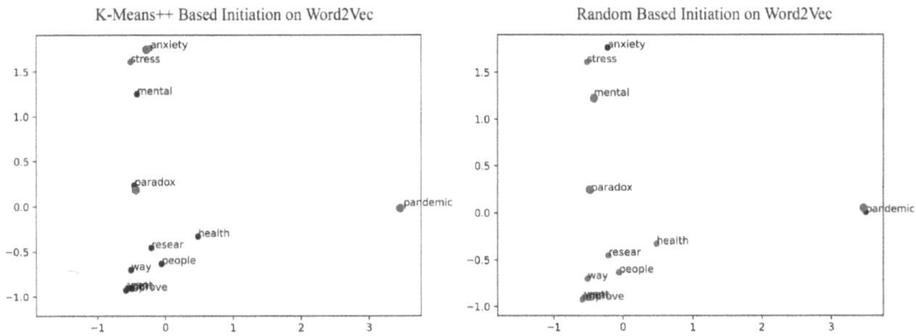

Figure 10.6 K-means clustering results from different conversion of word vectors.

tweet are more scattered. Fig. 10.6 is the sample of the clustering result after the words are converted into word vector, which we visualize after reducing the dimension using Principal Component Analysis (PCA).

4.3 Similarity measure

Cosine similarity score determines the similarity word context by measuring the distance of two vectors. Each word in a tweet that has been clustered is grouped into one. Each group is then calculated on the average of its word vector. From this process, a vector value is generated based on the calculation of a cluster with a certain context, so that three vectors are obtained. Each mean value is then calculated for its similarity score against the word vector of "mental health." Below are the results from each word vector techniques (Figs. 10.7–10.9).

Fig. 10.7 shows that the similarity score from Word2Vec is on the range 0,40–0,45 that the first cluster is scattered from 0,20 to 0,45, while the second cluster is on the range 0,401–0,405, and the third cluster is on the range 0,406–0,414.

Fig. 10.8 shows that the similarity score from ELMo is on the range 0,10–0,50 that the first cluster is scattered from 0,20 to 0,50, while the second cluster is on the range 0,446–0,450, and the third cluster is on the range 0,443–0,448.

Fig. 10.9 shows that the similarity score from BERT is on the range 0,65–0,75 that the first cluster is scattered from 0,5 to 0,75, while the second cluster is on the range 0,6785–0,6800, and the third cluster is on the range 0,6784–0,6794.

4.4 Evaluation

The last process in our model is evaluating the result of the target values and the predicted values. The suggested method's performance is assessed using a

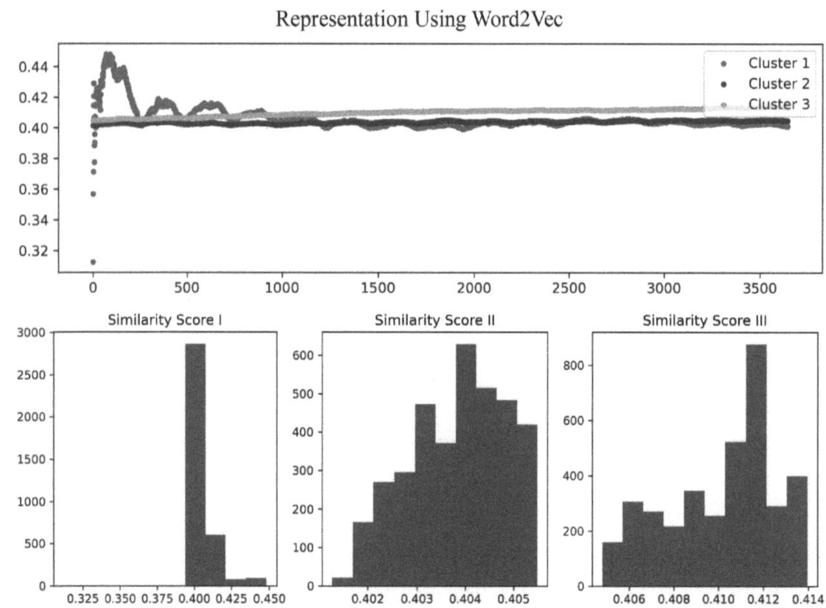

Figure 10.7 Word2Vec similarity measurement results.

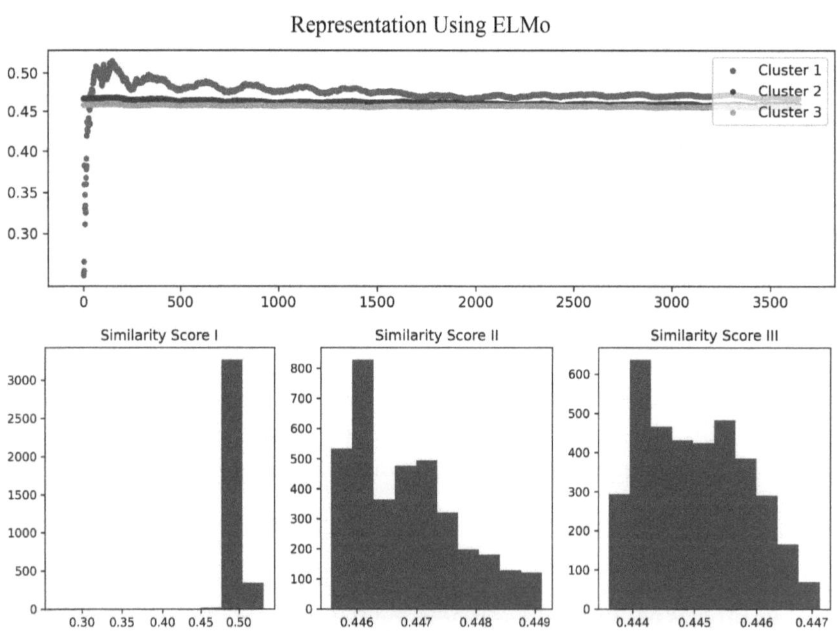

Figure 10.8 ELMo similarity measurement results.

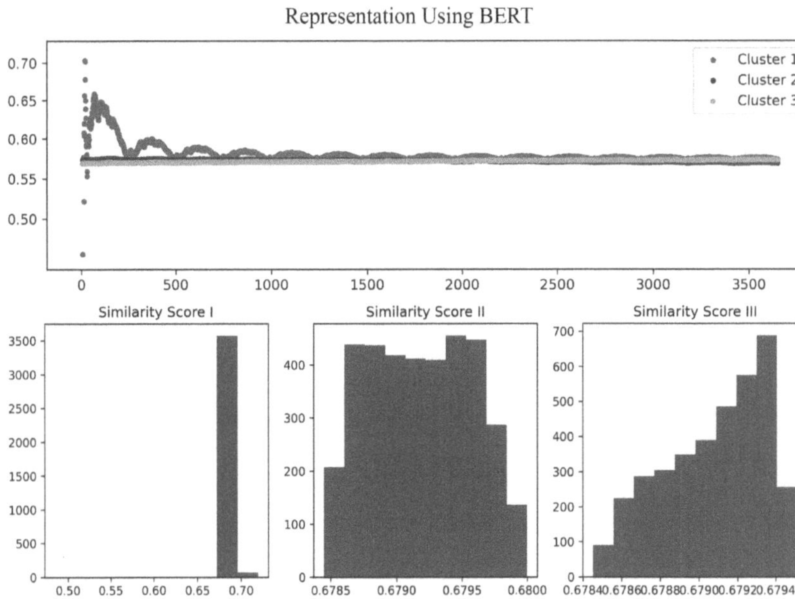

Figure 10.9 BERT similarity measurement results.

confusion matrix. The confusion matrix is a table that describes how well a classification performs on a training set where the true values are known. Below are the results from each word vector techniques.

The tables from the Word2vec, ELMo, and BERT results show that the thresholds should be obtained thoroughly for the better precisions. Word2-vec, ELMo, and BERT provide similarity scores with different density ranges. For Word2vec, it only takes a threshold value of 0.407 to get the highest accuracy. In contrast to ELMo and BERT, which must use a more detailed threshold of 0.4482 and 0.68008, respectively.

Fig. 10.10 and the result tables (10.3–10.5) show that higher the threshold, the more it will give number of FP. FP is the number of false classified of related tweets to mental health. It makes the recall scores get down. On the contrary, the lower thresholds that get from the testing, it will have a better recalls but increase in FN. FN is the number of false classified as unrelated tweets. Overall, BERT has the highest density in vector representation of words, and it provides a higher similarity point than the other two word embedding techniques. Also, BERT gets the highest accuracy 74%. This comes from the density of the word vectors, which is represented using BERT, so we can tune the threshold better than ELMo and Word2vec.

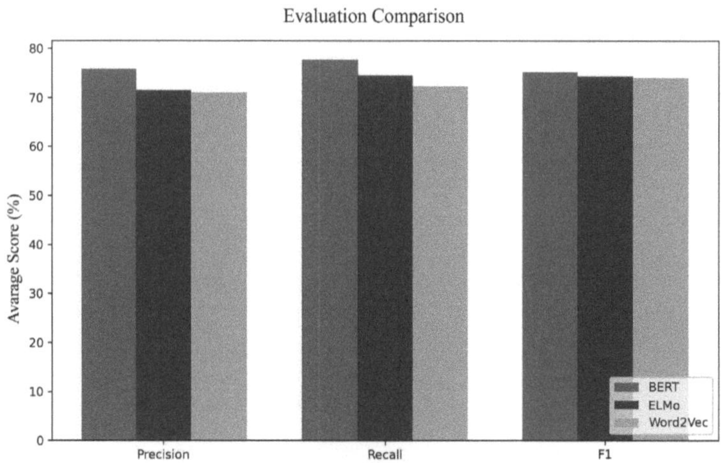

Figure 10.10 Evaluation comparison.

Table 10.3 Word2Vec results evaluation.

T	Precision (%)	Recall (%)	F1 (%)	Accuracy (%)
0.404	70	80	69	64
0.405	72	83	75	66
0.406	76	85	81	68
0.407	79	70	81	69
0.408	80	76	76	64
0.409	78	72	69	58

Table 10.4 ELMo results evaluation.

T	Precision (%)	Recall (%)	F1 (%)	Accuracy (%)
0.4479	69	79	69	68
0.4480	70	81	77	69
0.4481	71	76	80	70
0.4482	74	73	81	71
0.4483	73	70	76	68
0.4484	72	68	63	66

Table 10.5 BERT results evaluation.

T	Precision (%)	Recall (%)	F1 (%)	Accuracy (%)
0.68005	68	75	69	64
0.68006	70	88	71	68
0.68007	73	83	77	72
0.68008	74	67	78	74
0.68009	72	62	75	69
0.68010	69	59	74	66

5. Conclusion

Covid-19-related tweets are successfully streamed through Twitter API to get 3.645 tweets that could be used as the training set. In which, 69%, 54% are labeled as related to "mental health" and 30%, 45% are labeled as unrelated tweets. By evaluating the results, Word2vec is the most sensitive model for text classification. The model only takes the threshold value of 0.407 to get to the highest accuracy. In contrast, BERT has the least sensitivity, which it makes a better threshold tuning than ELMo and Word2vec. The model needs the threshold value of 0.68008 to get the best accuracy. BERT increases the accuracy from the Word2vec model up to 5%, in which it gets 74% of accuracy as the peak performance of the model.

References

[1] D. Xiangfeng, M. Bikdash, B. Meyer, From social media to public health surveillance: word embedding based clustering method for twitter classification, in: Southeast Con 2017, Charlotte, NC, 2017, pp. 1–7.

[2] E. Cambria, D. Rajagopal, D. Olsher, D. Das, Big social data analysis, Big Data Computing (2013) 401–414.

[3] M. Arumugam, Processing the textual information using open natural language processing (NLP), SSRN (2019).

[4] A. Mandelbaum, A. Shalev, Word embeddings and their use in sentence classification tasks, ArXiv (2016).

[5] S. Ghannay, B. Favre, Y. Estève, N. Camelin, Word embedding evaluation and combination, in: Proceedings of the Tenth International Conference on Language Resources and Evaluation (LREC'16), 2016, pp. 300–305.

[6] Y. Zi, S. Yuanyuan, On the dimensionality of word embedding, in: Proceedings of the 32nd International Conference on Neural Information Processing Systems (NIPS'18), 2018, pp. 895–906.

[7] T. Mikolov, I. Sutskever, K. Chen, G. Corrado, J. Dean, Distributed representations of words and phrases and their compositionality, in: Proceedings of the 26th International Conference on Neural Information Processing Systems, vol. 2, 2013, pp. 3111–3119.

[8] A. Trask, P. Michalak, J. Liu, sense2vec - a fast and accurate method for word sense disambiguation in neural word embeddings, ArXiv (2015).

[9] Y. Wang, Y. Hou, W. Che, T. Liu, From static to dynamic word representations: a survey, Int. J. Mach. Learn. Cybern. 11 (2020) 1611–1630.

[10] S. Wang, W. Zhou, C. Jiang, A survey of word embeddings based on deep learning, Computing 102 (2019) 717–740.

[11] M. Peters, M. Neumann, M. Iyyer, M. Gardner, C. Clark, K. Lee, L. Zettlemoyer, Deep contextualized word representations, in: Proceedings of the 2018 Conference of the North American Chapter of the Association for Computational Linguistics: Human Language Technologies, vol. 1, 2018, pp. 2227–2237.

[12] J. Devlin, M. Chang, K. Lee, K. Toutanova, BERT: pre-training of deep bidirectional transformers for language understanding, in: Proceedings of the 2019 Conference of the North American Chapter of the Association for Computational Linguistics: Human Language Technologies, vol. 1, 2019, pp. 4171–4186.

[13] K. Ethayarajh, How contextual are contextualized word representations? Comparing the geometry of BERT, ELMo, and GPT-2 embeddings, in: Proceedings of the 2019 Conference on Empirical Methods in Natural Language Processing and the 9th International Joint Conference on Natural Language Processing (EMNLP-IJCNLP), 2019, pp. 55–65.
[14] S.V. Xuan, T. Vu, S. Tran, L. Jiang, ETNLP: a visual-aided systematic approach to select pre-trained embeddings for a downstream task, in: Proceedings of the International Conference on Recent Advances in Natural Language Processing (RANLP 2019), 2019, pp. 1285–1294.
[15] L. Ge, T. Moh, Improving text classification with word embedding, in: 2017 IEEE International Conference on Big Data (Big Data), Boston, 2017, pp. 1796–1805.
[16] Y. Zhang, J. Lu, F. Liu, Q. Liu, A. Porter, H. Chen, G. Zhang, Does deep learning help topic extraction? A kernel k-means clustering method with word embedding, J. Inform. 12 (2018) 1099–1117.
[17] K. Kowsari, K. Jafari Meimandi, M. Heidarysafa, S. Mendu, L. Barnes, D. Brown, Text classification algorithms: a survey, Information 10 (2019).
[18] K. Khairnar, S. Pagare, P. Choudhari, S. Redgaonkar, An efficient text classification scheme using clustering, in: International Conference on Emerging Trends in Engineering, Science and Technology, Procedia Technology, vol. 24, 2016, pp. 11220–11225.
[19] D. Khurana, A. Koli, K. Khatter, S. Singh, Natural language processing: state of the art, current trends and challenges, ArXiv (2017).
[20] J.C. Collados, M.T. Pilehvar, From word to sense embeddings: a survey on vector representations of meaning, J. Artif. Intell. Res. 63 (2018) 743–788.
[21] A. Radford, K. Narasimhan, T. Salimans, I. Sutskever, Improving Language Understanding by Generative Pre-Training, 2018, p. 2.
[22] A. Vaswani, N. Shazeer, N. Parmar, J. Uszkoreit, L. Jones, A.N. Gomez, L. Kaiser, I. Polosukhin, Attention is all you need, in: Proceedings of the 31st International Conference on Neural Information Processing Systems (NIPS 2017), Curran Associates Inc., Red Hook, NY, USA, 2017, pp. 6000–6010.
[23] A.S. Halibas, A.S. Shaffi, M.A.K.V. Mohamed, Application of text classification and clustering of Twitter data for business analytics, in: 2018 Majan International Conference (MIC), Muscat, 2018, pp. 1–7.

CHAPTER ELEVEN

Predicting loneliness from social media text using machine learning techniques

Rishik Sood, Hrishav Varma, Kavita Pandey, Shikha Jain, Degala Sriram and Arshpreet Singh Guglani
Department of Computer Science & Engineering and Information Technology, Jaypee Institute of Information Technology, Noida, Uttar Pradesh, India

1. Introduction

In our daily life, everyone has experienced being alone. Sometimes, we also heard the sentence "I want to be alone" from so many people. This could be a wish when someone wants to introspect himself or it could be due to circumstances. The wish of a human being could be seen as a positive experience in terms of that he or she wants to explore himself in terms of his strengths and weaknesses. He wants to touch the taste of a relaxed feeling and a peace of mind. This kind of "Being alone" is defined in the positive scenario as solitude [1]. It has been observed in the history that our spiritual leaders, psychologists, and many more experience this solitude. They shared their feelings about their discovery in this journey and became inspirations for our society. It depicts one part of the story, or it can be said as positive part of the story of the sentence "I want to be alone" [2].

The other part of the story, i.e., in the negative side, someone feels lonely and wants to be alone. "Being alone" in the negative scenario is defined as loneliness [3]. The person who feels lonely starts avoiding social gatherings, interactions with the friends and family. They even start avoiding going out to the public places such as temple, park, etc. This could be due to several reasons such as grievance of near ones [4], sudden occurrence of chronic health conditions [5], a sudden loss of wealth [6], and many more. How these situations will be handled by an individual depends on several factors such as age, gender, personality, etc. It has been proven in the research that it is more in independent living and retired people [7,8]. Pandemic such as COVID-19 affected everyone across the globe in one way or the other.

Artificial Intelligence, Machine Learning, and Mental Health in Pandemics
ISBN: 978-0-323-91196-2
https://doi.org/10.1016/B978-0-323-91196-2.00011-9

As a result of this pandemic situation, the cases of loneliness as well as solitude have been increased. Sometimes the person wants to take a break for a short time and rejuvenate himself, which is acceptable. However, on the other hand, if the person is moving toward loneliness, which can lead to further mental health issues, needs to be detected at an early stage and treated in a proper manner.

In today's time, loneliness has become a pandemic, which leads to many psychological problems. One of the early studies shows that there is no relation between loneliness and depression. Neither loneliness causes depression nor depression causes loneliness [9]. However, their origin factors are same. Other group of researchers shows a strong correlation between loneliness and depression [10–12]. They prove loneliness as a resilient factor for depression [13]. The depressed people face severe health issues at a later stage in comparison to the people who are not feeling lonely or depressed. It has also been proved by one of the researchers that serious mental health consequences can be prevented if loneliness is detected at an early stage [7]. From this literature, it can be analyzed very clearly that differentiating between whether a person is actually feeling lonely or want a short break to relax is equally important and moreover its detection should be at an early stage. This chapter tries to answer this objective.

To find the answer, here, tweets would be classified into two categories, solitude and loneliness by using Natural Language Processing (NLP) and Artificial Intelligence (AI) techniques. The considered dataset, SOLO, is unstructured, which consists of around 3.8 million tweets. Another dataset, Sentiment140, is also used to create second class (comprises of solitude and other positive emotions). The datasets are preprocessed by using various preprocessing steps: mapping contracted words to full words, cleaning the tweets, lemmatizing the tweets, removing twitter tags, translating other languages to English, and removing image links and website links. The tweets are tokenized and the resulting sequences are embedded using GloVe and Word2Vec embedding. During the classification process, 80% of the dataset is considered as training dataset and remaining 20% is used as testing dataset. Four models, Random Forest, BiLSTM, GRU, and XGBoost have been applied for classification of tweets. Both Random Forest and XGBoost achieve an accuracy of 0.99, whereas GRU and BiLSTM achieve an accuracy of 0.9995.

Rest of the article is organized as follows. The next section discusses the various works related to the objective of the chapter. For better understanding of the readers, an overview of the techniques and used models is described in the followed Section 3. The proposed framework is discussed in Section 4. Implementation details are provided in Section 5, and it is followed by the discussion of important results and findings. The chapter ends with a conclusion note trailed by references.

2. Related work

As discussed above, the concepts of loneliness and solitude and the way they affect people are an important topic for research. Many of the current research studies around this theme have been limited to statistical and linguistic analysis. Few researchers have shown the importance of tweet data in analysis of loneliness and solitude, whereas other researchers studied the effects of loneliness on various age groups.The researchers also had shown the effect of social media on loneliness and solitude. Researchers have tried to find the answer of the following questions: how these things become aggravated during the pandemic time, and how an immediate attention can help toward mental health of people? Some of the important findings reported in the literature are presented as follows.

Pittman and Reich in 2016 [14] have shown the impact of social media platform on loneliness. The use of social media grows day by day. Thus, loneliness among these users is more in comparison to normal users. Their quantitative and qualitative analysis, as well as hypothesis testing, proved that image-based platforms can decrease the loneliness and increase the happiness as image-based platforms (for example: Snapchat, Instagram, etc.) offer a higher level of simulated social presence as compared to text-based platforms (for example twitter, yak-yak, etc.). Boursier et al. [15]. also studied the effects of excessive use of social media on loneliness during the COVID-19 pandemic. During pandemic, people feel lonely, thus, the use of digital technologies is increased to relive the stress and anxiety. They want to be a part of virtual communities, thus increasing social media usage. But the prolonged use of digital technologies further increases their anxiety. This often lands them in a vicious cycle. Galanaki [16] shows in a study that children are able to differentiate between the concepts of loneliness and solitude. They conducted interviews of 180 students comprising different grades and performed statistical analysis on it. It was found out that more than 2/3rd of the students often felt feelings of painful loneliness. This study also proved that girls' understanding toward the difference between loneliness and solitude is better in comparison to boys. To understand the concept of solitude, some level of maturity is required. This calls for more attention toward educating children about these concepts.

Badal et al. [17] did the study of loneliness on older adults of age 66–94, as they are more prone to loneliness due to loss of partners and friends, as well as declining of physical health and mobility. They interviewed these people and evaluated these interviews through NLP and Machine Learning techniques. Their results show that people with loneliness had longer responses to their questions and in their responses, more sadness has been reflected. According to their qualitative assessments, another important finding is that women are more likely to be lonely than men.

Hipson et al. [18] want to examine the language of solitude and loneliness on tweets. They analyzed the emotional content of 19 million tweets containing the words solitude, lonely, and loneliness. This corpus is named as SOLO (State of Being Alone) corpus. They assessed the sentiments of these words to get an idea of the context in which they are used. They found from their analysis that the words lonely and loneliness often have a negative sentiment associated with it, whereas words such as solitude denote a positive experience of voluntary aloneness. In another work done by Guntuku et al. [19], the authors collected 400 million tweets including tweets related to loneliness and a control corpus. Through the use of NLP, they were able to build a predictive model for loneliness. They also performed LDA to identify topics/themes among these tweets. These topics were used as input features to train a Random Forest model for this classification. There are a number of researchers [19–21] who all discuss loneliness in individuals based on the collected tweets. One of the main advantages to work on tweets is that twitter data is publicly available, and it is easier to access large amounts of data. These researchers performed linguistic analysis on them and provided their findings. Mahoney et al. [20] discussed in their article that from tweets analysis, we can find the loneliness among the users and timely support can be provided. Posting time of tweets, content of tweets, etc., can be used for analysis. Koh and Liew [21] mentioned in their article that how Twitter is a suitable platform for collecting data as compared to the traditional methods of interviews and surveys. Also, researchers can collect near real-time sentiments that reflect the perspectives and feelings of the community.

These studies have returned interesting analyses and findings about loneliness and solitude, but they fail to provide a method to identify and distinguish people on the basis of their state of loneliness. This is important as loneliness has adverse effects on mental and physical health, and some people might be at a very vulnerable stage. By knowing the state of loneliness timely, the adverse effects on mental and physical health can be avoided. The following section provides an overview of the methods and technologies used in the chapter.

3. Background

This section gives a brief overview of word embeddings (Word2Vec and GloVe) and classifiers (Random Forest, XGBoost, BiLSTM, GRU), which are used in the proposed framework.

3.1 Word embedding

Machine learning models do not understand the text. They can accept only numbers as input. To cater this need, text is converted into vector of real numbers using word embedding. Word embedding is the language model that extracts the semantic and contextual information from the text and preserves it in the form of numeric vector (as shown in Fig. 11.1). The similar words have closer vector representations and one word can have different vector representations. Neural networks, Probabilistic models, etc., have been used for getting the vector representation of a given word. The context of a word in a document, the relationship with other words, categorization of similar meaning words, word's syntactic similarity, etc., can be captured from the word embedding technique.Thus, this technique is also known as vector space model or distributed semantic model. The word embedding is needed as some deep learning and machine learning architectures can only process numeric data. It is widely used in feature extraction for text classification, clustering of documents, recommender systems. Some of the popular word embedding are one hot vector, TFIDF [22], LSA [23], Word2Vec [24], GloVe [25], Fasttext [26], and BERT [27]. In this chapter, we have used Word2vec and GloVe word embedding, so explained as follows.

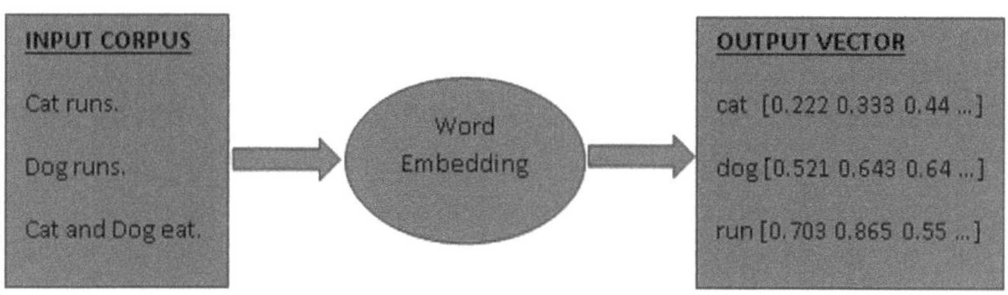

Figure 11.1 Generic input–output flow of word embedding.

3.2 Word2vec

Word2vec [24] is a prominently used word embedding technique proposed by Mikolov et al. in 2013. It is a vector representation of words encapsulating its context and meaning.Thus, the similar words will be kept together and dissimilar words will be kept at a distance. It is designed using one hidden and one output layer. It is an algorithm that takes text as an input and produce vector representation as an output. The Softmax Activation function is used only at the output layer. It collects the vocabulary from the dataset and generates a unique vector corresponding to each word in the dictionary. Broadly there are two types of Word2Vec models: Continuous Bag of Words (CBOW) and Skip-Gram. In CBOW, target word is predicted based on the context of neighboring words, whereas skip gram works in a reverse manner to CBOW. In skip gram model, context is predicted on the basis of current word. Context would be limited by a parameter called as window size. Both the architectures are good but as per the size of the dataset and speed, the one can be selected. CBOW is faster than skip gram but skip gram requires only a small amount of training data. On large datasets, skip gram produces better results. If we have 1000 words in the vocabulary list and we wish to generate a vector of size 300, the hidden layer will be represented by a matrix 1000×300. This matrix of hidden layer is actually the word vectors for each word.

3.3 GloVe

GloVe [25] stands for Global Vectors for Word Representation. It is another way of generating word embedding similar to Word2Vec. During vector representation, Glove considers both local statistics and global statistics, i.e., local and global context information of words, whereas Word2Vec considers on only local context information of words. GloVe is an unsupervised learning algorithm, which takes text corpus as input and maps each corpus word into a position in high-dimensional space. It is based on matrix factorization techniques. Firstly, cooccurrence matrix is constructed considering each word of the corpus and its context in a large corpus. Then, a large matrix obtained at step one is factorized to obtain a matrix with low dimension. Now, the vector of each word is represented by a row in the resultant matrix. Here, relationship among the words would be studied by analyzing the cooccurrence probabilities rather than the probabilities themselves. Ratio of the cooccurrence probabilities with numerous probe words would be calculated. Objective of GloVe learning is to learn word vectors in such a way that their dot product is equal to the log of the words cooccurrence probability.

3.4 Classifiers

The addressed problem in this chapter falls into a category of classification problem. Classification is a kind of supervised learning where inputs along with targets are provided. Based on the given data points and with the help of classifiers, the target class, i.e., loneliness and solitude would be predicted. This section provides an overview of the classifiers.

3.4.1 Random forest

Random forest classifier [28] is widely used in machine learning classification problems. It is a tree-based supervised learning algorithm. This algorithm is used for both classification and regression problems. Algorithm name contains the term "forest," and this term implies that there are many trees; only the difference is rather than actual trees there are many decision trees in a random forest algorithm. Each decision tree would be trained on different sample observations and provide a predicted value. All the predicted values will be averaged to provide the predicted value of Random Forest algorithm. The individual decision tree may face the problem of overfitting. However, by taking the average, this problem would be resolved. Random term in the algorithm implies two meanings. The first one is while building decision trees, random sample of training data points would be considered. Another context of random is while splitting the nodes, random subset of features would be considered.

The Random forest algorithm works as follows. First, we select random samples from the dataset. Based on the selected random samples, a decision tree would be created, which provides a predicted value. This predicted value will face the voting. The predicted result that gets the most votes will be the final predicted result. By considering a large number of decision trees, random forest provides high accuracy. One of the biggest advantages of random forest is ease in usability. Random forest algorithm helps us in finding the important features of any dataset. It is widely used in a variety of applications domains such as health care, agriculture, e-commerce, etc. In e-commerce, recommendations about any product or their services can be provided to the users. For identifying any disease or predicting the crop or pest value as per the environment conditions, this algorithm can be used.

3.4.2 XGBoost

It is one of the benchmark machine learning algorithms, which is used for tagged data [29]. Due to a number of advantages such as its performance, speed, option of parameter tuning, XGBoost is widely accepted by the research community. This algorithm is used for supervised learning problems. To achieve high accuracy, this model requires more training and tuning of the model in comparison to other models. XGBoost stands for "Extreme Gradient Boosting." The heart of XGBoost is Gradient boosting decision tree algorithm, which works on ensemble learning. It works on the principle of boosting weak learners.

It starts with the some initial prediction and calculates the errors for each observation. A new model will be built and the errors would be predicted. These predictions would be utilized to calculate new errors, and then next model will be built and associates them into an ensemble model. This cycle repeats until the building of new model continues. All previous models predictions would be added to make a prediction.

3.4.3 Bi-LSTM

Bi-LSTM [30] stands for Bidirectional Long Short Term Memory networks. As its name implies, it works in two directions, forward as well as backward. Actually it is an extension of traditional LSTM in the sense that two independent recurrent neural networks work together. One RNN works in forward direction, which remembers the past and predicts future and another RNN works in backward direction, which predicts the past from future. The advantage of this is that at any time stamp, it preserves information from both past and future, which results into faster learning.

Input sequence is processed in both the directions at the same time. The direct input sequence is provided to the recurrent layer of first neural networks and reversed input string is provided to the duplicate recurrent layer. Let us understand the working of Bidirectional LSTM with an example. Suppose we want to predict the missing word in the sentence and the given sentence is "I went to a _____ and then we did shopping."

In traditional LSTM, based on the context "I went to a," it will try to predict the missing word. Whereas in Bidirectional LSTM, we have Forward LSTM as well as Backward LSTM. Forward LSTM reads the information "I went to a" and Backward LSTM reads the information "and we did shopping." Based on the both the contexts, it is easy to understand and predict the missing word. Therefore, Bidirectional LSTMs perform better than traditional LSTMs.

3.4.4 GRU

GRU, Gated Recurrent unit [31], as its name implies, gates are added in the recurrent neural network. Actually these gates are added to solve the vanishing gradient problem of standard RNN. GRU utilizes one update gate and reset gate to decide what information to be passed to the output. These gates are actually the vectors. Reset gate decides how new input can be combined to the previous memory. How much of the previous state is to be kept further is decided by the update gate. Basic idea of using these gates is to learn the long-term dependencies. This learning property we have in LSTM also, therefore GRU can be said as a variant of LSTM. Update gate of GRU is actually the coupling of input and forget gate of LSTM. GRU and LSTM both produce comparable performances, but they have some important differences as well.

- Unlike LSTM, GRU does not require any memory unit to control information flow.
- There is no control in GRU; it can directly utilize all the hidden states.
- Training is faster and easier as there are less parameters in GRU.
- It also requires less knowledge to generalize.
- There are two gates in GRU, whereas LSTM utilizes three gates.

4. Proposed work

As discussed, there is a high need to detect the early symptoms of depression such as loneliness to avoid any unfortunate happening. At the same time, loneliness ("I am alone") should not be confused with solitude ("I want to be alone") or any other positive emotions. Hence, the objective of the chapter is to identify the hidden intention of an individual in a text of being alone. The social media text (tweets) is used to identify this hidden intention. Firstly, the tweets are preprocessed following various steps as explained below. Subsequently, the cleaned text is tokenized and processed using word embedding (Word2Vec and Glove) to obtain the numerical values for the textual data in the form of word vectors. Finally, obtained vectors are used as input for different classifiers (Random Forest, XGBoost, Bi-LSTM, and GRU) to classify the expression in the text as loneliness or other (i.e., solitude and other positive emotions). The overall flow of the proposed work is demonstrated in Fig. 11.2. The following section discusses the complete working.

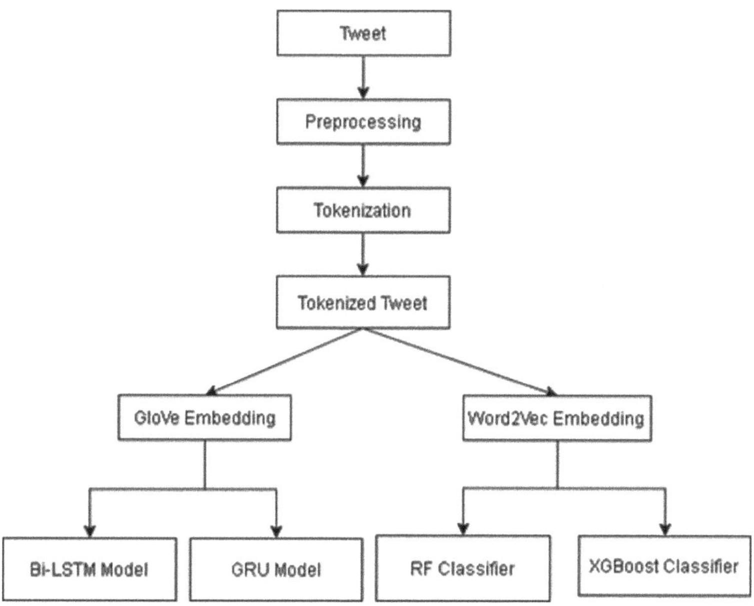

Figure 11.2 Work flow of the proposed work.

5. Implementation details

5.1 Dataset used

SOLO Corpus [18] stands for State Of Being Alone. It consists of 3.8 million tweets classified as solitude, lonely, and loneliness. In this corpus, they have done the classification based upon some carefully selected keywords in all three categories. For the proposed approach, random selections of 100k tweets from SOLO Corpus are used for "loneliness" classified tweets. Further, another corpus, Sentiment140 [32] is also used for second class, which represents solitude and other positive emotions. This corpus contains 1.6 million tweets. Random selection of 100k tweets from Sentiment140 not containing words such as lonely, alone, loneliness, etc., along with solitude tweets of SOLO corpus are taken as "other" classified tweets. If a person is expressing solitude or any other positive emotion, there is no need to worry and that is why we combined the solitude and positive emotion tweets under one class named "other." Table 11.1 shows the number of tweets after applying preprocessing and removing duplicates and invalid tweets. Moreover, 80%–20% Training and Testing splitting is done on the dataset.

5.2 Preprocessing

Preprocessing is a preliminary step that should be applied to raw text before applying any machine learning models. This step is very crucial for a machine learning model. Here, a number of steps are applied to clean the data and make it ready to be fed to the machine learning model. The steps are as follows:

At first, all the HTML tags, hyperlinks, links to images and other websites are removed from the raw tweets. Also, special characters, except #s, are removed. Twitter name tags are removed. It is done because these kinds of text generally do not contain any affect-related information. Subsequently, the accent characters are converted to English counterparts and slang words are replaced. It is followed by explanation of contracted words such as I'm, He'll, and so. It is done to make the text cleaner. Further, Emojis are converted to their meaning in words as it reveals lots of emotions. Then, whole text is converted to lowercase to ensure uniformity. The number words are converted to their numeric counterparts. To get the readable text, the text is checked for spelling as well. Sometimes, people use some

Table 11.1 Number of tweets details.

		Tweets	Training data	Testing data
Classes	Loneliness	90,349	72,280	18,069
	Other	96,770	77,416	19,354

words from their native language to express their feelings and hence machine translation is also used to preserve such words. Once the text is cleaned and become readable, it is tokenized and root word of each token is obtained using lemmatization process. Since, for BiLSTM and GRU, it is preferred to have tokens of same size, each token is padded. After following all these steps, text becomes ready to be given as input to word embeddings.

5.3 Word embedding used

After preprocessing, text is converted to numeric vector using the two word embedding techniques: GloVe and Word2Vec. This is an important step as machine learning model cannot process textual data directly.

5.4 GloVe embedding

While applying GloVe, training is performed on aggregated global word-word cooccurrence statistics from a corpus, and the resulting representations showcase interesting linear substructures of the word vector space.

Glove embedding matrix matches and stores the tokenized index of the word present in training vocabulary with the corresponding 100-dimensional glove vectors. The size of the embedding matrix is {Training_-Vocabulary_Size x 100}. That means, each word is represented by a vector of size 100. This matrix is then used as weights for the embedding in the embedding layer of the classifier model. For example, 100 dimension GloVe word vector representation for "lonely" is,

[−0.35021, −0.37695, 0.047034, 0.69498, −0.29744...].

Box 11.1 represents the implementation details of the Glove embedding layer.

BOX 11.1 Glove embedding layer implementation details

Embedding (len (word_index) +1,EMBEDDING_DIMENSIONS, embeddings_initializer = Constant (embedding matrix),input_length = MAX_length, trainable - = False)

5.5 Word2Vec embedding

While implementing Word2Vec, Skipgram is used where we take the target word as input and try to predict the context of the word. The implementation of Word2Vec is shown in Box 11.2. Cleaned and normalized tweets are tokenized and fed into the Word2Vec model.

BOX 11.2 Word2Vec embedding layer implementation details
model_w2v = gensim.models.Word2Vec (tokenized_tweet, vector_size = 500, widow = 5, negative = 20, workers = cores −1, compuete_loss = True, epochs = 100, callbacks = [callback()])

After 100 epochs of processing on the data, a word vector of size 500 is obtained. We take the average of all the words present in one tweet to get a vector that represents the whole tweet. For example: 500-dimension Word2Vec word vector representation for "lonely" is,

[−1.31013, −1.03854, 9.69931, −5.462834, 1.062949...].

5.6 Classification models

The proposed method uses four binary classifiers in combinations with the above stated two word embeddings. The classifiers BiLSTM and GRU are used with GloVe embedding, whereas Random Forest and XGBoost are used with Word2Vec embedding. The hyperparameter details of all four models are provided in Table 11.2.

Table 11.2 Hyperparameter details.

Model	Specifications
GloVe + BiLSTM	Embedding layer Dropout layer Bidirectional LSTM layer (64 units) Dropout layer Dense layer (32 units, activation = relu) Output layer (2 units, activation = softmax) Optimizer = Adam Loss = Categorical cross-entropy
GloVe + GRU	Embedding layer Dropout layer GRU layer (64 units) Dropout layer Dense layer (32 units, activation = relu) Output layer (2 units, activation = softmax) Optimizer = Adam Loss = Categorical cross-entropy
Word2Vec + random forest	N_estimators = 100 Split criterion = Entropy
Word2Vec + XGBoost	Loss = Deviance Max_depth = 6 N_Estimators = 100

6. Results and discussion

The proposed models are evaluated using the confusion matrix, F1 score, accuracy, precision, and recall. The confusion matrix summarizes the performance of the classification algorithm. It tells about the number of exact matches. F1 score, accuracy, precision, and recall are the statistical methods of evaluation of and algorithm qualitatively and quantitatively. The confusion matrix is illustrated in Fig. 11.3. The class 0 represents the class "Loneliness" and class 1 represents "Others." As it can be observed that True-Positive and True-Negative for all four models show the decent figures. Out of all these models, GloVe with BiLSTM and GloVe with GRU demonstrate the better results as compared to other models.

Table 11.3 presents the comparative results of all the four models implemented for the classification of tweets as Loneliness versus Others. It is observed that out of all four models, F1 score and accuracy of BiLSTM and GRU with GloVe are showing the comparable and excellent results. Since, in the given model, recall of class 1 (i.e., Loneliness) is more important than that of class 0, GloVe with BiLSTM model is preferred over all other models.

GloVe + BiLSTM		
	Predicted 0	Predicted 1
Actual 0	0.51747%	0.00013%
Actual 1	0.00032%	0.48207%

GloVe + GRU		
	Predicted 0	Predicted 1
Actual 0	0.51755%	0.00040%
Actual 1	0.00005%	0.48199%

Word2Vec + Random Forest		
	Predicted 0	Predicted 1
Actual 0	0.47835%	0.02253%
Actual 1	0.02090%	0.47820%

Word2Vec + XGBoost		
	Predicted 0	Predicted 1
Actual 0	0.49189%	0.00586%
Actual 1	0.00777%	0.49447%

Figure 11.3 Confusion matrix.

Table 11.3 Testing results.

		Class 0		Class 1		
	F1 micro	**Precision**	**Recall**	**Precision**	**Recall**	**Accuracy**
GloVe + BiLSTM	**0.99955**	**0.99938**	0.99974	0.99972	**0.99934**	**0.99955**
GloVe + GRU	**0.99955**	0.99923	**0.99989**	**0.99989**	0.99917	**0.99955**
Word2Vec + random forest	0.98639	0.98445	0.98822	0.98828	0.98636	0.987564
Word2Vec + XGBoost	0.95656	0.95812	0.955	0.95501	0.95813	0.95656

Bold represent the higher value results.

7. Conclusion

Due to pandemics, most of the businesses shut down. The people working in IT industry, Education sector, etc., are working from home. The markets are closed and people are forced to stay in door for their safety. Therefore, people get adapted to a mechanical lifestyle. As they are not meeting to their friends and family members, they feel affected by small issues, which also make them very emotional and sensitive. Due to all these, they are unable to control their tensions and getting effected to various psychological disorders. In these disorders, depression due to loneliness becomes a pandemic in modern times, which requires immediate attention.

This chapter presents the techniques to recognize the state of loneliness of an individual using the web text (tweets). In total, 200k tweets are picked from the SOLO corpus and Sentiment140 dataset to perform experimentation and classification in two categories: Loneliness and Others. Firstly, a sequence of preprocessing steps is applied to clean the raw tweets. Subsequently, word embeddings such as GloVe and Word2Vec are applied to obtain the word vectors. These word vectors are further used by classifiers BiLSTM, GRU, Random Forest, XGBoost to detect whether an individual is actually feeling lonely or is talking about only solitude or other positive emotions. Interesting results are obtained, which show that BiLSTM and GRU with GloVe embedding demonstrate the best accuracy and F1 score. Also, high recall for loneliness class is obtained using BiLSTM with Glove model.

The proposed application can help an individual, his relatives, or medical professionals to detect depression at an early stage and provide timely support. Moreover, the application can be further extended to detect all levels of depression. It can also be used to detect other mental disorders among people.

References

[1] C.R. Long, J.R. Averill, Solitude: an exploration of benefits of being alone, J. Theor. Soc. Behav. 33 (1) (2003) 21–44.

[2] D.E. Christie, The work of loneliness: solitude, emptiness, and compassion, Angl. Theol. Rev. 88 (1) (2006) 25–46.

[3] J.T. Cacioppo, L.C. Hawkley, L.E. Crawford, J.M. Ernst, M.H. Burleson, R.B. Kowalewski, et al., Loneliness and health: potential mechanisms, Psychosom. Med. 64 (3) (2002) 407–417.

[4] R.S. Kovarsky, Loneliness and disturbed grief: a comparison of parents who lost a child to suicide or accidental death, Arch. Psychiatr. Nurs. 3 (1989) 86–96.

[5] L. Deckx, M. van den Akker, F. Buntinx, Risk factors for loneliness in patients with cancer: a systematic literature review and meta-analysis, Eur. J. Oncol. Nurs. 18 (5) (2014) 466–477.

[6] C.L. Niedzwiedz, E.A. Richardson, H. Tunstall, N.K. Shortt, R.J. Mitchell, J.R. Pearce, The relationship between wealth and loneliness among older people across Europe: is social participation protective? Prev. Med. 91 (2016) 24–31.
[7] K.B. Adams, S. Sanders, E.A. Auth, Loneliness and depression in independent living retirement communities: risk and resilience factors, Aging Ment. Health 8 (6) (2004) 475–485.
[8] J. Stern, Loneliness, Solitude and Inclusion for Leaders. Leadership and Religious Schools: International Perspectives and Challenges, 2013, pp. 109–126.
[9] D.G. Weeks, J.L. Michela, L.A. Peplau, M.E. Bragg, Relation between loneliness and depression: a structural equation analysis, J. Person. Social 39 (6) (1980) 1238–1244.
[10] B.M. Hagerty, A. Williams, The effects of sense of belonging, social support, conflict, and loneliness on depression, Nurs. Res. 48 (4) (1999) 215–219.
[11] R. Mushtaq, S. Shoib, T. Shah, S. Mushtaq, Relationship between loneliness, psychiatric disorders and physical health? A review on the psychological aspects of loneliness, J. Clin. Diagn. Res. 8 (9) (2014) WE01.
[12] T. Liu, G.H. Wong, J.Y. Tang, S. Lu, D. Leung, L. Sze, et al., Detection of depression using the UCLA three-item loneliness scale in older Chinese, Innov. Aging 3 (Suppl. 1) (2019) S530–S531.
[13] E. Erzen, Ö. Çikrikci, The effect of loneliness on depression: a meta-analysis, Int. J. Soc. Psychiatr. 64 (5) (2018) 427–435.
[14] M. Pittman, B. Reich, Social media and loneliness: why an Instagram picture may be worth more than a thousand Twitter words, Comput. Hum. Behav. 62 (2016) 155–167.
[15] V. Boursier, F. Gioia, A. Musetti, A. Schimmenti, Facing loneliness and anxiety during the COVID-19 isolation: the role of excessive social media use in a sample of Italian adults, Front. Psychiatr. 11 (2020).
[16] E. Galanaki, Are children able to distinguish among the concepts of aloneness, loneliness, and solitude? Int. J. Behav. Dev. 28 (5) (2004) 435–443.
[17] V.D. Badal, S.A. Graham, C.A. Depp, K. Shinkawa, Y. Yamada, L.A. Palinkas, et al., Prediction of loneliness in older adults using natural language processing: exploring sex differences in speech, Am. J. Geriatr. Psychiatr. 29 (8) (2021) 853–866.
[18] W.E. Hipson, S. Kiritchenko, S.M. Mohammad, R.J. Coplan, Examining the language of solitude versus loneliness in tweets, J. Soc. Pers. Relat. 38 (5) (2021) 1596–1610.
[19] S.C. Guntuku, R. Schneider, A. Pelullo, J. Young, V. Wong, L. Ungar, et al., Studying expressions of loneliness in individuals using twitter: an observational study, BMJ Open 9 (11) (2019) e030355.
[20] J. Mahoney, E. Le Moignan, K. Long, M. Wilson, J. Barnett, J. Vines, S. Lawson, Feeling alone among 317 million others: disclosures of loneliness on Twitter, Comput. Hum. Behav. 98 (2019) 20–30.
[21] J.X. Koh, T.M. Liew, How loneliness is talked about in social media during COVID-19 pandemic: text mining of 4,492 Twitter feeds, J. Psychiatr. Res. (2020), https://doi.org/10.1016/j.jpsychires.2020.11.015. ISSN 0022-3956.
[22] T. Joachims, A probabilistic analysis of the rocchio algorithm with TFIDF for text categorization, in: Carnegie-mellonunivpittsburgh pa dept of computer science, 1996.
[23] S.T. Dumais, Latent semantic analysis, Annu. Rev. Inf. Sci. Technol. 38 (1) (2004) 188–230.
[24] T. Mikolov, I. Sutskever, K. Chen, G.S. Corrado, J. Dean, Distributed representations of words and phrases and their compositionality, in: Advances in Neural Information Processing Systems, 2013, pp. 3111–3119.

[25] J. Pennington, R. Socher, C.D. Manning, GloVe: global vectors for word representation, in: Proceedings of the 2014 Conference on Empirical Methods in Natural Language Processing (EMNLP), 2014, pp. 1532–1543.
[26] A. Joulin, E. Grave, P. Bojanowski, M. Douze, H. Jégou, T. Mikolov, Fasttext. Zip: Compressing Text Classification Models, arXiv preprint arXiv:1612.03651, 2016.
[27] J. Devlin, M.W. Chang, K. Lee, K. Toutanova, Bert: Pre-training of Deep Bidirectional Transformers for Language Understanding, arXiv preprint arXiv:1810.04805, 2018.
[28] T.K. Ho, Random decision forests, in: Proceedings of 3rd International Conference on Document Analysis and Recognition, vol. 1, IEEE, August 1995, pp. 278–282.
[29] T. Chen, C. Guestrin, Xgboost: a scalable tree boosting system, in: Proceedings of the 22nd Acmsigkdd International Conference on Knowledge Discovery and Data Mining, August 2016, pp. 785–794.
[30] S. Zhang, D. Zheng, X. Hu, M. Yang, Bidirectional long short-term memory networks for relation classification, in: Proceedings of the 29th Pacific Asia Conference on Language, Information and Computation, October 2015, pp. 73–78.
[31] R. Dey, F.M. Salem, Gate-variants of gated recurrent unit (GRU) neural networks, in: 2017 IEEE 60th International Midwest Symposium on Circuits and Systems (MWSCAS), IEEE, August 2017, pp. 1597–1600.
[32] A. Go, R. Bhayani, L. Huang, CS224N Project Report, Stanford, Twitter Sentiment Classification Using Distant Supervision, vol. 1, 2009, p. 12.

CHAPTER TWELVE

Perceiving the level of depression from web text

Sankalp Singh Bisht, Herumb Shandilya, Vaibhav Gupta, Shriyansh Agrawal and Shikha Jain
Department of Computer Science & Engineering and Information Technology, Jaypee Institute of Information Technology, Noida, Uttar Pradesh, India

1. Introduction

Depression is classified as affective disorder with three levels as mild, moderate, and severe [1]. When a person suffers with mild depression, he feels lonely persistently. Slowly and gradually, as the person moves toward moderate depression, he starts feeling worthless and guilty. If timely help is not provided, it may lead to suicidal ideations or even suicidal attempts. This phase is commonly known as severe depression.

On an average, all around the world, more than 264 million people [2] are approximated to get diagnosed with depression. The major method of diagnostic analysis is face to face clinical interviews. But the downside to this issue is that nearly 75% of patients [3] do not want to consult the doctors and psychiatrists, thus leading the disease of depression to advance stages.

During the recent times of ongoing technical revolutions, Artificial Intelligence has come out as a strong tool for any kind of technical analysis over data, involving the concepts of Machine Learning and Natural Language Processing. The process involves extracting data, such as tweets, records, metric from publicly available sources, corpuses or performing large-scale surveys, integrating crowdsourcing of resources. The availability of social media data, such as those of Facebook posts, Twitter tweets data, is a rich source for performing analysis and provides for a lot of data that is available to researchers, statisticians, clinicians for doing their research studies in the field of medical diagnosis, thus resulting in more informed and well-equipped medical fraternity. Alongside this, continuous negative emotions affect the people negatively, and its excess, even a smaller amount can lead to something more dangerous such as suicide. Mental illness is on a continuous rise among the new generations [4]. Among 80%–90% of

Artificial Intelligence, Machine Learning, and Mental Health in Pandemics
ISBN: 978-0-323-91196-2
https://doi.org/10.1016/B978-0-323-91196-2.00008-9

suicides reported, the person suffered from some kind of mental illness [5,6]. Depression is the most common mental illness, and due to its nonrecognition and denial, it is highly unreported, and as a result, it is difficult to track solely on the base of medical records or surveys.

Thus, the paper presents the techniques to identify whether an individual is in depression or not. If yes, then, the levels of depression as mild (i.e., loneliness), moderate (i.e., depressive), and severe (i.e., suicidal thoughts) are recognized. The paper has used the textual data collected from social media such as Twitter and Reddit. A number of machine learning algorithms (word embeddings and classifiers) are applied to perceive the affective disorder. This application can help the individual in early detection of depression without any human intervention and seek medical help. Moreover, it also provides an insight about the feelings of the individual to the medical practitioners, which, in turn, can help them provide better decision-making.

The rest of the paper is organized as follows: Section 2 gives insight to the related work done by researchers in the similar field. Section 3 presents the background knowledge in brief. Section 4 explains the proposed approach and its implementation in detail. The results are explained in Section 5, followed by conclusion in Section 6.

2. Related work

Many researchers across the globe worked toward early detection of depression and suicidal thoughts. Review of some of the relevant papers is presented here. Stephen et al. [7] focused on dividing "depression" as a mixture of eight feelings, namely, anger, anticipation, disgust, fear, joy, sadness, surprise, and trust. They calculated the scores based on these feelings and took weighted mean for calculation of "net depression score." For some particular cases, they also analyzed the user's tweeting patterns, over hour ranges, day ranges, and weekly ranges, to get a correct magnitude about the depression level. Singh et al. [8] achieved very good results for depression detection, on different sorts of Machine-Learning-based models, including RNN, GRU, and CNN. In the research, they also considered characters in tweet texts, which were ignored by previous researches. They embedded the characters, and used it in GRU model, and the results were outstanding, which shows that depiction of characters is important while taking note of levels of depression of a user. In 2019, the authors [9] proposed the machine-learning-based algorithms to detect the presence of words related to feeling of depression in one's tweets and got about 72% accuracy. They removed hyperlinks, and characters, which have led to false classification, and using that information can actually increase the efficiency of the model.

In 2020, Alsagri et al. [10] implemented Decision Tree, Naïve Bayes, and Support Vector Machine (with different kernels) over different combinations of account measures (as-is and normalized) and sentiment features (mixed, average and none). The accuracy ranged from 65% to 75%, over whole set, and numeric for "as-is" account measures with nonsparse embeddings gave the best result. As a whole, the results were better when measures were not normalized and features of tweets were categorized for relevance.

In 2016, the authors [11] collected the data from participants' Twitter account to analyze if they are feeling suicidal or not using decision tree algorithm. They used the Depressive Symptom Inventory—Suicide Subscale (DSI-SS), The Interpersonal Needs Questionnaire (INQ), and Acquired Capability for Suicide Scale (ACSS) scales to assess facets of Joiner's Interpersonal Theory of suicide: thwarted belongingness, perceived burdensomeness and used 2015 version of Linguistic Inquiry and Word Count software (LIWC) to build a feature vector consisting of the LIWC variables, together with a target class label: suicidal, nonsuicidal (as determined by the DSI-SS).

Authors [12] in this research study collected and analyzed the linguistic behavior before and after a suicide attempt from a novel dataset of social media data of different users. Data was collected for the people who publicly stated on Twitter that they have tried to take their own life and provided enough evidence for the casual observer to determine the date of their suicide attempt. Most of them were between the age of 15 and 29. Subsequently, they employed semisupervised learning techniques and demonstrated that quantifiable signals relevant to suicide can be found in social media data with simple analysis.

In 2018, the research [13] aimed the creation of an automated model for analysis and estimation of suicide risk from social media data and a person's digital life, (i.e., Facebook, Twitter, Instagram, Reddit, Tumblr), wearable (e.g., Fitbit, Jawbone), and other technology (e.g., Strava, Runkeeper). They examined how this could be used to improve existing screening for suicide risk within the healthcare system. Further, the ethical and privacy concerns of creating a system for suicide risk screening were explored. Data was collected from users of OurDataHelps.org, all the three genders (male, female, nonbinary). It was observed that there are quantifiable signals present in the language used on social media that machine learning algorithms can use to separate users who would go on to attempt suicide from those who would not with relatively high precision. Moreover, the machine learning algorithms depend on a wide swath of subtle clues, rather than a few indicative phrases.

Researchers also used [14] online social websites: Reddit, SuicideWatch, and Twitter with a focus on understanding and detecting the suicidal thoughts in online user content. They performed a thorough analysis of the content, the language preferences, and the topic descriptions to understand the suicidal thoughts from a data mining perspective. Six different sets of informative features were extracted. A number of preprocessing steps followed by six supervised learning algorithms were applied and compared to detect suicidal ideation within the data.

In 2019, another researcher [15] addressed the early detection of suicide ideation through deep learning and machine-learning-based classification approaches applied to Reddit social media. It employed a hybrid approach of Long Short-Term Memory and Convolutional Neural Network (LSTM-CNN) to evaluate and compare with other classification models. The experiment showed the combined neural network architecture with word embedding techniques can achieve the best relevance classification results. Additionally, the results support the strength and ability of deep learning architectures to build an effective model for a suicide risk assessment in various text classification tasks.

In 2020, the authors [16] proposed an algorithm termed "Suicide Artificial Intelligence Prediction Heuristic (SAIPH)" capable of predicting future risk to suicidal thought by analyzing publicly available Twitter data. They used data from twitter of Canadians in their 20s.The algorithm consisted of a tiered process to achieve two objectives. The first objective was to generate a method to classify SI cases from controls, and the second objective was to generate a method to assess when flagged individuals are likely to be at risk. For objective one, the algorithm structure involves first converting text-based tweet content into scores representative of psychological constructs using neural networks and subsequently training a random forest on the neural network derived data in a training set of cases and controls to predict case status. For objective two, tweet level random forest prediction scores generated over a user's timeline are evaluated for alterations in the frequency of high scores relative to the user's average pattern.

After doing the thorough literature survey, it is observed that early detection of level of depression accurately using the social media posts can help the individual in correct diagnosis without any human intervention. Moreover, it can also provide additional information about the feelings of the individual to the medical practitioners, which can help them in giving better medical help. According to World Health Organization (WHO), feeling lonely is one of the initial symptoms of depression. However, researchers have not given much attention to loneliness detection. Moreover, they are working either to detect only depression or the suicidal thought. Nevertheless, loneliness, depression, and suicidal thoughts are interlinked and should be analyzed collectively.

3. Background

This section presents basic information about various word embeddings and classifiers, which are used in the subsequent sections.

3.1 GloVe

GloVe [17] stands for global vectors. It is a word embedding, which captures both global statistics and local statistics of a corpus, in order to come up with word vectors. The GloVe model is different from the standard Word2Vec model, which only captures the local statistics of the corpus. Further, they are trained in different manner and hence lead to word vectors with subtly different properties. GloVe model is based on global word to word cooccurrence counts leveraging the entire corpus. Word2vec on the other hand leverages cooccurrence within local context (neighboring words).

GloVe is based on matrix factorization techniques on the word-context matrix. Here, firstly a large matrix of size as words corresponding to context of cooccurrence information is constructed, i.e., for each "word" we count how frequently we see this word in some "context" in a large corpus. The number of "contexts" is of course large, since it is essentially combinatorial in size. The matrix is then factorized to yield a lower-dimensional (word x features) matrix, where each row now yields a vector representation for the corresponding word. In general, this is done by minimizing a reconstruction loss. This loss tries to find the lower-dimensional representations, which can explain most of the variance in the high-dimensional data.

3.2 BERT

Bidirectional Encoder Representation from Transformers (BERT) [18] is another word embedding used for handling Natural Language Processing (NLP)-related problems, based on Machine Learning, particularly, using the concept of Transformers. The model is pretrained and was introduced by Google, by Jacob Devlin and his team in 2018. Based on usage statistics since 2019, Google has been using this technique to have a better understanding for user searches. The English language BERT, which was originally introduced, has two models, namely BERT (Base), with 12 Encoders and 12 Bidirection self-attention heads, and BERT (Large), with 24 Encoders and 16 Bidirectional self-attention heads, both of which are pretrained on unlabeled data extracted from BookCorpus (800M words) and English Wikipedia (2500M words).

While BERT has been pretrained on Wikipedia, it can be fine-tuned on custom datasets, which made it our first choice to use for this task. Words are problematic because plenty of them are ambiguous, polysemous, and synonymous. BERT is designed to solve ambiguous sentences and phrases that are made up of lots and lots of words with multiple meanings.

BERT has its roots originating from pretraining contextual representations including ULMFit, ELMo, Generative Pre-Training and Semisupervised Sequence Learning. Marking a difference from previously existing techniques, BERT is an unsupervised language representation and deeply bidirectional and is pretrained using only a plain text corpus. BERT takes into account the context for each occurrence of a given word, while context-free models such as word2vec or GloVe generate a single word embedding representation for each word in the vocabulary.

3.3 RoBERTa

RoBERTa [19] stands for Robustly Optimized BERT Pretraining Approach. It was presented by researchers at Facebook and Washington University. The objective of this new word embedding was to optimize the training of BERT architecture in order to take lesser time during pretraining. RoBERTa uses 160 GB of text for pretraining, including 16 GB of Books Corpus and English Wikipedia as used in BERT. The additional data included Common Crawl News dataset (63 million articles, 76 GB), Web text corpus (38 GB), and Stories from Common Crawl (31 GB). It works over BERT's language masking strategy, where the system aims to predict intentionally hidden parts of text, while the samples of language are unannotated. Implemented in PyTorch, RoBERTa alters the primary hyper-parameters of BERT, it deprecates the next-sentence pretraining objective and increases the learning rates and size of mini-batches. Thus, these alterations result in improvement of masked language modeling objective, compared to BERT, and finally leads to improved downstream task performance. The training of RoBERTa was done on a higher magnitude order of data, as compared to BERT, and also the training time was tremendously increased. This leads to more general representations for downstream tasks compared to BERT.

3.4 DistilBERT

DistilBERT [20] works on concept of learning a distilled (approximate) version of BERT, thus retaining 97% of performance while using only half of the number of parameters. On the basis of specifications, DistilBERT does not employ token-type embeddings and retains only half of the number of layers, as compared to Google's BERT. DistilBERT uses the concept of distillation, which results in the approximation of the Google's BERT, that is, it renovates the large neural network by a smaller neural network. The main idea behind the concept of distillation is that once when a large neural network has been trained completely, then the full output distributions of the model can be approximated by using a smaller neural network. This technique is quite similar to the posterior approximation. Kullback–Leiber divergence is used in this model, which is one of the important and most used optimization functions for posterior examination in Bayesian Statistics.

3.5 XLNet

XLNet [21] emphasizes on improved training methodology, uses large volume of data, and employs high computational resources, to attain the results It is a large-scale bidirectional transformer, just like BERT, but it gives results that are better than prediction metrics of BERT, on 20 language tasks. BERT neglects dependency between the masked positions and suffers from a pretrain-fine tune discrepancy. XLNet overcomes the limitations of BERT thanks to its autoregressive formulation.

To improvise the training process, XLNet makes use of permutation language modeling, where in random order, all the tokens are predicted. As compared to BERT, which makes use of masked language model, only the masked tokens (that are 15%) are predicted. This is being compared to the traditional existing language models, in which all the tokens were to be predicted in the sequential order instead of random order. This utilizes the capability of model to learn bidirectional relationships, and thus, it handles the relations and dependencies between the words in a better way. In addition to these specifications, Transformer XL was used at the position of base architecture, which showed good level of performance, while the permutation-based training was not performed. During the training of

XLNet, over 130 GB of textual data was used, while 512 TPU chips were used, which ran for 2.5 days. Both of these metrics are much larger than BERT.

3.6 LSTM/BiLSTM

LSTM (Long Short-Term Memory) [22] is an Artificial Recurrent Neural Network, which has feedback connections. It is specially designed and used for sequences of data, such as speech, audio, and video. A single unit of LSTM contains a cell, an input gate, an output gate, and a forget gate. The cell memorizes the values, over specified time constraints while the three gates regulate the flow of information with respect to the specified cell.

A Bidirectional LSTM, or BiLSTM [23], is a sequence processing model that consists of two LSTMs: one taking the input in a forward direction, and the other in a backward direction. BiLSTMs effectively increase the amount of information available to the network, improving the context available to the algorithm (e.g., knowing what words immediately follow and precede a word in a sentence).

3.7 GRU/BiGRU

GRU (Gated Recurrent Unit) [24,25] is an advancement of LSTM, but with a simpler architecture as these do not have a cell, these just have hidden state operator. Due to a smaller number of parameters, they are faster to train as compared to LSTM units.

GRU is an improved version of standard recurrent neural networks. To solve the vanishing gradient problem of a standard RNN, GRU uses, so-called, update gate and reset gate. These two vectors decide what information should be passed to the output.

A Bidirectional GRU or BiGRU [26] is a sequence processing model that consists of two GRUs: one taking the input in a forward direction, and the other in a backward direction. It is a bidirectional recurrent neural network with only the input and forget gates. Implementation of GRU is similar to above. With the help of a bidirectional variant, the model learns the context in both senses, which helps to make decisions.

4. Proposed approach

The objective of the proposed approach is to perceive the level of depression (mild, moderate, and severe) using the textual dataset collected from the social media posts (Reddit, Twitters). In this paper, we considered

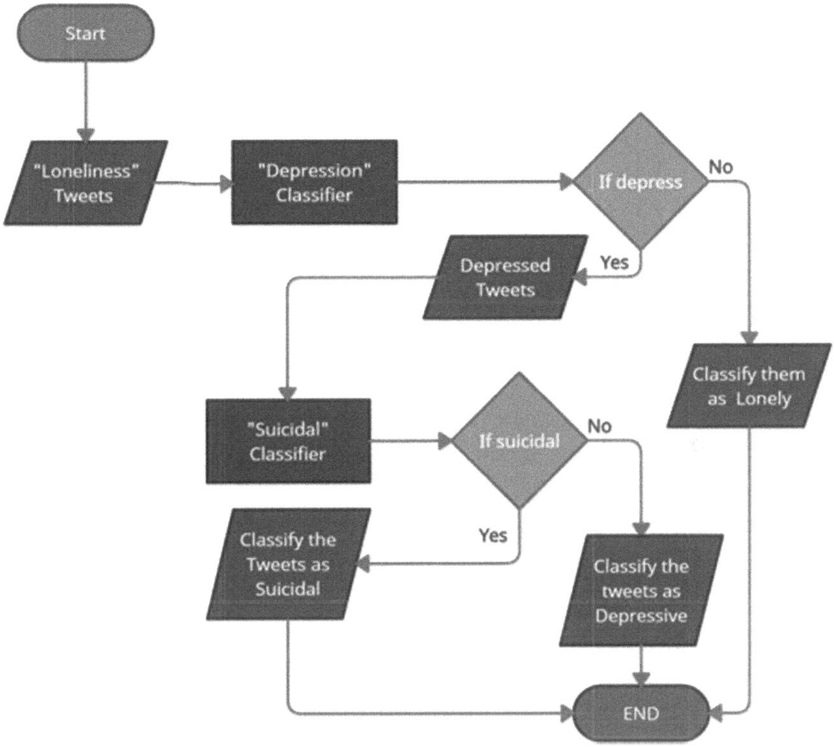

Figure 12.1 Flow of proposed approach to detect the level of depression.

that if a person is feeling lonely, he is experiencing mild depression. Similarly, the term depressive is used to represent moderate depression and suicidal thoughts are representing the severe stage of depression. Machine learning models such as LSTM, BiLSTM, GRU, BiGRU along with different combinations of word embeddings (variants of BERT, XLNET, and GloVe) are implemented to get three level of classification as shown in Fig. 12.1. This work is in continuation of the previous chapter where tweets are classified as loneliness versus others (means solitude and all other positive emotions).

So, we receive the tweets that are classified as lonely by a classifier used in previous chapter. The task performed in this chapter is to create a further pipeline of checking if the given tweets are depressive in nature and if that is true are they also suicidal. Therefore, at every stage, we have a binary classifier. The purpose of this study is to identify the stage of depression for an individual without intruding in his life.

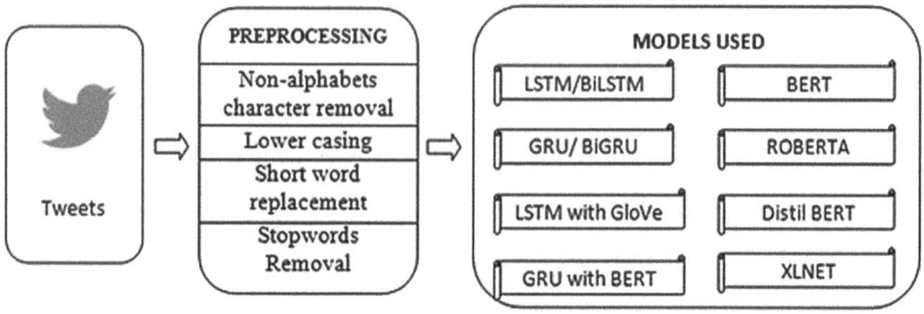

Figure 12.2 Steps of proposed approach.

Various datasets are used at different stages of the implementations. For classifying the loneliness posts, SOLO corpus [27] is used. This dataset labeled millions of tweets under three classes: solitude, lonely, loneliness. Subsequently, a dataset comprises more than 10k tweets, which are classified as depressive and nondepressive. Finally, Reddit posts are used for suicidal thought classification. In this dataset, more than 5k posts are collected under two classes: nonsuicidal and suicidal. Fig. 12.2 illustrates the different steps applied while carrying out level of depression detection. At both the levels (depressive/nondepressive and suicidal thought/nonsuicidal thought), same steps are carried out. In total, eight models are simulated. Models 1–8 are used for suicidal/nonsuicidal thought classifications. Models 5–8 are used for depressive/nondepressive classifications. With each model a gradient clipper was used to tackle the problem of exploding gradients.

4.1 Preprocessing

Keeping in mind the nature of the model, minimal preprocessing is carried out to avoid any loss of information. The steps of preprocessing followed are: nonalphabet characters removal, lower-casing, short words replacement, and stop-words removal. Subsequently, tokenization and lemmatization are done before feeding the data to machine learning models.

4.2 MODEL 1: BERT

BERT is a Transformer-based encoder that reads the entire sequence of words at once. Therefore, it is considered bidirectional. This characteristic allows the model to learn the context of a word based on all of its surroundings (left and right of the word).

Before feeding word sequences into BERT, 15% of the words in each sequence are replaced with a [MASK] token. The model then attempts to predict the original value of the masked words, based on the context provided by the other, nonmasked, words in the sequence. In technical terms, the prediction of the output words requires:

1. Adding a classification layer on top of the encoder output.
2. Multiplying the output vectors by the embedding matrix, transforming them into the vocabulary dimension.
3. Calculating the probability of each word in the vocabulary with SoftMax.

We first load the pretrained BERT-base-uncased tokenizer as the transformer has already been trained with a specific vocabulary, which means we need to train with the exact same vocabulary and also tokenize our data in the same way that the transformer did when it was initially trained.

There are few special tokens that need to be initialized and added to torchtext. They are [CLS], [SEP], [PAD], [UNK]. Their index can be taken directly from tokenizer and passed into torchtext.Torchtext along with a pretrained tokenizer function can handle many tasks from preprocessing. Like convert tokens to their index, build vocabulary. Vocabulary for the text is handled by the tokenizer while vocabulary for the labels is built from training text using torchtext. Batches are divided in size of 64. The activation function is Tanh, which helps to regulate the values flowing through the network. The Tanh function squishes values to always be between −1 and 1. The loss function added was BCELoss, which creates a criterion that measures the Binary Cross Entropy between the target and the output. Adaptive Moment Estimation is used as optimization function, which is an algorithm for optimization technique for gradient descent.

4.3 MODEL 2–4: other transformer-based models

Next three simulated transformer-based models are: Roberta, DistilBERT, and XLNet. These models initialized with pretrained weights and used that to retrain over our dataset. The classification layer was attached at the end to get the results in the desired format followed by sigmoid activation. We have used AdamW as optimizer and BCELoss as loss metric. In all these four models (MODEL 1–4), hyper-parameters are kept same for consistency (as shown in Table 12.1).

4.4 MODEL 5: LSTM/BiLSTM

We used these models because they are explicitly designed to avoid the long-term dependency problem. Remembering information for long periods of time is practically their default behavior, not something they struggle to learn. We have used Adam optimizer, and the criterion used was BCE with LogitsLoss.

4.5 MODEL 6: GRU/BiGRU

The GRU controls the flow of information like the LSTM unit, but without having to use a memory unit. It just exposes the full hidden content without any control. We wanted to use this approach as lengths of tweets capped at 280 characters. GRU is more computationally efficient. For BiGRU, the Bidirectional parameter was set to true. Both the models have BCE with LogitsLoss as the loss function.

4.6 MODEL 7: LSTM with GloVe

Here, LSTM is fed with the output obtained from the GloVe embedding. With the GloVe embedding, the vocabulary is created directly from twitter-based trained GloVe layer. When we have used the GloVe layer the parameters are directly taken from the embedding; thus the require_grad is set to false and the model is not trained for those parameters. Pretrained-GloVe embedding used in here is trained on Twitter (27 billion tokens, 1.2M vocab, uncased 100 dimensional vectors).

4.7 MODEL 8: GRU with BERT

In this model, since the embedding is taken directly from the BERT pre-trained model, there is no need to change or update them and thus require_-grad is set to false for every parameter, which is included in BERT. Now, for the feed forward layer, we have chosen to go with BiGRU. The implementation of BiGRU is similar to above but instead of using an embedding layer to get embeddings for our text, we will be using the pretrained transformer model. Another difference from the above GRU implementation is the use of BCE with logitloss as a criterion, which is sigmoid layer combined with the BCELoss in one single class. These embeddings will then be fed into a feed forward to produce a prediction for the sentiment of the input sentence.

A method of regularization called dropout is used. Dropout works by randomly dropping out (setting to 0) neurons in a layer during a forward pass. The probability that each neuron is dropped out is set by a hyper-parameter and each neuron with dropout applied is considered independently. This process is used to combat overfitting.

Hyper-parameter and fine-tuning are needed after creation of the model. The parameters are specified in Table 12.1.

Table 12.1 Specification of the hyper-parameter of all models.

MODEL 1: BERT	learning_rate = 2e-5 epsilon = 1e-8 batch_size = 32 epochs = 5
MODEL 2: Distil-BERT	learning_rate = 2e-5 epsilon = 1e-8 batch_size = 32 epochs = 5
MODEL 3: ROBERTA	learning_rate = 2e-5 epsilon = 1e-8 batch_size = 32 epochs = 5
MODEL 4: XLNET	learning_rate = 3e-05 epsilon = 1e-8 batch_size = 32 epochs = 5
MODEL 5: LSTM/BiLSTM	embedding _dim = 100 hidden_dim = 8 output_dim = 1 n_layers = 2 bidirectional= True for BiLSTM False for LSTM dropout = 0.5 epochs = 6
MODEL 6: GRU/BiGRU	sent_length = 30 batch_size = 20 output_dim = 2 hidden_dim = 16 n_layers = 2 dropout = 0.2 lr = 1e-4 epochs = 15 bidirectional= True for BiGRU False for GRU clip = 10
MODEL 7: LSTM with GloVe	embedding _dim = 100 hidden_dim = 8 output_dim = 1 n_layers = 2 bidirectional= True dropout = 0.5 epochs = 6
MODEL 8: GRU with BERT	hidden_size = 100 embedding_dim = 100 n_layers = 2 dropout = 0.3 learning_rate = 0.001 batch_size = 64 spatial_dropout = False

5. Results

Tables 12.2 and 12.3 and present the comparative results of both the classifications (depressive/nondepressive and suicidal thought/nonsuicidal thought) using all eight models. It is observed that as the complexity of the model increases, the result also gets changed. The single (UNI) variant model like LSTM, GRU did not perform as well as their bivariate version, which clearly states that reading the context both ways will help the model to understand and build up better parameters to guess. On adding GloVe embedding to these models, the accuracy increases as the context is already defined. Since BERT outperforms the GloVe embedding when it comes to understanding context the model with BERT architecture and feeds forward network as GRU outperforms every model in accuracy for the suicidal/nonsuicidal dataset. In this dataset, it is also important to note that the information is sensitive and identifying which cases are nondepressive is severely important and thus class-0 precision matters, which are why the XLNET model is given preference over others. Figs. 12.3A–F and 12.4A–F illustrate the comparative graphs of both the classifications.

6. Conclusion

Depression is one of the deadly mental disorders in today's world, and unfortunately, it is increasing at a very high rate. Moreover, it is difficult for any individual and his family to accept it. As a result, it goes untreated for a long time in most of the cases. However, early detection of depression can soothe the situation to a great extent. Considering web text as an important source of raw data, which encapsulates the affect information of an individual, we proposed a novel approach to perceive the level of depression from texts (especially tweets) taken from web. The proposed approach considers the tweets that are already classified as "Loneliness" and process them. It first classifies whether the given text is depressing or not and if it is depressing, then it is further classified whether it is suicidal or not suicidal. This way tweets are analyzed to check the level of depression as moderate or severe when people start thinking of suicide. The simulation is carried out using four different models for depressive/nondepressive classification and eight models are used at suicidal/nonsuicidal thought classification. It is observed that GRU with BERT outperformed all the models and showed the accuracy of 99% and 97%. Since class 1, which represents depressive in first classifier and suicidal is second classifier, is an important class to be focused on, it

Table 12.2 Results of depressive/nondepressive classifications.

		F-1 micro	Recall micro	MCC score	Class-0 precision	Class-0 recall	Class-1 precision	Class-1 recall	Accuracy
MODELS	Uni-LSTM	0.887	0.887	0.633	0.89	0.99	0.9	0.52	0.89
	Uni-GRU	0.506	0.506	−0.122	0.75	0.56	0.16	0.3	0.51
	Bi-LSTM	0.987	0.987	0.963	0.99	1	0.99	0.95	0.99
	Bi-GRU	0.878	0.879	0.682	0.96	0.88	0.66	0.87	0.88
	LSTM (GloVe)	0.957	0.957	0.871	0.96	0.99	0.94	0.85	0.96
	GRU (BERT Embed.)	0.986	0.986	0.959	0.98	1	1	0.94	0.99

Table 12.3 Results of suicidal/nonsuicidal thoughts classifications.

		F-1 micro	Recall micro	MCC score	Class-0 precision	Class-0 recall	Class-1 precision	Class-1 recall	Accuracy
MODELS	Uni-LSTM	0.887	0.887	0.756	0.83	0.86	0.92	0.9	0.89
	Uni-GRU	0.901	0.901	0.789	0.85	0.89	0.94	0.91	0.9
	Bi-LSTM	0.914	0.914	0.818	0.85	0.93	0.96	0.91	0.91
	Bi-GRU	0.928	0.928	0.845	0.89	0.91	0.95	0.94	0.93
	LSTM (GloVe)	0.935	0.935	0.839	0.91	0.86	0.95	0.97	0.94
	GRU (BERT Embed.)	0.974	0.974	0.938	0.94	0.98	0.99	0.97	0.97
	BERT	0.969	0.969	0.933	0.94	0.97	0.98	0.97	0.97
	Roberta	0.955	0.955	0.904	0.92	0.96	0.98	0.95	0.96
	DistilBERT	0.938	0.938	0.864	0.92	0.9	0.95	0.96	0.94
	XLNET	0.963	0.963	0.919	0.97	0.92	0.96	0.99	0.96

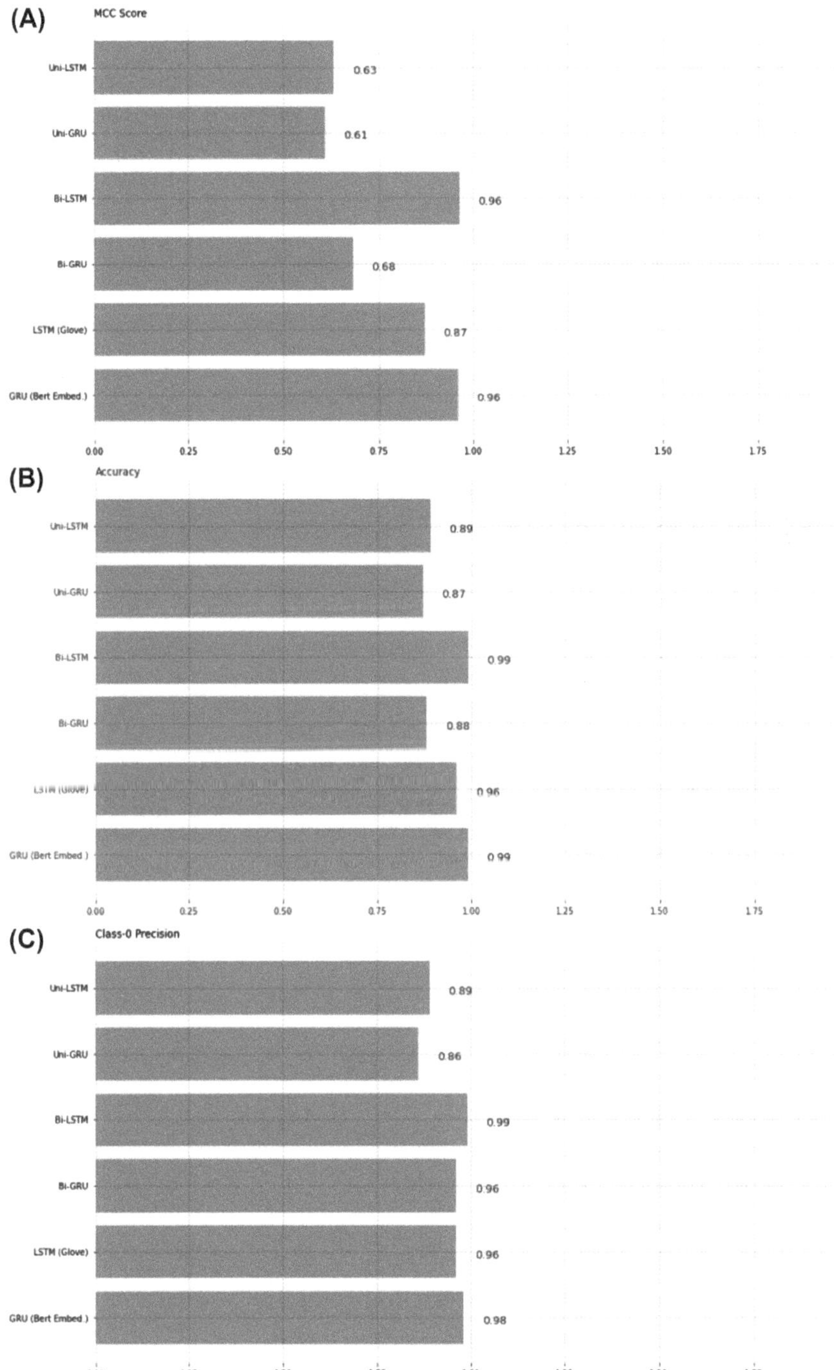

Figure 12.3 Graphs of depressive/nondepressive classifications.

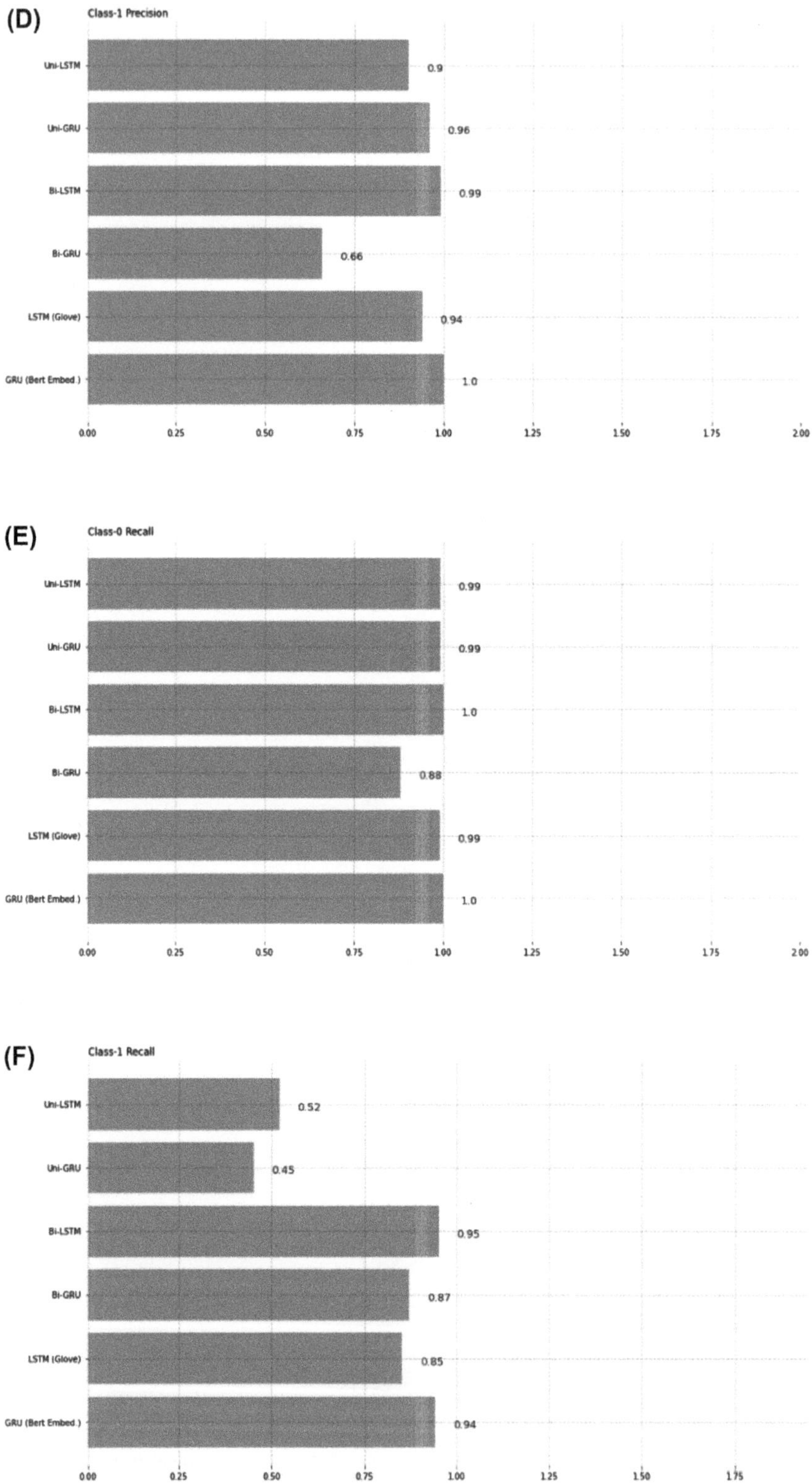

Figure 12.3 (*continued*).

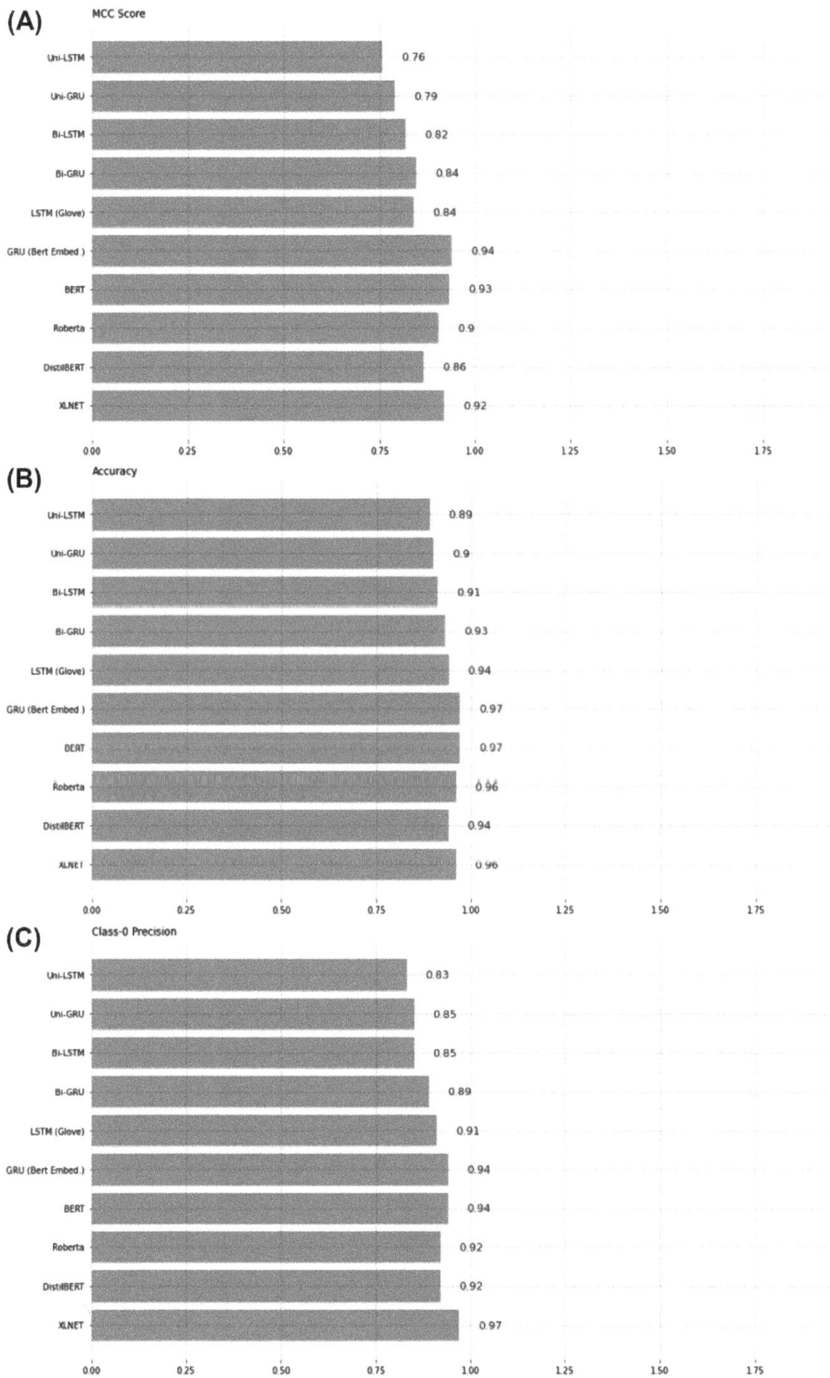

Figure 12.4 Graphs of suicidal/nonsuicidal thought classifications.

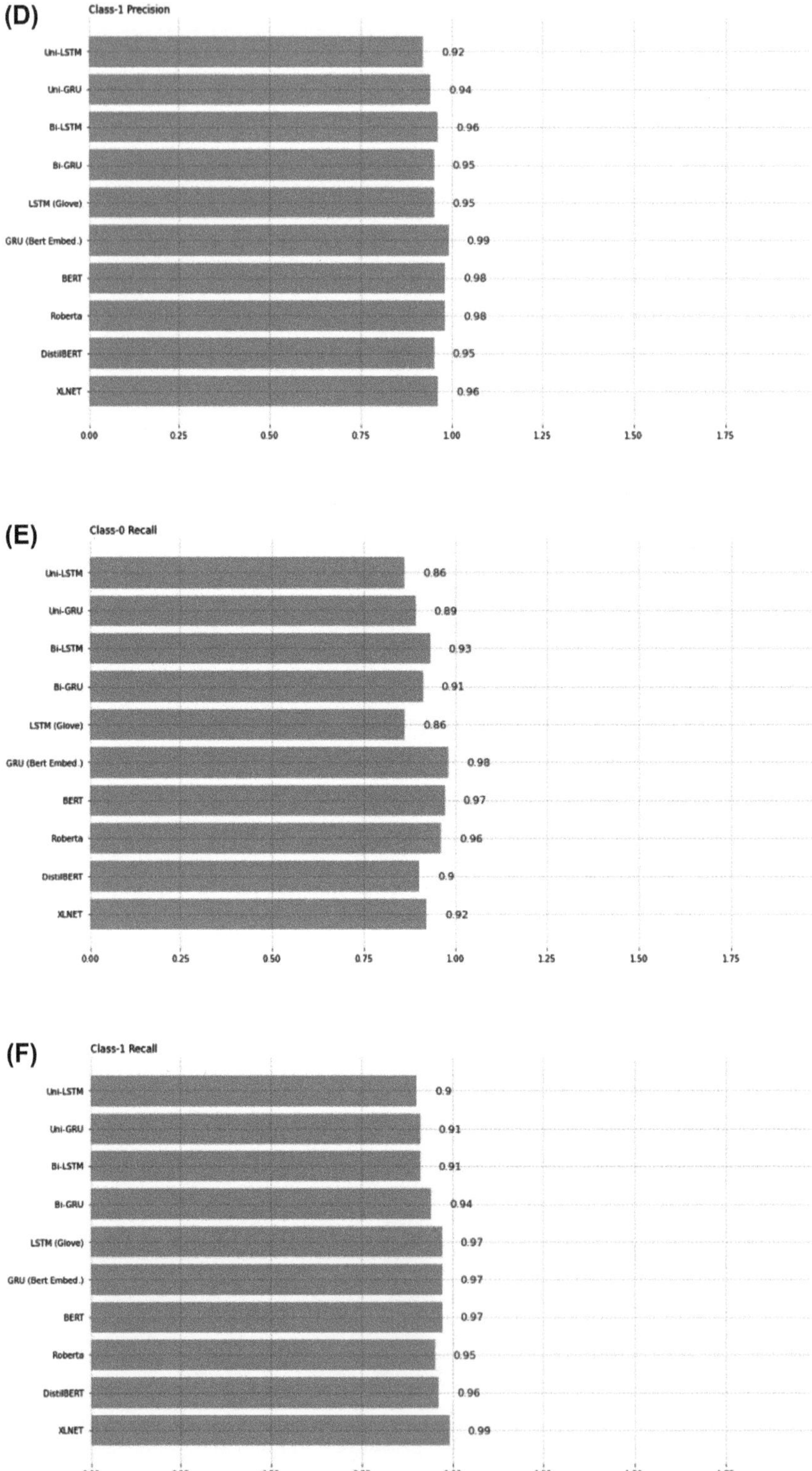

Figure 12.4 (*continued*).

is found that for class-1 recall with XLNet gave the best result for suicidal dataset with class-1 recall being 0.99 and GRU with Bert Embeddings giving 0.94 class-1 recall for depression dataset. This application can help the individual in early detection of depression without any human intervention and seek medical help. In future, the proposed model can be converted into a mobile application, which can help an individual in identifying the mental health status.

References

[1] National Collaborating Centre for Mental Health (UK), The classification of depression and depression rating scales/questionnaires, in: Depression in Adults with a Chronic Physical Health Problem: Treatment and Management, British Psychological Society, 2010.

[2] https://www.who.int/news-room/fact-sheets/detail/depression. (Accessed date: 30 July 2021).

[3] S.R. Johnson, Addressing behavioral health to improve all health, Mod. Healthcare 47 (22) (2017) 10−14.

[4] S. Bethune, Gen Z more likely to report mental health concerns, Mon. Psychol. 50 (1) (2019) 20.

[5] S. Shahtahmasebi, Examining the claim that 80−90% of suicide cases had depression, Front. Pub. Health 1 (2013) 62.

[6] T. Schmutte, M. Costa, P. Hammer, L. Davidson, Comparisons between suicide in persons with serious mental illness, other mental disorders, or no known mental illness: results from 37 US states, 2003−2017, Schizophr. Res. 228 (2021) 74−82.

[7] J. Stephen, P. Prabu, Detecting the magnitude of depression in Twitter users using sentiment analysis, Int. J. Electr. Comput. Eng. 9 (2019) 3247, https://doi.org/10.11591/ijece.v9i4.pp3247-3255.

[8] D. Singh, A. Wang, Detecting Depression through Tweets, Standford University, CA, 2016, pp. 1−9, 9430.

[9] M. Hemanthkumar, A. Latha, Depression detection with sentiment analysis of tweets, Int. Res. J. Eng. Technol. 6 (5) (2019).

[10] H.S. AlSagri, M. Ykhlef, Machine learning-based approach for depression detection in twitter using content and activity features, IEICE Trans. Inform. Syst. 103 (8) (2020) 1825−1832.

[11] S.R. Braithwaite, C. Giraud-Carrier, J. West, M.D. Barnes, C.L. Hanson, Validating machine learning algorithms for Twitter data against established measures of suicidality, JMIR Mental Health 3 (2) (2016) e21.

[12] G. Coppersmith, K. Ngo, R. Leary, A. Wood, Exploratory analysis of social media prior to a suicide attempt, in: Proceedings of the Third Workshop on Computational Linguistics and Clinical Psychology, June 2016, pp. 106−117.

[13] G. Coppersmith, R. Leary, P. Crutchley, A. Fine, Natural language processing of social media as screening for suicide risk, Biomed. Inf. Insights 10 (2018), 1178222618792860.

[14] S. Ji, C.P. Yu, S.F. Fung, S. Pan, G. Long, Supervised learning for suicidal ideation detection in online user content, Complexity 2018 (2018).

[15] M.M. Tadesse, H. Lin, B. Xu, L. Yang, Detection of suicide ideation in social media forums using deep learning, Algorithms 13 (1) (2020) 7.

[16] A. Roy, K. Nikolitch, R. McGinn, S. Jinah, W. Klement, Z.A. Kaminsky, A machine learning approach predicts future risk to suicidal ideation from social media data, NPJ Digi. Med. 3 (1) (2020) 1−12.

[17] J. Pennington, R. Socher, C.D. Manning, GloVe: global vectors for word representation, in: Proceedings of the 2014 Conference on Empirical Methods in Natural Language Processing (EMNLP), October 2014, pp. 1532–1543.
[18] J. Devlin, M.W. Chang, K. Lee, K. Toutanova, Bert: Pre-training of Deep Bidirectional Transformers for Language Understanding, arXiv preprint arXiv:1810.04805, 2018.
[19] Y. Liu, M. Ott, N. Goyal, J. Du, M. Joshi, D. Chen, V. Stoyanov, Roberta: A Robustly Optimized Bertpretraining Approach, arXiv preprint arXiv:1907.11692, 2019.
[20] V. Sanh, L. Debut, J. Chaumond, T. Wolf, DistilBERT, a Distilled Version of BERT: Smaller, Faster, Cheaper and Lighter, arXiv preprint arXiv:1910.01108, 2019.
[21] Z. Yang, Z. Dai, Y. Yang, J. Carbonell, R.R. Salakhutdinov, Q.V. Le, Xlnet: generalized autoregressive pretraining for language understanding, Adv. Neural Inf. Process. Syst. 32 (2019).
[22] H. Sak, A.W. Senior, F. Beaufays, Long Short-Term Memory Recurrent Neural Network Architectures for Large Scale Acoustic Modeling, 2014.
[23] S. Zhang, D. Zheng, X. Hu, M. Yang, Bidirectional long short-term memory networks for relation classification, in: Proceedings of the 29th Pacific Asia Conference on Language, Information and Computation, October 2015, pp. 73–78.
[24] R. Dey, F.M. Salem, Gate-variants of gated recurrent unit (GRU) neural networks, in: 2017 IEEE 60th International Midwest Symposium on Circuits and Systems (MWSCAS), IEEE, August 2017, pp. 1597–1600.
[25] J. Howard, S. Ruder, Universal Language Model Fine-Tuning for Text Classification, arXiv preprint arXiv:1801.06146, 2018.
[26] R. Lu, Z. Duan, Bidirectional GRU for Sound Event Detection. Detection and Classification of Acoustic Scenes and Events, 2017.
[27] S. Kiritchenko, W.E. Hipson, R.J. Coplan, S.M. Mohammad, SOLO: A Corpus of Tweets for Examining the State of Being Alone, arXiv preprint arXiv:2006.03096, 2020.

Technologies for vaccinating COVID-19, its variants and future pandemics: a short survey

Saurabh Jain[1], Priyanka Chawla[2], Keshav Kaushik[1] and Adarsh Kumar[1]
[1]Department of Systemics, School of Computer Science, University of Petroleum and Energy Studies, Dehradun, Uttarakhand, India
[2]Lovely Professional University, Jalandhar, Punjab, India

1. Introduction

Multiple COVID-19 strains are observed during recent times in both developed and developing countries. With the availability of COVID 19 vaccines, its distribution is started with a systematic plan in various geographical regions of this world. In Ref. [1], the COVID-19 distribution system is discussed. The major subsystems of this distribution system are shown in Fig. 13.1. This system has a vaccine production, supply, and distribution process. This involves multiple parties that deliver the raw materials, medical equipment, medical kits, and other medical supplies. All of these stakeholders are associated with the central distribution system. In parallel, the vaccine tracking system is also developed to handle the federal government

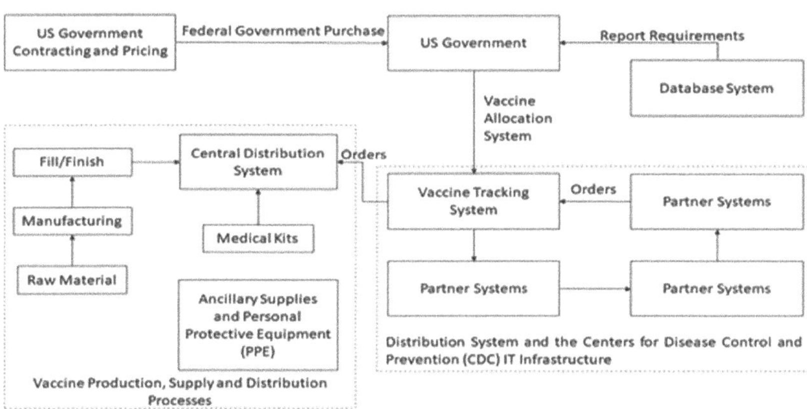

Figure 13.1 COVID-19 vaccine distribution system in India.

Artificial Intelligence, Machine Learning, and Mental Health in Pandemics
ISBN: 978-0-323-91196-2
https://doi.org/10.1016/B978-0-323-91196-2.00010-7

requirements, partner systems, on-site vaccine handling, and vaccine tracking details.

The different federal government has taken different initiatives for handling COVID-19 distribution system. For example, the electronic Vaccine Intelligence Network (eVIN) [2] system is used by the Indian government for real-time vaccine tracking, management, and collecting the status. This system is used for improving immunization coverage in various regions. This system is used for stocking and storage of COVID-19 vaccine across 10,500 vaccine cold chain points in 12 states. This network is found to be useful in implementing the federal government plans to vaccinate old age people at the first stage. This system uses mobile phones and cloud data services for tracking the vaccine conditions and collecting other data. In conclusion, IT infrastructure is in practice for handling the COVID-19 vaccine distribution scenario. Similarly, practices are expected to be integrated with futuristic healthcare services to avoid last-minute arrangements. Fig. 13.2 shows the distribution practices adopted in the United States [3]. In this system, special arrangements are made to handle COVID-19 vaccination drives. In this system, there are multiple administrative sites for commercial partners and federal governments to track the COVID-19 vaccine orders. These sites include pharmacy, LTC, home health, Indian health services, and other federal entity sites. In addition to these administrative

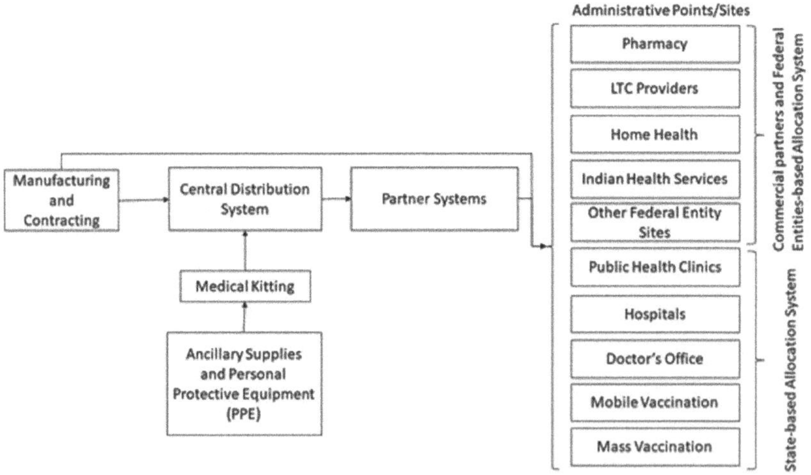

Figure 13.2 COVID-19 vaccine distribution system in the United States. *Credits: Courtesy from the Factory to the Frontlines The Operation Warp Speed Strategy for Distributing a COVID-19 Vaccine. https://www.hhs.gov/sites/default/files/strategy-for-distributing-covid-19-vaccine.pdf.*

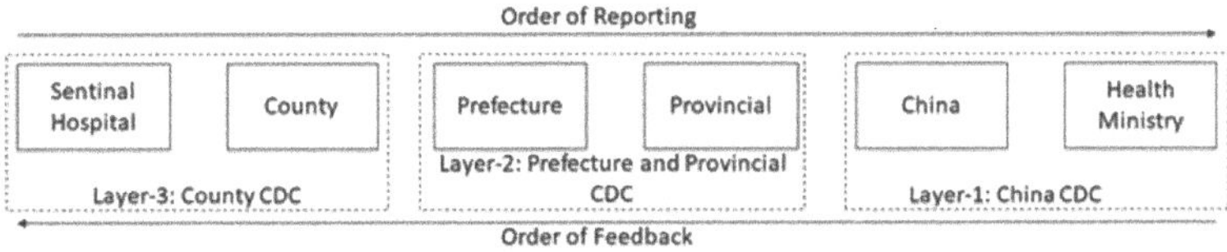

Figure 13.3 Centers for Disease Control and Prevention (CDC) system in China. *Credits: Courtesy S. Sun, Z. Xie, K. Yu, B. Jiang, S. Zheng, X. Pan, COVID-19 and healthcare system in China: challenges and progression for a sustainable future, Glob. Health 17 (1) (2021) 1–8.*

sites, there are other sites administrated by local entities. For example, public health clinics, hospitals, doctor's office, mobile vaccination, and mass vaccination drives. All of these administrative sites are attached to manufacturing and contracting units for effective control. The whole system is interconnected with a central distributed system that has partner systems for effective distribution, administration, and management. The central distribution system is well connected with manufacturing and medical kitting points for order tracking and distribution. Fig. 13.3 shows the Centers for Disease Control and Prevention (CDC) system in China [4]. In China, there is a three-layer system to report and collect feedback. In reporting, three layers (China CDC, prefecture and provincial CDC, and county CDC) system helps in medicine and related service operations and management. The complete system is not transparent for in-depth study. However, a clear set of functionalities and responsibilities at a high level shows that in-depth functionalities could be designed for effective management.

Chen et al. [5] discussed the WHO-EPI (Expanded Program on Immunization) vaccine distribution plan. Fig. 13.4 and Fig. 13.5 shows two examples of WHO-EPI plans for vaccine distribution in developing countries. To have better healthcare drives, the following are the important points that should be considered during a pandemic or other situations [2,4,6]:

- Improved stock availability: During multiple COVID-19 strains, it has been observed that lack of COVID-19 vaccine stocks increases the number of COVID-19 cases. With the availability of the COVID-19 vaccine in November 2020, various strategies are implemented in different countries to distribute the COVID-19 vaccine. In Ref. [6], distribution strategies are briefly discussed for the United Kingdom. Here, mobile team-based strategies are proposed to have the vaccination for care homes and prisons. With the analysis of risk assessment for COVID-19 in UK population, the necessity of COVID-19 vaccination in rapid mode increases.

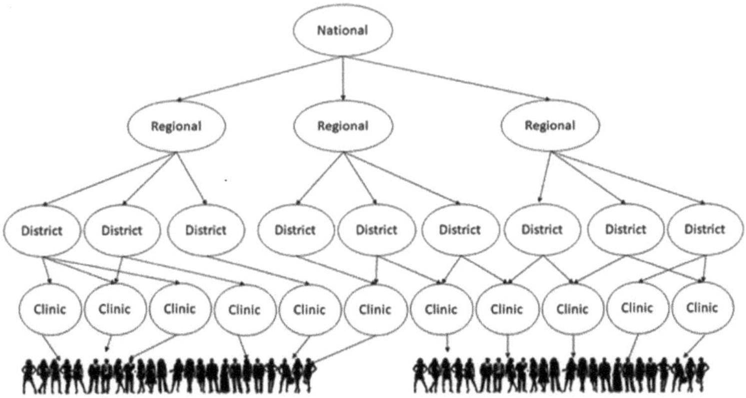

Figure 13.4 WHO-EPI vaccine distribution network for developing countries (example 1). *Credits: Courtesy S.I. Chen, B.A. Norman, J. Rajgopal, T.M. Assi, B.Y. Lee, S.T. Brown, A planning model for the WHO-EPI vaccine distribution network in developing countries, IIE Trans. 46 (8) (2014) 853–865.*

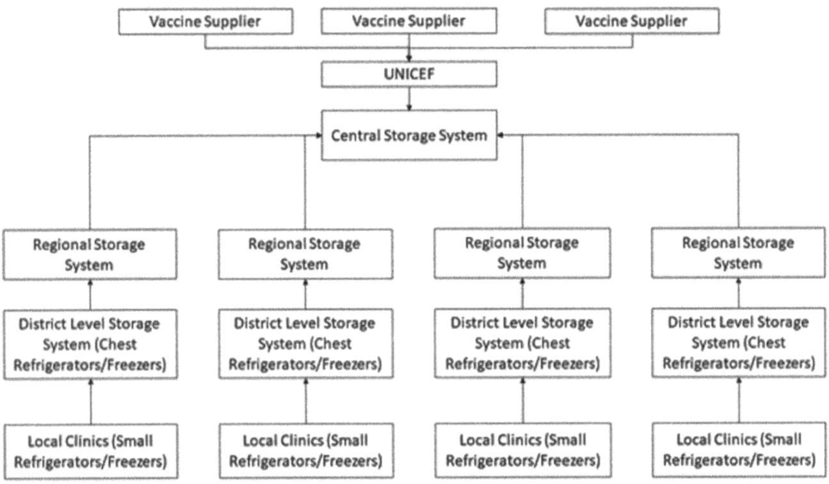

Figure 13.5 WHO-EPI vaccine distribution network for developing countries (example 2).

- Real-time data accessibility and visibility: In Ref. [6], few statistics are presented for the United Kingdom. Similar statistics are existing for almost every country having a large population.
- Efficient vaccine logistics management: Illahi and Mir [7] identified that there is a need for epidemiologists and transport planners to work together in handling the COVID-19 pandemic situations where

epidemic logistical and supply chain frameworks and models are required to be planned for vaccine distribution as well. Further, a holistic and integrated approach is required in the healthcare sector that should be capable of making necessary arrangements in sourcing the essential commodities and preparing the distribution plans. These distribution plans play a vital role in reducing the COVID-19 risks in the population. It is recommended that without replenishment parameters logistics and supply chain management frameworks are weak. Thus, there is a strong need to incorporate this parameter in distribution planning.

- Technology development, manpower and skill development, and capacity building: In addition to logistics arrangement, manpower safety and training are equally important. A large number of people have to be vaccinated daily. Without medical staff safety and training, it is not an easy job. A large number of developed and developing countries are facing this issue. Proper planning is required to vaccinate a large number of people. This planning includes arranging frontline workers, preparing their timetables and duty charts, training them for safety and vaccination, etc. All of these planning and arrangement will optimize the healthcare services.
- Large-scale implementation: World population is 7.9 billion, and vaccinating the majority of them needs large-scale planning. Thus, there is a need to constantly monitor the vaccination activities and implementation plans. Thus, it is recommended to use specific indicators and indices [6]. These indicators or indices can simplify the tasks by dividing them into multiple churns. Large-scale planning is also necessary because it is difficult to avoid mass gathering in large-populated countries. In these countries, many political and social gathering activities happen frequently. Thus, there is a need for robust models that can preplan the strategy to handle vaccination at a large scale.
- Information broadcasting: Preparation of vaccination plans, arranging logistics, training the frontline workers about the logistical operation, making records, and updating the patient information require information broadcasting. A reliable mode of information broadcasting is necessary to inform every stakeholder about the necessity of their role.
- Coordination and reverse logistics: Vaccination records collected from local units to regional or district level units and further transfer to central place maintain the record of every patient. This way of handling the vaccination plan helps in arranging the resources in a well-planned manner. This transfer of information requires coordination.

Coordination in a hierarchical way can handle the transfer of information in a much efficient way.

- Assumptions and parameter selection in research and planning: In preparing vaccination preplans, various assumptions and parameters are selected to observe the progress. However, there is a need to consider parameters and assumptions closer to realistic conditions. The closer realistic conditions create a more accurate picture and optimize the cost as well.

Among others, the present COVID-19 distributed system faces various challenges that can be partially or completely handle through advanced technologies. Some of these challenges are briefly explained as follows.

- A large number of developing countries do not have sufficient cold storage and its distribution system for vaccine preservation and distribution. It has been observed that temporary arrangements are made to handle COVID-19 distribution. Thus, a reusable cold storage facility, its maintenance, secure operation, and accessibility are require to handle COVID-19, its new strains, and future pandemic situations.
- Lack of medical or healthcare databases for quick medicine research and testing is necessary. All this is possible if the healthcare data of all patients in disconnected healthcare services is securely collected, stored, and processed through efficient, effective, and optimized approaches.
- Healthcare services with increases in health issues increase the costs as well. This cost can be minimized with the use of technologies, its proper usage, and considering it as a replacement to traditional practices. For example, on-site patient/doctor visits can be avoided with remote-data collection.

This chapter is organized as follows. Section 2 introduces the importance of crowdsourcing, its challenges, and the necessity of using mobile and other digital devices-based crowd computing environments for vaccination distribution. Section 3 describes the importance of the Internet of Things (IoT) in vaccine preservation and distribution system. Section 4 explains the recent trends in handling COVID-19 vaccination drives, the importance of technologies in it, and how cybersecurity can ensure physical and system security in different scenarios. Section 5 briefly explains the usage of parallel and distributed computing architectures for COVID-19 handling. Section 6 explains the usage of postquantum cryptography in the healthcare system for ensuring system security. Section 7 explains the importance of drones and robotics to handle the COVID-19 vaccination system. This section emphasizes the recent work done to handle medical operations and healthcare drives that required contactless drives for human safety and security. Section 8 explains the usage of blockchain technology in healthcare record-keeping and secure retrieval. Section 9 explains the recent research challenges identified in the COVID-19 vaccines distribution system, initiatives, and the importance of technologies for optimizing the medicine distribution processes. Finally, a conclusion is drawn in Section 10.

2. Crowdsourcing in COVID-19

Crowdsourcing with the help of digital devices and cloud infrastructure is an effective solution for handling real-time applications requiring distributed approach for data handling. Vaccination distribution and patient management is a distributed system approach where patients from different geographical locations are identified, medicines are arranged, medicines are made available to local hospitals or zones for vaccination, patients registration for vaccination is performed, and patients are vaccinated with records kept in secure databases. This whole system has various challenges such as [6]:

- **Data security**: Data security is a major challenge in healthcare. Patient's historical data, present information, and medical prescriptions are important that need to be placed in a secure position. In COVID-19 cases, two doses at different time intervals are given to patients. Handling a large number of patients with multiple doses increases the complexity of the healthcare sector especially in those countries where healthcare services are scarce.
- **No standard approach of patients data collection and analysis**: In a large population, it is difficult to identify patients in an automated way. There is a need to integrated human efforts with technology to speed up this scenario. Human initiation with a technology-enabled solution is possible through crowd computing. Crowd computing can ease the jobs of patients identified through human involvements, data collection, processing, analysis, and storage.
- **Lack of systemic way of vaccination distribution and record-keeping**: Presently, the healthcare system is having a traditional vaccination distribution system. During COVID-19 times, it has been observed that special conditions are required to preserve or distribute the medicine. For example, it requires cold storage while in the store or distribution stage, nurses vaccinating COVID-19 medicines require surgical grade sand, alcohol wipes, syringes, needles, masks, gloves, and

other medical equipment at the place before starting the campaign. Thus, "how to distribute vaccines" and "safely vaccinating the patients" are major challenges in the COVID-19 distribution system.
- **Medicine's long-term efficacy and possible side effects**: The rapid and very short time development of COVID-19 medicines creates mistrust in a large section of the population that it may have long-term efficacy and possible side effects. Thus, this creates mistrust among people. To handle this mistrust and reflect the true statistics among people, crowdsourcing can play a vital role. Information computed and displayed at end-users mobile or digital devices enhances the crowd computing capabilities and shows true results that can be verified easily by anyone.
- **Optimizing vaccination distribution system**: The vaccine distribution system can be optimized with resource reusage. Resource availability and reusage can help in transferring the required information, establishing coordination among frontline workers, storing the information, and broadcasting plans. In the present digital world, all of these important tasks can be solved easily with mobile-based crowdsourcing.

3. Internet of Things (IoT) network for vaccination and its distribution

IoT plays important role in vaccination [8]. Using IoT technology, various use-cases can be prepared. For example, a sensor-based IoT network can help collect the vaccine data at any time to a remote location. This data is important for patients to trust and accept the vaccine. Likewise, information about patients, vaccine procurement environment, vaccine quantity, availability, etc., can be measured using IoT networks. Various other scenarios that can take advantage of IoT network include [9–12]:
- It is very much convenient to use an IoT network to track the vaccines. In a scenario, where a large number of patients have to be handled, IoT networks can remotely monitor patient situations and help in preparing the vaccination plan for them.
- IoT networks can be scaled up and Industrial IoT networks can be created to implement the healthcare plan at a large scale.
- Healthcare 4.0 involves IoT as a major unit in establishing the interconnection. This interconnection may be useful for doctors, patients, staff members, and healthcare services providers. In case of scarcity of resources, an IoT-based solution is very much helpful in establishing the

interconnection, performing better coordination, and timely sharing the information.

- IoT networks help trace every piece of equipment and its condition at any time. Thus, in a pandemic situation, it will be much easier to trace any healthcare equipment.

4. Cybersecurity and IoT for vaccination and its distribution

The COVID-19 epidemic was a once-in-a-lifetime event that changed millions of people's lives around the world, ushering in what has come to be known as the modern standard in terms of social conventions and how we live and function. Compared to having a profound effect on environment and culture, the crisis has resulted in a number of unusual cyber-crime-related events that have impacted society and businesses. The heightened anxiety caused by the pandemic increased the likelihood of cyber-attacks advancing, leading to a spike in the number and range of cyber-attacks. Pharmaceutical firms must defend their valuable intellectual property, supporting evidence, and supply chains against cyber-attacks after developing COVID-19 vaccinations in a relatively short time it takes to build drug therapies. The leading vaccine manufacturers of the world produced novel vaccines spectacularly, showing the strength of global cooperation between pharmaceutical business leaders. Since the IP underlying COVID-19 vaccines and their associated supply chains is an advantage that cyber threats have already attempted to acquire, it requires cutting-edge cybersecurity technology and systems. Spear-phishing attacks were carried against the international companies that fund the international cold chain required for vaccine delivery. Credential harvesting attempts have been made against organizations worldwide in minimum six countries recognized today to gain access to confidential vaccine distribution and delivery records.

4.1 The rise of cyber-attacks during COVID-19

As COVID-19 spread around the world, it spawned a second major threat to an innovation society: a series of unjustified, as well as focused, cyber-crime and cyber-attacks promotions. There have been reports of scams acting as elected authorities (e.g., the WHO) and alliances, exploiting financing platforms, conducting PPE fraud, and pledging COVID-19 solutions after the outbreak. These types of scams are targeted at the general public, as well as the millions of people who work from home (WFH). WFH has brought to light a new set of cybersecurity challenges and issues that companies and individuals have never faced before. In Ref. [13], from a cyber-crime perspective, the COVID-19 pandemic reflects the broad range of cyber-attacks that happened across the globe during the disease outbreak. To expose the modus operandi of cyber-attack activities, cyber-attacks are studied and viewed in the form of major global events. Concerning what appeared to be major variations between the start of the epidemic in China and the very first COVID-19-related cyber-attack, the study shows how attacks become more common over time, to the point that three or four separate cyber-attacks were reported on several occasions. The COVID19 outbreak has triggered a great deal of panic, depression, and a major shift in our manner of living. Companies have had to respond to the need for working remotely on a large scale and at a rapid pace. The COVID19 outbreak has triggered a great deal of panic, depression, and a major shift in our manner of living. Companies have had to respond to the need for working remotely on a large scale and at a rapid pace. Many businesses [14] have been forced to reorganize their existing infrastructure and processes that were put in place in a panic to allow people to WFH without the necessary training or training. None of these companies or organizations had prepared for such a significant and rapid transformation in such a short period of time. In Ref. [15], the authors like to point this out during the outbreak, healthcare institutions were one of the most common targets of cyber-attacks. The outbreak has also raised questions about cybersecurity, especially in light of the current standard of encouraging workers to operate from home (WFH), the challenge of state-sponsored attacks, and a spike in phishing and ransomware. Although WFH has included reduction of security threats relating to healthcare, we however have presented different realistic methods to reduce the risks of cyber-attacks. It is critical for healthcare organizations to strengthen the protection of their critical data and infrastructure by adopting a robust cybersecurity strategy. The drug companies have lost $14 billion [16] due to cyber theft in intellectual property, according to the United Kingdom Office of Data Security and Privacy Guarantee (IP). Anyone with insider access is blamed for 53% of pharmaceutical IP thefts and associated hacks, according to the UK Office of Data Security and Information Assurance. According to a recent Proofpoint survey, the total cost of a data failure in the pharmaceutical industry is expected to be $5.06 million, with one of the highest remediation costs of $10.81 million in all industries. According to CISA's study, cybercriminals are targeting

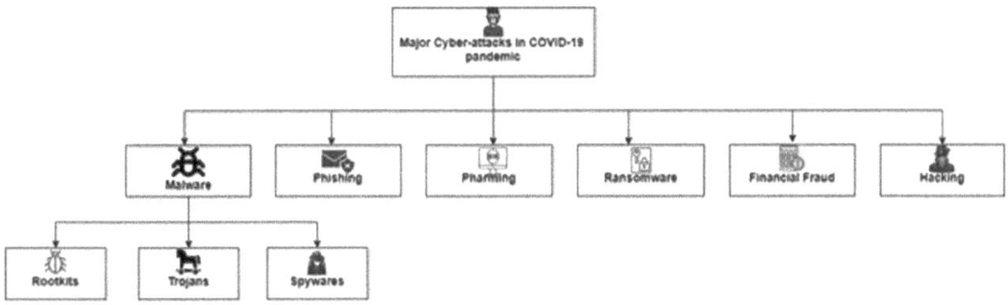

Figure 13.6 Major cyber-attacks in COVID-19 pandemic.

COVID-19 supply chains in a more coordinated, multifaceted way. There is evidence that state-sponsored cybercriminals aim to travel laterally across networks to perform cyber-attacks and obtain additional sensitive information from target ecosystems for potential campaigns. Phishing is the first target for cybercriminals, preceded by ransomware delivery, registration of new COVID-specific domain names, and a relentless quest for vulnerable danger surfaces. The condition has been compounded by the lack of substantial advances made to maintain infection prevention and follow-up. Blockchain technology is increasingly being cited as a tool to assist with numerous aspects of various applications. This paper stresses the role of blockchain in avoiding pandemics in the future. In Ref. [17], the various applications of blockchain technologies that can aid in the fight against COVID-19 are discussed. Various cyber-attacks have happened during the COVID-19 pandemic and have affected cyberspace to a great extent. Some major cyber-attacks are shown in Fig. 6 starting with Malware attacks and phishing-related cyber frauds that have dominated during the COVID-19. Individual people with hacking expertise and cybercriminals hoping to offload vaccination connections are the most probably perpetrators. Their skills will be unpredictable but on the lower end of the spectrum. There seems to be profit to be gained, but it is not as tempting or easy as other forms of cybercrime. The end goal is to undermine the scheduling system's [18] legitimacy by allowing unwanted improvements or additions to the waiting list.

4.2 Cyber threats of COVID-19 vaccines: prevention and containment

Unless one or any company is involved in the vaccine supply chain, you can assess your protection and improve your defenses as necessary. Phishing or online threats are the two most likely types of violence. The Department of Justice Coronavirus Answer web page is a valuable guide for individuals who wish to read more about COVID-19 fraud and how to deter or fight it. It is a smart idea to double submission with state or local health agency websites, as well as the Centers for Disease Control and Prevention before you try to share medical or financial details online (CDC). Never send personal and financial details over unreliable Internet networks such as email or social media. One note of advice, though: do not waste too much time seeking to grasp how attackers think. Moreover, if we fully comprehended their motivations and strategies (which we do not), they would change over time. The key is to identify the most possible types of attacks that each process and resource could encounter and then create protections around him or her. Generally, cybercrime is a crime that is reliant on the Internet. Cybercrime is a kind of crime that is made possible by the Internet. During COVID-19 lockdown, most of the users were engaged on the Internet that leads to an increase in the cyber-attack surface. Various measures can be taken in the containment of the supply chain for COVID-19 vaccines. Some of the prominent ones are as below:

- To close down cyber-attackers exploiting traditional security flaws, a Zero-Trust-based methodology to securing any endpoint in the pharmaceutical manufacturer's R&D, Clinical Testing, Production, and Supply chains are needed. Currently, pharmaceutical firms and a slew of distribution companies are seeing a much higher than the anticipated explosion of endpoints. Whenever it comes to protecting endpoints, traditional server operating systems' trustworthy and unsecured accounts are a time sink—and have proven inefficient amid Security Operations teams' great attempts.
- In vaccine supply chains, evaluate and distributor's security preparation, specifying minimum thresholds of commitment to security requirements that provide a single, cohesive security model for all organizations. It is critical to get any supplier network participant on the very same security framework while building a safe vaccine supply chain. This move guarantees transparency, clearer duties and obligations, and a consistent understanding of protected responsibilities and access rights.
- Privileged Access Management (PAM) should be prioritized in the vaccine supply chain to ensure access controls access to confidential data, beginning from IP. According to CISA's study, several efforts have been made to capture sensitive information, which often has limited access rights and is frequently left available. PAM must be implemented immediately to tighten protections on all of these sensitive accounts across the supply chain, providing only just-in-time access to classified IP, delivery and logistics data, vaccination schedules, and other data.

- It is a given that Multi-Factor Authentication (MFA) be enforced around the entire vaccine supply chain. MFA is a close to zero option for authenticating registered accounts since usernames and passwords are insufficient. MFA is made up of two or three elements that can verify your identity based on what you know (code works, passwords, PINs), what you have (predefined pins, a smartphone, tokens systems that generate pins), or what you are (a mobile phone, tokens machines that generate pins or predefined pins), or what you are (a mobile phone, tokens devices that produce pins or predefined pins) (fingerprints, biometrics, iris, facial recognition, and face scans).
- Now is the time for Unified Endpoint Security (UES) to become the industry norm across all drug supply chains. To prevent cyber-attacks from stealing IP, shipping data, and important logistics data, vendors that can quickly process vast volumes of data to identify completely undiscovered threats are required today. Complete Software's strategy for exploiting its specific durability, flexibility, and information capabilities is one to keep an eye on. Through depending on their Endpoint Resilience program, which provides decisions on a data connection to any entrepreneur's endpoint, they offer cohesive endpoint protection.

4.3 Challenges in cybersecurity and IoT in the distribution of COVID-19 vaccine

Throughout COVID-19, nationally and internationally governing agencies have emphasized the critical need for healthcare professionals and institutions to defend themselves from cyber-attacks, acknowledging that an increasing number of cyber-criminals are looking to exploit the medical sector's weaknesses [19]. This involves a tendency to steal IP rights, such as evidence relevant to the creation of the COVID-19 vaccine, simulation, and innovative therapies. Healthcare professionals and universities must also ensure that they are aware, secure, and ready to respond to any cyber threat. In Ref. [20], the aim is to identify cybersecurity problems such as social media online bullying and recommend strategies for strengthening information protection of government institutions during an outbreak. Deductive reasoning and exploratory research were used to assess the proof. The COVID-19 outbreak has exposed society's dependency on computer technology, as well as the need for appropriate cybersecurity to safeguard remote employees and the tools they use. Additional comparisons between COVID-19 and cybersecurity risks may be established well beyond direct connection. Although the effects of COVID-19 could be more severe than those of cybersecurity, this report [21] analyses the parallels, including the difficulties people face in managing risk and responding to these challenges. A greater understanding of the similarities will help us shape our impact on future to cybersecurity development and reaction to cybersecurity threats. The cybersecurity framework at home may not have the same degree of protection as in organizations, and the cybersecurity threat landscape extends if the house is built under a digital infrastructure (connected devices) framework. This environment may be one of the factors why the number of incidents has risen by more than 35% [22]. VPN systems are used to encrypt teleworking correspondence, but security breaches exploit flaws in home people and devices, reducing the efficacy of VPN deployments. Attackers have focused on social engineering attacks that reap the benefits of the panic caused by the COVID-19 epidemic to increase the effectiveness of their threats. This paper [23] proposes an IoT-based approach for preventing touching different items and surfaces in workplaces. qToggle is the name of the system, which offers a platform for quickly and easily interconnecting mobile devices and equipping them with information to help automate certain office tasks. ESP8266/ESP8285 processors, Raspberry Pi boards, and wearable sensors are included in the majority of qToggle units. Users can monitor a variety of equipment and instruments using a smartphone device. Intruders aim to leverage people's apprehension of the infection, the flaws involved with data acquisition sensors and IoT computers, and their eagerness to pursue solutions or defenses. In Ref. [24], we will look at the forms of cyber-attacks that have been attributed to the COVID-19 outbreak. We will use Neural Networks to explore information about phishing attacks. This study examines a variety of technological and socio-economic factors. We will also look at how states react to such attacks in terms of defensive measures. End-User, Device or Sensors, and Cloud are the three layers we describe. Since the methodological and technical platforms used are so complex, various vaccines are expected to be best suited to different segments of the human population. Furthermore, whether and to what degree the ability of the vaccines under consideration, as well as unrelated vaccines such as BCG, may enhance immunological fitness by teaching innate immunity to pathogen-agnostic defense and SARS-CoV-2 [25], remains unclear. Due to the short production time and the innovation of the equipment used, these vaccines will be released with a slew of unsolved issues that will only be resolved over time. Technical questions about producing millions of vaccines, as well as ethical issues about providing these vaccines to even the poorest countries, are looming roadblocks. On November 18, Pfizer/BioNTech [26] announced tentative effectiveness findings for their COVID-19 vaccine, confirming levels of 95%. Moderna declared 95% effectiveness on November 16, and the Oxford and AstraZeneca community confirmed protection and immunogenicity along a broader spectrum of groups 2 days later. We require transparency around vaccine delivery and execution as the focus shifts to deployment. Collaboration across diverse networks of government, businesses, healthcare professionals, and the public would be critical to success.

5. Parallel and distributed computing architecture using IoT network for vaccination and its distribution

As discussed in Section 1, vaccination distribution plans are distributed in nature. According to WHO-EPI integration for vaccine distribution in developing countries, vaccines are made available to local regions by distributing them from national-level distribution centers to regional distribution centers. Thereafter, it is made available in local regions. In such distributed environment, digital technologies play an important role. Vaccine-related data storage, processing, and computation require digital devices to make the process faster, efficient, and secure. Herem parallel and distributed computing architecture plays important roles. Architecture including fog, edge, cloud, and serverless computing architectures can help the process to compute/process the information at a much faster rate. In Refs. [12,27,28], similar architecture usage is explained for different applications during COVID-19 times. Different use-cases for parallel and distributed scenarios are as follows.

- A hierarchical distributed network can utilize the computing services to securely compute, store, and transmit the data at different ends. This computing architecture can utilize crowdsourcing platform services to arrange resources and manage network services at different places. This proposal will make it easy for the local center to arrange resources that are nearby and reliable and utilize the computing services.
- The edge, fog, and cloud-integrated computing resources provide distributed services. These distributed services can work throughout the application life cycle. The parallel processing facility can help in collecting the patient data, storing securely in the database, retrieving as and when required, sharing wherever it is convenient and necessary to make it available and update it with vaccination records.
- Parallel and distributed environments are well known to ensure fault-tolerant environments. This feature is important for healthcare services.

Healthcare services need patient data availability as and when required. Thus, parallel and distributed processing if synchronizing the data with nearby computing centers and ensuring fault-tolerant feature, then it is much convenient for healthcare services to ensure the availability of patient data.

- In nearby times, it is expected that patient-centric healthcare services will be given more importance compared to specialization-based services. In patient-centric healthcare services, the availability of patient data is largely important. A parallel and distributed environment can ensure this service much conveniently and easily.
- A parallel and distributed processing-based approach is more efficient and cost-effective compared to federated computing. In this approach, resources can be arranged to perform distributed computing. Arrangement of resources can make distributed computing easier for health care as well. The reusability of resources makes this program suitable for healthcare and cost-effective as well.

6. Postquantum cryptography solutions for futuristic security in vaccination and its distribution

In [29], quantum computing importance and issues are addressed. Here, it has been found that quantum computing can fail many security algorithms. Thus. advanced security approaches are required to be designed keeping quantum-based cryptanalysis into consideration. Postquantum cryptography is one such aspect that considers lattice-based cryptography, isogeny-based cryptosystem, code-based cryptography, multivariate cryptosystem, and supersingular elliptic curve isogeny cryptography. In addition to this, quantum key distribution over a longer distance with minimum energy consumption is another major issue of postquantum cryptography. In the healthcare system, patient data is important from a patient-centric healthcare system. Data security in transmission, storage, and processing stages can be ensured using postquantum cryptography aspects from a futuristic point of view. Integration of quantum and postquantum cryptography aspects with other technologies is equally important. Some of this technology integration and its importance are discussed as follows [29–31].

- Quantum computing with blockchain technology ensures the provision of peer-to-peer, distributed, decentralized, and transparent processes for much real-time application. Besides, fast computing processing through quantum gates and circuits can be made possible. Blockchain technology provides the ability to end nodes to inherit the properties of the network and create the ability to secure the network with fast computation approaches. Besides, a well-planned continuous attack analysis can secure the environment against futuristic attacks.

- Integration of quantum computing with IoT networks increases the chances of implementing various real-time applications at a large scale. For example, health care is a critical sector. There is a strong need to integrate a high computing environment with health care for making it enhance to large-scale integration. Likewise, integration of the internet of vehicles with a high computing environment can solve various traffic-related issues in overcrowded cities.
- Quantum computing with artificial intelligence can speed up the classification and categorization processes. In these processes, AI and machine learning algorithms can be executed at a much faster rate to address the application challenges. If system execution and output generation are made fast with quantum computing algorithms, then system response and efficiency in real-time scenarios can be improved.
- Quantum computing with cloud/fog/edge or serverless computing environment can ensure the availability of computing environments closer to its usage. Availability of a fast computing environment close to the application can guarantee that system will operate in real time, and there are minimal chances of any lag in generating the output. This improves the QoS and the importance of application in daily usage as well.
- In addition to the above-integrated environment, quantum computing is expected to be integrated with many other technical aspects as well. This includes DevOps, smart cities, the Digital world, game engines, augmented/virtual reality, mainframes, automated vehicles, and many more. Thus, it is possible to design a simple system and integrate it with fast computing (such as quantum computing). This will ensure security without special cryptography primitives and protocols as well. For example, Fig. 13.7 shows an example of a simple interface that involves user, interface, and backend system. Here, simple queries are exchanged between these three parts. With this integration, simple queries can be considered in the software design category. Additionally, if quantum computing aspects are integrated with the simple design, then system response time can be minimized. This will avoid a large number of attacks as well.

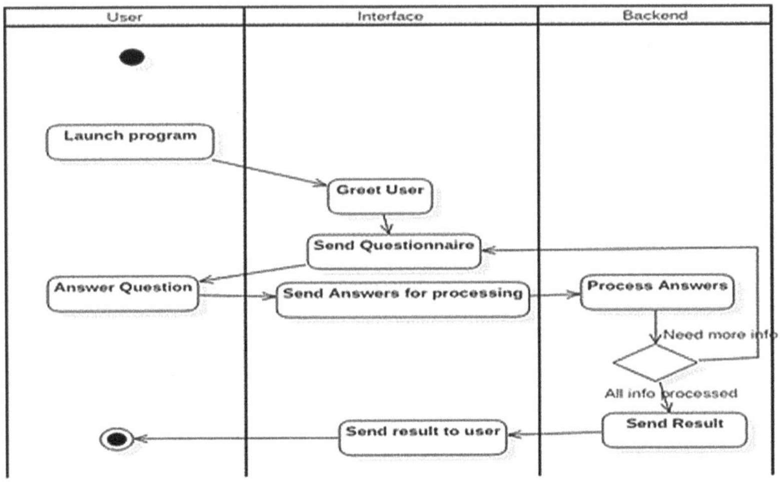

Figure 13.7 Simple user interface design for system accessibility.

7. Drone and robotics operation management using IoT network for vaccination and its distribution

In [32–34], drone-based approaches are proposed in recent times. The drone-based approaches are found to help handle COVID-19 situations. Here, thermal images are collected and these images are further used for identifying the COVID-19 cases. In past, drones are used in medical transportation. In multidrone movement and operation control activities, the movement of drones and associated activities play important roles. Here, associated activities involve collecting the data, avoiding collisions, ensuring necessary healthcare services, and many more. In drone movement, various strategies have been proposed in recent times [30]. Figs. 13.8–13.11 show examples of some of these strategies. Fig. 13.8 shows a distance-based strategy where drones can be used to distribute the vaccine in contact-free campaigns. In this strategy, drones move at a constant distance to avoid a collision. Here, LiDAR sensors are used to avoid collisions with other objects. Drone movement is possible for ensuring a collision-free environment without LiDAR sensor as well provided the area of movement is well known and movement strategies are well planned. For example, Fig. 13.9 shows zone-based movement. Here, the area of drone movement is well known and divided into symmetric zones. Each zone is monitored by a single drone. Thus it is very efficient to control the drone movement and decide the movement strategies with preplanned zone designs. All of these

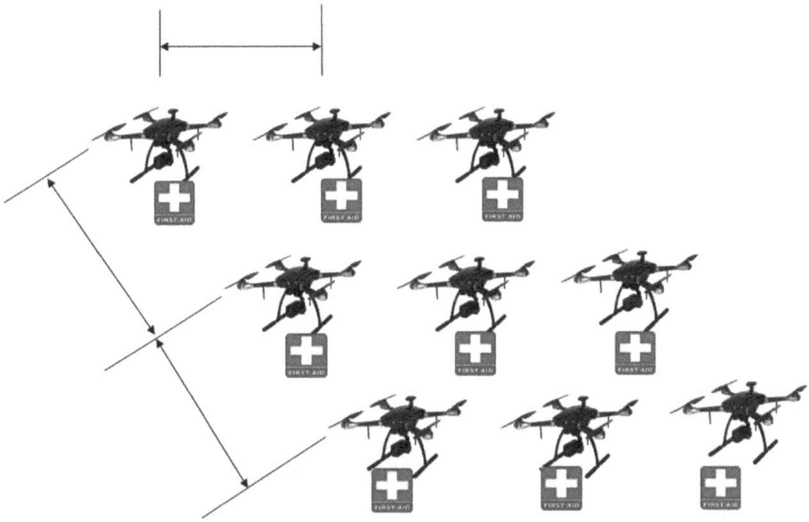

Figure 13.8 Distance-based drone movement.

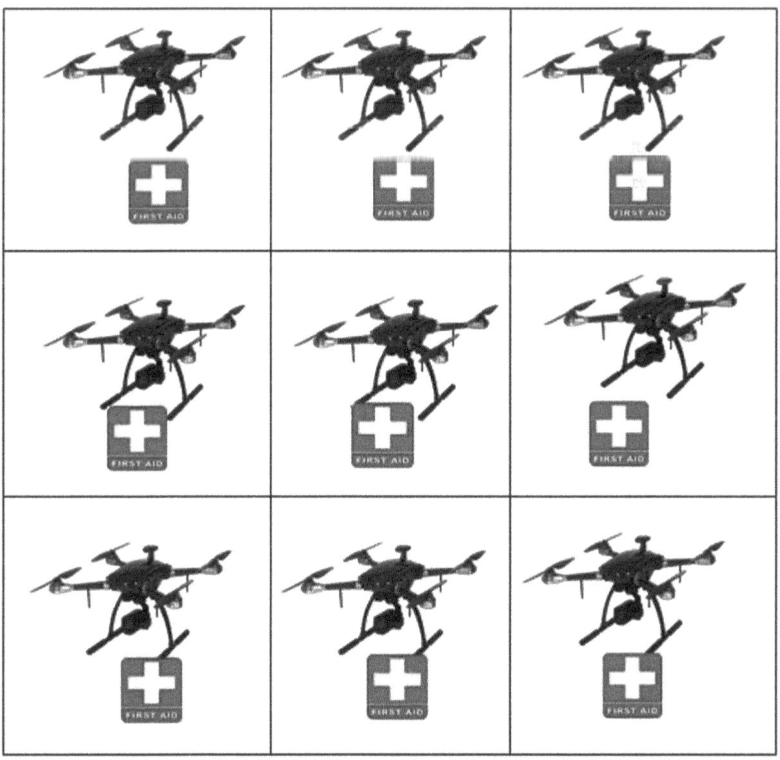

Figure 13.9 Zone-based drone movement.

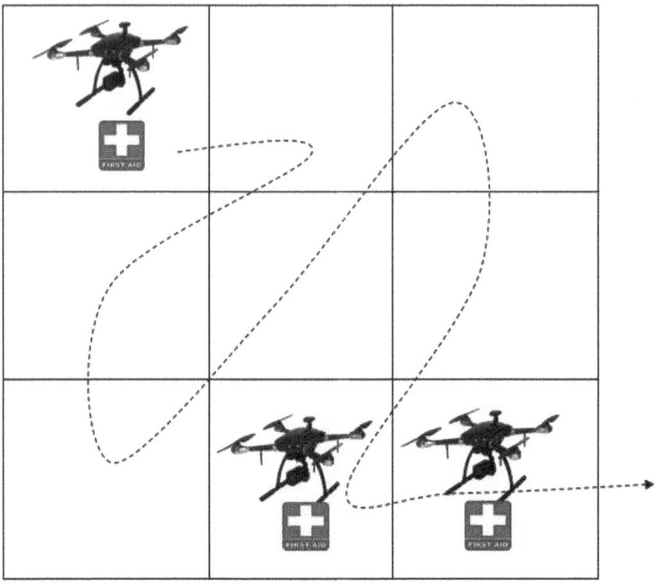

Figure 13.10 Zig-zag drone movement.

zone designs are symmetric. However, this strategy can allow asymmetric zone division as well. Thus, the major advantage of this design is that drones can utilize this strategy to move and cover any preplanned area. Fig. 13.10 shows the zig-zag movement strategy. Here, drones are allowed to move in a zig-zag manner. Here, it is mandatory to divide the movement area into the symmetric zone and follow the zig-zag drone movement strategy. This strategy allows a lesser number of drones to cover the complete area compared to zone-based drone movement (as shown in Fig. 13.9). Fig. 13.11 shows the serial drone movement where drones are moving in one direction after the constant time interval to avoid a collision. Here, different strategies can be deployed for drone movements. In one strategy, the drone can move row-by-row at different times. For example, a complete area is divided into nine zones with a 3×3 matrix. In this 3×3 matrix, there are three rows. In each row, if drones are moving after constant time interval but with the different start time for each row, then a collision can be avoided, drones can be reused, and a complete area can be covered. The major challenges in integrating drones and robotics with the healthcare sector are [30,32–34]:

- Drones create a noisy environment. To increase drone and robotics usage in the healthcare sector, noiseless drones should be used or preferred. Thus, preference should be given to design the noiseless drones.

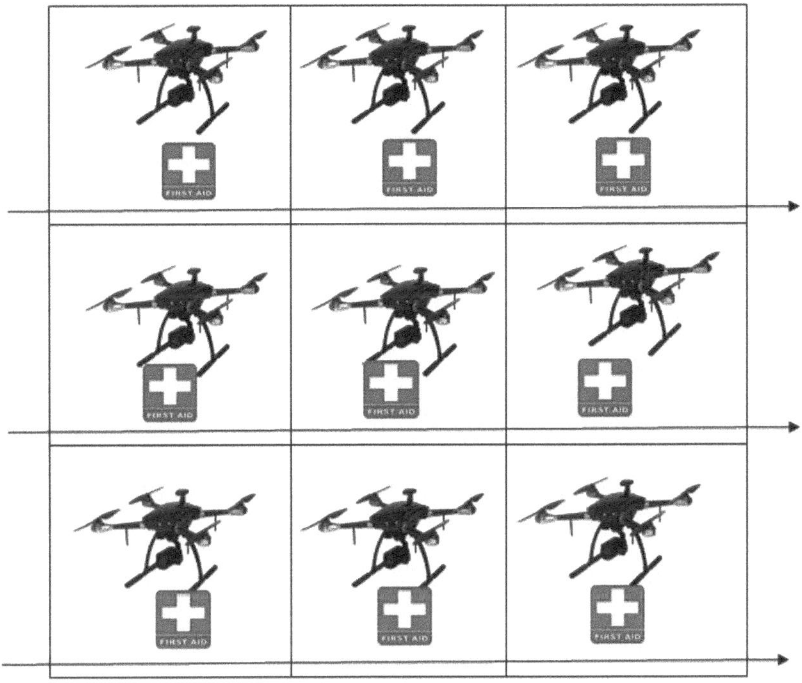

Figure 13.11 Single direction zone movement.

- Energy-efficient drones with improved working time are required to be designed. In addition to noise reduction, energy consumption plays important role in embedded designs. There is a strong need to reduce energy consumption and improve the working time such that maximum benefits can be taken using these devices at minimum cost.
- Presently, there is no standardization on the movement of drones in different geographical regions because of safety and privacy concerns. Thus, there is a need to add this issue at large scale and solutions are required to be proposed for standardizing the drone movement policies and strategies.

8. Blockchain technology and IoT for vaccination and its distribution

Patients' data has become an essential element for industrial health care. The growth in healthcare data is accompanied by the need to process it in a protected way. Healthcare industry infrastructure includes connected devices and software programs that communicate with computer networks. The use of the IoT and blockchain technology will greatly affect the market for the healthcare industry. IoT and the blockchain-based healthcare infrastructure will improve the efficiency of data processing, create new business opportunities, provide data transparency and security.

8.1 Role of Internet of Things in healthcare system

The IoT is the internetworking of billions of physical devices such as lights, home appliances, phones, etc., and other things that are embedded with computers, processors, circuits, sensors, and network connectivity that enable communication between different devices and data collection as well as sharing between these devices. The IoT allows surroundings to be sensed and devices to be accessed across the existing infrastructure remotely (as shown in Fig. 13.12), which creates more opportunities for the direct union of the physical being into digital systems and results in even better performance and correctness [35]. IoT is an emerging technology that has a variety of uses and applications, which has helped humankind to change something without being physically present at that location. IoT in health care has a lot of advantages. There are wearables, implants, sensors, and devices that can be monitored remotely from any geographical location. IoT has given a boom to a lot of sectors with new applications and remote

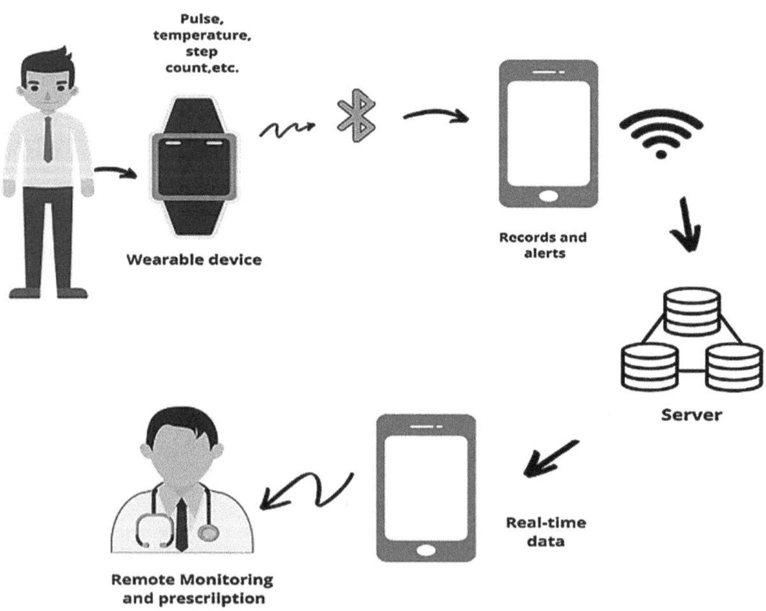

Figure 13.12 Patient remote monitoring.

monitoring capabilities to make humans life easier. Where there are advantages, there are disadvantages too. Presently, a single user carries several devices with him, which makes keeping track of anyone device difficult. People are surrounded with devices in their homes, offices, and public places. Therefore, to keep track of every device on a network, there are software applications that let the user monitor all the devices inside the network and if the device allows, outside the network [36].

This technology is spreading like a disease all over the world and has already connected billions of devices until now and has filled the gap between the physical and the digital world. It has improved the productivity of industries and societies. There are many research areas where IoT is growing its roots rapidly. Some of them are:

- Smart homes
- Smart cars
- Health care
- Agriculture
- Industries
- Transportation

Before the introduction of the IoT, we were accustomed to finding the remote of the Air Conditioner, reaching for the switch to turn on/off the light, searching for the keys of the car or keys for our home. Similarly, doctors were accustomed to limited visits and phone calls for interacting with patients. There was no way to remotely monitor the patient's vitals and health continuously and make further recommendations according to the data. IoT devices have made remote monitoring possible in the healthcare sector, which unlocks the potentials of keeping the patients safe and healthy and giving the power to physicians to give better care. It has also increased the engagement of doctors and patients and the interactions have become easier and efficient. Remote Monitoring of patient's health keeps the patient's visits and long stay inside the hospital at a minimum to reduce the risks of readmission. IoT has also reduced healthcare costs significantly and has improved treatment outcomes [37].

IoT has done wonders in the field of health care. It has improved the quality of patient monitoring and testing by monitoring patients remotely. It majorly benefits the patients who live in remote areas and face difficulties in reaching out to doctors and get themselves treated with proper testing and infrastructure. IoT devices can sense various human activities periodically and can provide all the data to the doctor that eases the need to visit them every day or two, especially for aged people who are required to get themselves monitored periodically. Doctors and relatives can know their locations in case of medical emergencies and can reach out to them easily using that same IoT healthcare wearable device. There are already many smart healthcare wearable devices that involve different microcontrollers, sensors, and actuators for smart monitoring of patients. They are available in many forms such as clothing, accessories, insulin pumps, and now even pills that contain sensors and can track the person who has swallowed it [38].

Several medical embedded devices are also available such as pacemakers that are directly implanted inside the human body and can track the working of the human heart and can predict heart attacks at an early stage. Such IoT wearable devices are controlled and accessed using mobile apps and send messages and notifications in case of any abnormality with periodically monitored data of the patient. This data can be shared with the doctor or health service provider immediately so that they can know about the patient's abnormal health without the help of any staff and even before the patient visits them.

IoT wearable devices can even help young adults to monitor their daily physical activities that they generally record to maintain the balance. All this data can be collected and can be shared among various devices, but one of the major issues it faces is the security. To handle patients remotely, the infrastructure requires secure data sharing since health data is private, and this data may even contain the location of the patient that raises the risk of exposure. The current system involves centralized architecture for data sharing that is not secure in all cases so it can be solved by using Blockchain technology.

8.2 Benefits and safety challenges in patient-centric healthcare systems

IoT has many advantages over healthcare systems. These advantages can be categorized with the healthcare staff, patient, hospital, doctor, pharmacist, etc. IoT has changed how a patient's vitals are monitored. Various devices that are in the form of wearables such as fitness bands and other connected devices or sensors such as Blood Pressure Monitor, glucometer, heart rate cuffs, etc., which give the patients some personalized attention as these devices can be further configured to give us calculated data of calories, appointments, peak rate, etc. Healthcare sector has been adopting IoT for the betterment of doctors and patients to provide utmost care and service. Surgical implants and devices are being used to provide patients a better life than they had imagined [39].

There are a lot of cases being reported having cybersecurity issues, accessing, and controlling a user's home appliances, etc. Managing security on these many nodes is a lot more difficult as every device keeps sending the data, which can be intercepted by hackers to gain access on the network. With the development of technology, hacking is relatively a lot easy. Cybersecurity is an important and required sector to prevent unauthorized access to user's data and to keep the privacy options safe and secure. Several major issues are [40,41]:

- Lack of access to healthcare system—Though there is a lot of development in the field of health care, but the people in rural areas do not have a proper access to the healthcare technology as most of them are available in the urban areas, and the people in the rural areas could not manage to come to the urban areas every time.
- Adherence to the treatment—The healthcare providers do not have proper equipment to monitor whether their patients are sticking to the treatment that is prescribed to them and are following it properly or not. Due to the lack of knowledge in patients, they might not be able to properly stick to the exercises that are prescribed, which increases the risks and chances of hospitalization.
- Expenses—Rising cost of health care is a major issue as the expenses in health care have increased to a great extent in the recent years.
- Privacy—Privacy of data in health care is an important thing to be taken care of as the patients expect that their personal data would be protected and would remain confidential. Since IoT-based healthcare devices lack the privacy of data, so it is important to take care of the privacy of the data of the patients.
- Security—IoT has changed the way how the things work and is used in almost every field and in health care too, but the IoT applications and the data received from the IoT-based devices are not secure, which is one of the major challenges faced by IoT in health care.

8.3 Blockchain technology and its architecture

Some of the important blockchain technology aspects and architecture are briefly explained as follows.

- Blockchain technology was first practically introduced in 2008 by an unknown person known as Satoshi Nakamoto[42]. Blockchain technology was used in Bitcoin, which is a currency to verify the transactions between sender and receiver.

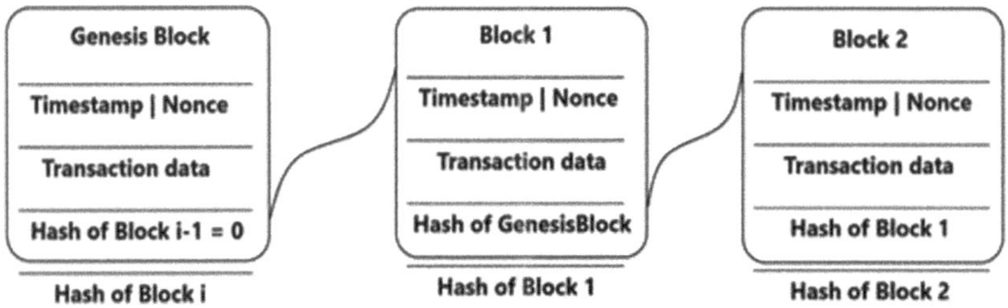

Figure 13.13 Blockchain architecture.

- Blockchain is a linear data structure like a doubly linked list connected with each other with hashes, a block is defined by its hash and the hash of the block is made with of the previous block, this prevents anyone to modify or delete any block in the transaction. The first block is called the Genesis block, also called the Block 0, from Genesis block, blocks are added, and a chain is formed. Fig. 13.13 shows an example of blockchain architecture.
- The first block, which is the origin, is known as the Genesis block. As there is no previous block, the hash of the previous block will be 0. The identification of each block is done by using a hash value, which is like a fingerprint that is unique for each block. The Blockchains generally check the hashes of each block after a certain amount of time. If there is any change in the block, then it can be detected and located because of the avalanche effect that follows. So, if the change in the hashes is unacceptable in the system, then it would be impossible for anyone to make any changes because not only the hash of the manipulated block but the blocks associated will also change, thus making each Block of the Blockchain system immutable [43,44].

There is a mining competition so that it can be decided which machine will add the block to the transaction. Consensus algorithms help in deciding which machine will add the block. Fig. 13.14 shows a reward-based blockchain approach that give rewards to miners on successfully putting a challenges or solving it. There are many consensus algorithms such as Proof of Work (PoW), Proof of Elapsed Time (PoET), etc. Data of the block includes the nonce of the block, difficulty, and timestamp of the block. A nonce is a random number whose hash must be smaller than the target hash to reach the consensus. The difficulty is the number of zeroes that must be before a hash to reach the consensus, for PoW, whereas it is the random time wait associated with each machine in PoET [44,45]. A timestamp is when a transaction has happened, and a block is added in the chain.

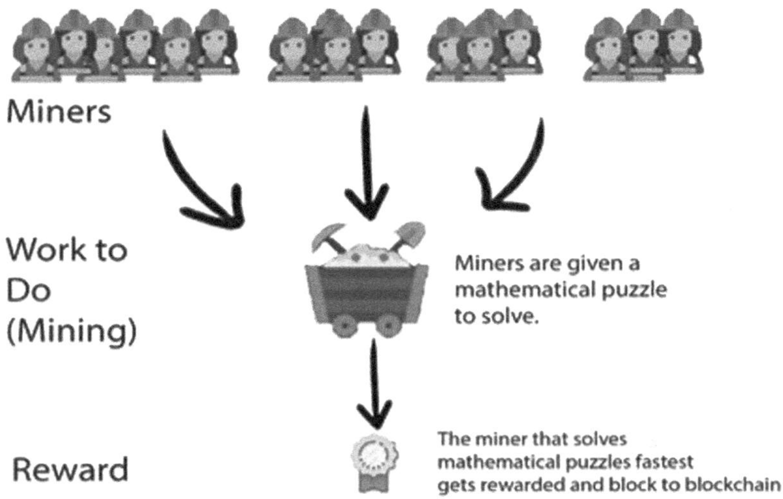

Figure 13.14 Mining process in blockchain technology.

Merkle Tree root is used for summarizing the integrity of all the transactions efficiently. Each transaction hash is paired and concatenated and then hashed again till a single root hash is generated, this root hash is called as Merkle Tree root.

While a blockchain is an excellent architecture for securing IoT networks, the methods and computations it uses do not support wearable devices and daily sharing of data with different hospitals. One of the main disadvantages of blockchain is that it uses a lot of electricity just for generating one block, which in health care could just be data of one test or an operation prescribed medicines, which is a good example of limited scalability. Most of the blockchain networks that function around the world use PoW, which doubles hashes on every nonce, so every time a nonce is received by the machine, it double hashes and disregards it if it is not less than the length of the target hash, which consumes a lot of electricity to compute, for one machine, to reach a consensus many machines compute nonce, turning it into a heavy machinery game. The providers also to increase their chances of consensus use many machines just to have one consensus. To prevent the disadvantages of blockchain to affect the idea, a lightweight private blockchain is considered, in which practical Byzantine Fault Tolerance is used, which applies to our blockchain to reach consensus, the Byzantine Fault Tolerance system helps in low overheads and increases the performance of PoW [46].

A blockchain will enable the patient only to share their blocks and can decide which blocks to share with the hospitals. Many healthcare systems have been exploited by the hospitals and hackers can access that data from the hospital about the patient. To avoid analysis and data privacy of patients, this mode of blockchain has been chosen. A private blockchain is a chain of blocks that is owned by a user or group that has the password or cryptographic key to access it. Since blockchain is decentralized, and every block has the information of all the transactions, but in a cryptographic hash that cannot be undone to get the data, hence all the blocks will be separated by their respective hospitals and the main server will be dedicated, which will contain all the info of all the blocks of the chain, meaning blockchain, which will be private and only the user will be having the cryptographic passkey for that chain. The user can choose to share the data on the blocks with the hospitals, this way the doctor can only view the data of the user and cannot change it since if they change it, the original data will be in the cloud along with other blocks that have been in the miner's machine. This way, low overhead occurs, computation power is being used less, and performance is also high, following the privacy of the user [47].

8.4 Various frameworks for healthcare systems using blockchain technology

Within the healthcare industry, various blockchain-based solutions have been proposed that connect doctors, hospitals, and patients and provide improved privacy protection and efficient processing of data in healthcare systems.

Dwivedi A. et al. [48] have proposed an architecture that gives an almost perfect solution to security and privacy threats and taking care of the IoT constraint factor. In this work, the author introduced an efficient mixed architecture that includes the benefits of the blockchain, private key, public key, and many other lightweight cryptographic concepts to develop an EMR management that keeps focusing on patient access control. This paper also focuses on concepts to reduce their risks such as modification attacks, DoS, etc. However, the focus has been on answering the resource constraints of IoT. Rathee G. et al. [49] have focused a secured healthcare framework using blockchain. Blockchain has been used to provide transparency and secrecy among the intermediates, patients, and to document each activity made by IoT devices. This proposed healthcare framework shows the Blockchain's usefulness for efficiently applying the transparency and security of a patient's record, between customer and provider can do shipment process and document accessibility using Blockchain. Further, using blockchain in health care, a patient's record information, medical shipment process, or intermediates activity can be captured from IoT objects between customer and provider. Any illegal activity would be easily traceable using Blockchain that will be in between provider and customer. Dea-woo Prak et al. [50] have discussed the world cybersecurity agreement to collect and share the information related to cybersecurity all over the world for national cybersecurity using Blockchain technology. The authors analyzed the security of Blockchain and designed a hyper ledger Blockchain system for it by using the proof-of-stake consensus and linked all the information related to cybersecurity to the hyper ledger using the national cybersecurity center. Meet Shah et al. [51] elaborated a system to encrypt the user's file and stored it across multiple peers inside the network. The authors used an InterPlanetary File System (IPFS) protocol, which creates a hash value and indicates the path of the files. The system uses AES 256 bit encryption algorithm to encrypt the data and maintain the confidentiality of data. The authors claimed that the system not only solves the security issue by the distributed cloud system but also ensures that the peers can rent their underutilized storage and could earn cryptocurrency as a result. Aanchal Yadav et al. [52] have mentioned how Blockchain can be used to solve many problems related to health care. The authors have mentioned that the increase in the expenditure on drug discovery and patient recovery and the third-rate and fake medicines, all these problems can be solved by using Blockchain technology as it does not involve any third party or intermediaries. In this paper, the authors have reviewed the usage of Blockchain in patient data management, supply chain, etc. Agbo C. et al. [53] reported systematic research on healthcare applications using Blockchain. The authors have presented an overview of Blockchain mentioning all the use cases of Blockchain in health care. They also focused on what limitations came when Blockchain applications were developed and what are the challenges and security risks faced by Blockchain. The research shows that there are many applications of Blockchain in health care, and many of them have already been developed. Ajao et al. [54] have proposed an architecture for the efficient monitoring and securing of products based on petroleum distributed records using efficient Blockchain that implements a decentralized ledger database. The authors propose a system using blockchain that will prevent tampering, fraudulent activity, and corruption of transactions and a geolocation tracking and monitoring of petroleum volume level in real time. Bamakan S. et al. [55] have discussed an overview of various consensus algorithms with their disadvantages and advantages and propose an analytic framework having four categories to characterize based on consensus algorithms' performance including algorithms' securities and vulnerabilities, degree of decentralization, the profitability of mining, and algorithms throughput. Also explaining the challenges and future research directions of this field. Priyanka S. et al. [56] have proposed a cost-effective wearable cardiorespiratory monitoring device that can display data in real time on a phone or computer screen. The authors display data based on four parameters: respiration rate, heart rate, peripheral capillary oxygen saturation that can help in monitoring a heart patient. Using the data, heart attacks can be predicted, and patients can be saved. Leila Ismail et al. [57] discussed a lightweight blockchain architecture for healthcare data management by creating clusters of participants and creating a copy of the ledger to each cluster with the help of a canal, a method to have secure and confidential transactions. The authors also propose a solution to avoid forking that is available in Bitcoin Blockchain architecture. The authors also present an analysis that shows why their architecture is much more efficient than Bitcoin Blockchain architecture.

8.5 Markle root tree (MRT) for COVID-19 vaccination

With new computing techniques, encryption is far more advanced today than it was ever before. Hashing techniques were developed to be used for indexing and locating items on a database because of the ease of usage. Hashing was used as a comparison technique that then was implemented as an encryption method to authenticate messages due to its comparability. Hashing is used in encrypting and decrypting digital signatures. Now, the hash function in use can help the digital signature mechanism to generate a message digest. This message digest is compared with the received message digest value, which then uses the same hash function to generate the hash value and compare it to the received hash value. If the hash values match, the message was likely transmitted without error. What makes this technique secure is the near impossibility of determining the original number on a hashed value, unless the algorithm is known. There are a set of requirements that a hash function has to satisfy to be called a cryptographic hash function, they are [35]:

1. It must be easy to take the message and put it through a hash function and receive output.
2. The hash value or the hash should not be reversible, i.e., there should be a zero possibility of reaching the original message by reverse-engineering the hash.

3. It should be deterministic. The hash value received at the output should not change with time. For every input, there must be a determined constant output hash value.
4. Any minor or major changes in the message should warrant a different hash value and should have no resemblance to the hash value of any other message that is remotely similar.
5. Last but not least, two messages should never produce the same hash value. It must be computationally infeasible to have two messages produce the same hash value.

This technique of hashing has various hashing algorithms that are used to implement it. These hashing techniques were implemented to a large extent in the formation of the blockchain or Bitcoin technology. It was a key part of how transactions worked and how the basis of security and authentication was established in every transaction.

8.5.1 The need for Merkle tree

Digital signatures have already been proposed a long time ago[36], and their sole use is to authenticate digital messages or documents, thereby assuring the receiver that the message was sent through a genuine source and is unaltered [37]. A Merkle tree includes all transactions, which in turn is useful in comparing the fingerprints of transactions. Here, all sets of transactions are collected to generate the fingerprints. As a result, its verification of fingerprints helps provide information whether a particular transaction is added to a block or not [38]. Digital signatures were based on conventional encryption algorithms, but there is a lack of convenience of systems [36]. The second advantage is of reduced computational costs instead of using modulo N(natural number). A Merkle tree is similar to a binary tree, i.e., each node will have a maximum of two nodes. A Merkle tree is a binary tree with its root node being the Merkle root. This Merkle root is obtained by hashing two transaction hashes(from the leaf node position) together to make another combined hash, which is then hashed again till it converges at one point at the root node also called the Merkle root. This Merkle root is a part of the block header of every block that is transmitted or "Mined" during the process of bitcoin mining. This Merkle key then completes the block header and serves as an authenticity key for future reference. Once established in a block, the Merkle root cannot be changed. If changed, all the users in the mining process will get to know that the data has been tampered with and will hence be ruled unauthentic. To check the authenticity of the user(or the transaction), we start from the Merkle root and then

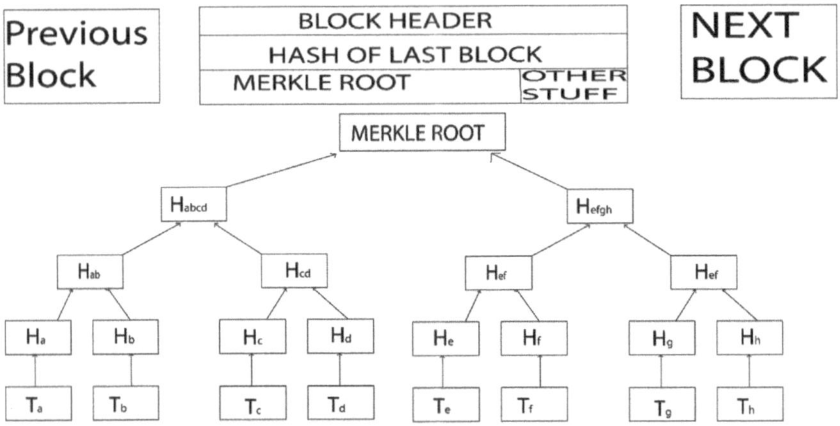

Figure 13.15 Pictorial representation of Merkle tree.

traverse down the tree, if we reach the leaf node(i.e., transaction), then it is considered as authentic. Hashing is a one-way function (as mentioned above) and even a minor change will change the whole hash for the entire transaction or the document. Fig. 13.15 shows an example of Merkle tree. Consider a block comprising of eight transactions, each of which has a unique transaction ID say T_A through T_G. Each of which has a unique hash value after being hashed (h_a to h_g). These hash values or hashes are the leaf nodes of the binary tree we are building. The hashes are then taken in pairs and hashed again, which then results in forming parent nodes such as h_{ab}, h_{cd}, h_{ef}, h_{gh}. These are then taken in pairs and hashed again. This process continues till we arrive at one hash value at the top of the binary tree, which is called the Merkle root. The tree obtained is called the Merkle tree.

Following are the steps that can be used to create a Merkle tree:

1. Create a custom hashing algorithm.
2. Consider a few transactions or documents in a block and use the hashing algorithm on them.
3. Combine the obtained hash values or hashes and make them into pairs.
4. Hash the obtained pairs and continue the process upward.
5. Once there comes a point where there is only one hash value remaining, i.e., once we obtain the root node, stop.
6. This root node is called the Merkle root. And our tree obtained in the process is called the Merkle tree.
7. This unique Merkle root is then placed in the block header that serves as a unique identity to transactions in the block.
8. Any transaction in the block can then be authenticated by traversing through the branch that it is in using the Merkle root.

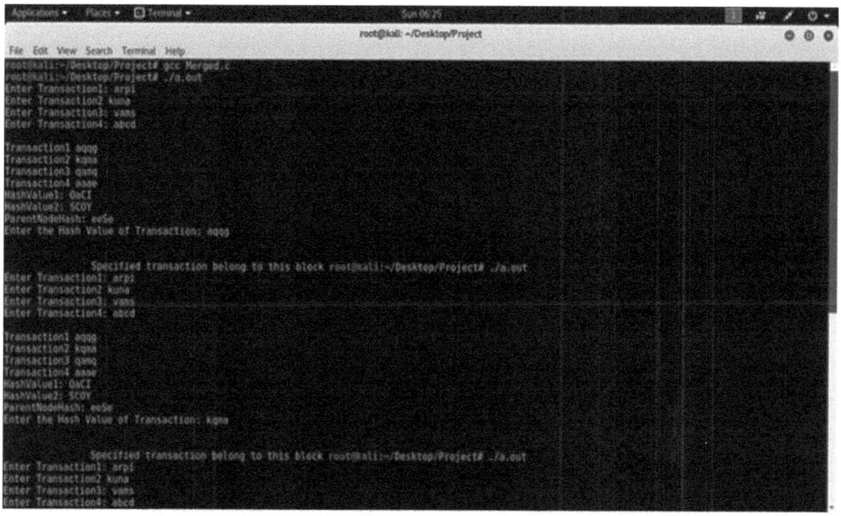

Figure 13.16 Blockchain simulation for vaccination drive.

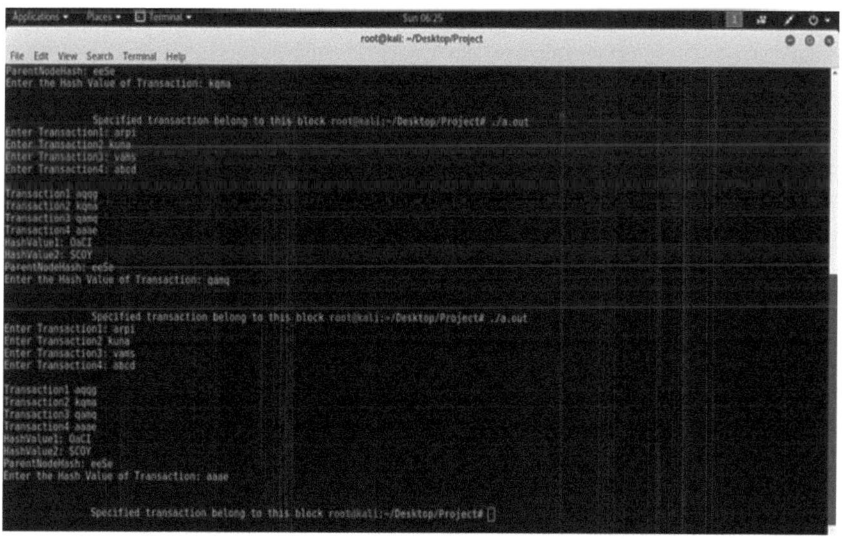

Figure 13.17 Blockchain verification in the simulation process.

9. If the transaction is found on the branch, then it is authentic. Or else, it is not.

Fig. 13.16 and Fig. 13.17 show an example of a blockchain simulator designed using python and an object-oriented concept. In this blockchain implementation, user can enter their data and can see the simulation of various activities performed using blockchain-like performing a transaction, selection of users, transferring the funds between blockchains, generating hash values, generating private, public and shared keys, applying encryption/decryption and digital signature operations using a common key, and many more. This blockchain simulation is designed to keep vaccination distribution into consideration because the simulated operations are useful for distribution plans.

9. Research challenges in vaccination and its distribution

In research challenges, the selection of parameters and assumptions for planning the vaccination driver requires more realistic scenarios [6]. Variation in these assumptions and parameters are required to be verified with realistic results before applying. Likewise, various challenges need to be investigated in this program. This includes designing a framework that adapts the dynamic situations. It has been observed that multiple COVID-19 strains are observed in various countries. These strains are getting the COVID-19 form more severe compared to previous versions. Thus, there is a strong need to preplan the activities and arrange frontline workers. Arranging these workers and providing training for their safety and logistic operation require coordination. A preplanned coordination strategy with digital technologies is more helpful in handling the situations. Other challenges include:

1. Make plans to publicly endorse the vaccine and its importance through real-time studies and trusted people.
2. Planning, executing, and analyzing the vaccine drives in a systematic way and as per the directions of world-renowned organizations.
3. Transforming the vaccination plans and decisions into a well-accepted public act. This act should give the right to people that necessities can be ensured for them.
4. Federated COVID-19 protection and promotion efforts are made by both government organizations and individuals in both developed and developing countries. However, multiple strains and an increase in the number of cases show that self-protection is primary concern compared to other approaches.

9.1 Mental health during COVID-19 times and vaccine for stress relief

As COVID-19 has affected a large number of people socially, mentally, economically, and physically, it is important to identify the effects and possible remedies. This section shows the recent studies on mental health care for a different set of people including the general public. Following studies are presented to study and analyze the impact of COVID-19 during recent times.

- Walton et al. [58] conducted the study to analyze the mental effects on medical staff and doctors. This is a theoretical discussion and development-based study to analyze the effects on medical staff and detailed the guidelines for organization, team, and individuals. This study is important to consider because COVID-19 has created huge pressure on healthcare members and infrastructure throughout the world. In this work, various stress indicators during COVID-19 are identified. This includes physical, behavioral, emotional, and cognitive indicators. Further, a set of support practices are detailed for the pandemic situation.
- Gruber et al. [59] studied the behavior of 3000 participants during COVID-19. Results are graphically drawn and statically discussed for various factors such as happiness, life satisfaction, self-esteem, and depressions. Results found that dose of nature is important for life, and it can give much more valuable support to handle mental health. Factors such as "duration of greenspace usage" are identified and analyzed. This factor is considered under dose of nature and associated with improving mental health. Overall, this study is found to be very useful and helpful in reducing mental health.
- Thapa et al. [60] study the importance of healthcare briefly. Here, factors such as "psychological wellbeing of pregnant women" are emphasized only for bringing the audience's attention toward health care in COVID-19. The short form of this article has covered large but important aspects that need to be stressed upon. This includes stress, anger, confusion for maternal health. However, there is a need to extend this study for more in-depth analysis.

Likewise, there are other studies conducted in recent times [58–63] to study the mental health and need for vaccines to remove stress in current times. Table 13.1 shows a comparative analysis of such studies. It has been identified in these studies that physical exercise and the dose of nature are more important compared to vaccination. Short of vaccine, its harmful and unknown facts are major reasons of not able to make the trust of people. Further, there is a need to have strong research and innovation findings in the future for handling current and future pandemics.

9.2 Vaccination storage facility shortage, Indian scenario and mental health

The emergence of the recently discovered book COVID19 has thrown the entire planet into chaos. From the last 4 months, a large group of people have been affected. People are considering infected persons' avoidance,

Table 13.1 Comparative analysis of mental health studies conducted during COVID-19 times.

Author	Year	A	B	C	D	E	F	G	Major observations	Major shortcomings
Walton et al. [58]	2020	✓	✗	✓	✓	✓	✓	✗	This work has studied the recommendations, practices, and supports for healthcare providers and individuals.	This study lacks provide statistical details and facts. This work can be extended to have an in-depth indicator analysis to find concrete proofs for stress.
Gruber et al. [59]	2020	✓	✗	✓	✓	✗	✓	✗	A statistical analysis of sociodemographic and lifestyle variables is analyzed. Results show that dose of nature is found to be much useful in stress removal during COVID-19.	This work can be extended to apply machine learning-based approaches for analyzing the data. The machine learning-based models can give more in-depth analysis and outlier detection.
Thapa et al. [60]	2020	✗	✓	✓	✗	✗	✓	✗	This work is a short survey of maternal health and associated parameters. Here, factors like stress, anger, and confusion during pregnancy and COVID-19 are discussed.	This work can be extended to include a statistical-based discussion to emphasize the importance of the identified factor.

Antunes and Frontini [61]	2021	✗	✓	✓	✗	✗	✓	✗	This is a short survey article to identify the parameters that affect mental health. Here, the importance of physical activities is also discussed.	This work can be extended with in-depth analysis and surveys. Further, a statistical-based analysis can be useful to analyze the facts rather than theoretical discussions.
Soga et al. [62]	2021	✗	✓	✓	✓	✗	✓	✓	This work has prepared psychological symptoms and discussed the need to find innovative solutions. Here, clinical approaches and policy issues are also discussed which need research attention.	An in-depth analysis of research directions, associated datasets, studies, and frameworks are yet needed to be explored. This work proposes a set of directions but needs to have some research base to accept the work on real-ground.
Huang et al. [63]	2021	✓	✓	✓	✓		✓	✓	This work discussed the issues to health workers and young people during COVID-19 times. The need to measure psychological consequences for the high-risk population is explored.	This work covers an in-depth analysis of psychological factors associated with mental health. Statistical analysis is also performed. However, this work can be extended to perform a comparative analysis with existing studies to find the best approach. .

Note: A: Medical staff mental health condition discussions, B: General public mental health discussion, C: Support discussions during COVID-19, D: Major injury discussions E: Minor Injury Discussions, F: Survey article, G: Vaccine for Stress Relive.

vaccination, medical treatment, and other safeguards. To combat the spread of the virus, the authorities of most nations, including India, have already implemented a number of measures such as lockdown, social distance, and the suspension of schools, universities, and religious gatherings, among others. The cold chain is a technique for carrying and preserving vaccinations at temperatures between 2 and 8°C. The cold chain starts when the vaccine is made, proceeds to the province or territorial vaccine dissemination facility and vaccination service provider, and concludes when the vaccine is given out. All employees must be educated in vaccine storage and cold chain management, according to vaccine suppliers. Employees learning should be facilitated by using the NSW Health Vaccine Storage and Cold Chain Management digital training session to equip staff to successfully manage the cold chain. The vaccine cold chain issue is just the latest example of the pandemic's disproportionate impact on the underprivileged, who are more likely to live and work in overcrowding, which allows the virus to spread, have limited access to medical oxygen, which is essential for COVID-19 treatment, and whose healthcare systems shortage labs, materials, and professionals to conduct large-scale laboratory tests. A vaccine bottle is only valid for 6 hours after being pierced to provide a dosage, after which it must be destroyed, necessitating careful onsite cold storage and vaccination procedures. As its COVID19 vaccine will most likely be in low supply in many regions during early deployment, vaccination workers will need to prevent deterioration and wastage, which can account for up to 30% [64] of the availability. The necessity for booster dosages, the use of diluents, and availability to vulnerable people, such as healthcare professionals, children, and the old, all provide additional challenges to the cold chain in remote regions.

The AstraZeneca Plc vaccine, made by the Serum Institute of India, or the Covaxin shot, created by Bharat Biotech International, a private firm located in Hyderabad, are used in India's local vaccination program. Due to the extreme absence of accurate data, India's authorization of the Bharat Biotech injection, which was created with government-backed research institutions, was received with considerable condemnation from experts. In 2019, the worldwide vaccination marketplace was predicted to be worth Rs. 2.3 lakh crores [65], accounting for 2% of the worldwide pharmaceuticals industry. In contrast, India's vaccine market was valued at Rs. 9500 crores in 2020 and is predicted to increase at a CAGR of 18% to reach Rs. 256.5 billion crores by 2026. In Ref. [66], a research is conducted on 662 individuals from throughout India, finding that over 80% of them were concerned with COVID-19-related thoughts. Sleep problems, social networking anxiety, and worry about catching COVID-19 were indicated by 12.5%, 36.4%, and 37.8% of individuals, respectively. Surprisingly, more than 80% of participants said they needed mental health treatment.

10. Conclusion and future directions

With the COVID-19 vaccine development, various distribution strategies are planned in different geographical regions of this world. These activities involve advanced technologies and frontline medical workers to make the distribution plan successful. In addition to this, various suppliers and distributors are involved in this program. Integration of all stakeholders and making a secure distribution plan require well-prepared models or frameworks. These frameworks should be dynamic and accept the changes with change in real-time conditions. This work has outlined the distribution strategies designed so far in COVID-19 vaccination distribution. Here, more emphasis is drawn on the use of technologies. For example, the importance of crowdsourcing is discussed for resource availability, sharing, and reusage. Besides, IoT, parallel and distributed processing, Healthcare 4.0 services, drones, robotics, and blockchain technologies and their usage in vaccination plans are discussed. Here, the focus is drawn toward the integration of multiple technologies and providing an efficient solution that largely focuses on optimizing the cost and providing better healthcare services, especially during pandemic times. This work can be extended in various other directions including proposing frameworks that integrate the proposed solution over large-scale implementation. Further, vaccination case studies can be prepared once the implemented program is found to be successful.

References

[1] COVID-19 and Influenza Vaccine Distribution Stakeholder Considerations, 2020. https://avalere.com/insights/covid-19-and-influenza-vaccine-distribution-stakeholder-considerations.

[2] Real-Time Vaccine Logistics Data to Improve Immunization Coverage Through the Electronic Vaccine Intelligence Network (eVIN). https://www.undp-capacity development-health.org/en/capacities/focus/innovation-and-technologies/digitizing-the-supply-chain/the-electronic-vaccine-ntelligence-etwork-evin-in-india/.

[3] From the Factory to the Frontlines The Operation Warp Speed Strategy for Distributing a COVID-19 Vaccine. https://www.hhs.gov/sites/default/files/strategy-for-distributing-covid-19-vaccine.pdf.

[4] S. Sun, Z. Xie, K. Yu, B. Jiang, S. Zheng, X. Pan, COVID-19 and healthcare system in China: challenges and progression for a sustainable future, Glob. Health 17 (1) (2021) 1–8.

[5] S.I. Chen, B.A. Norman, J. Rajgopal, T.M. Assi, B.Y. Lee, S.T. Brown, A planning model for the WHO-EPI vaccine distribution network in developing countries, IIE Trans. 46 (8) (2014) 853–865.

[6] M.C. Mills, D. Salisbury, The challenges of distributing COVID-19 vaccinations, EClinicalMedicine 31 (2021).

[7] U. Illahi, M.S. Mir, Maintaining efficient logistics and supply chain management operations during and after coronavirus (COVID-19) pandemic: learning from the past experiences, Environ. Dev. Sustain. (2021) 1–22.

[8] A. Kumar, R. Krishnamurthi, A. Nayyar, A.K. Luhach, M.S. Khan, A. Singh, A novel Software-Defined Drone Network (SDDN)-based collision avoidance strategies for on-road traffic monitoring and management, Veh. Commun. 28 (2021) 100313.

[9] M. Goyal, A. Kumar, Sustainable E-infrastructure for blockchain-based voting system, in: Digital Cities Roadmap: IoT-Based Architecture and Sustainable Buildings, 2021, p. 221.

[10] S. Jain, K. Kaushik, D.K. Sharma, R. Krishnamurthi, A. Kumar, Sustainable Infrastructure Theories and Models, in: Digital Cities Roadmap: IoT-Based Architecture and Sustainable Buildings, 2021, p. 97.

[11] P. Srikanth, A. Kumar, A trustworthy partner selection for MMOG using an improved three valued subjective logic uncertainty trust model, PalArch's J. Archaeol. Egypt/Egyptol. 18 (4) (2021) 5677–5698.

[12] A. Kumar, M. Elsersy, A. Darwsih, A.E. Hassanien, Drones Combat COVID-19 Epidemic: Innovating and Monitoring Approach, in: Digital Transformation and Emerging Technologies for Fighting COVID-19 Pandemic: Innovative Approaches, 2021, pp. 175–188.

[13] H.S. Lallie, et al., Cyber security in the age of COVID-19: a timeline and analysis of cyber-crime and cyber-attacks during the pandemic, Comput. Secur. 105 (2021) 102248, https://doi.org/10.1016/j.cose.2021.102248.

[14] S. Furnell, J.N. Shah, Home working and cyber security – an outbreak of unpreparedness? Comput. Fraud Secur. 2020 (8) (2020) 6–12, https://doi.org/10.1016/S1361-3723(20)30084-1.

[15] B. Pranggono, A. Arabo, COVID-19 pandemic cybersecurity issues, Internet Technol. Lett. 4 (2) (2021) e247, https://doi.org/10.1002/itl2.247.

[16] 10 Ways Cybersecurity Can Protect COVID-19 Vaccine Supply Chains - Business 2 Community, 2021. https://www.business2community.com/cybersecurity/10-ways-cybersecurity-can-protect-covid-19-vaccine-supply-chains-02392668. (Accessed 30 March 2021).

[17] K. Kaushik, S. Dahiya, R. Singh, A.D. Dwivedi, Role of blockchain in forestalling pandemics, in: Proceedings – 2020 IEEE 17th International Conference on Mobile Ad Hoc and Smart Systems, MASS 2020, 2020, pp. 32–37, https://doi.org/10.1109/MASS50613.2020.00014.

[18] Cybersecurity Threats to the COVID-19 Vaccine – Talk IoT, 2021. https://talkiot.co.za/2021/02/17/cybersecurity-threats-to-the-covid-19-vaccine/. (Accessed 31 March 2021).

[19] M. Muthuppalaniappan, K. Stevenson, Healthcare cyber-attacks and the COVID-19 pandemic: an urgent threat to global health, Int. J. Qual. Health Care 33 (1) (2021) 1–4, https://doi.org/10.1093/intqhc/mzaa117.

[20] S.M. Toapanta Toapanta, J. Alfredo Espinoza Carpio, L.E. Mafla Gallegos, An Approach to Cybersecurity, Cyberbullying in Social Networks and Information Security in Public Organizations During a Pandemic: Study Case Covid-19 Ecuador, 2020, https://doi.org/10.1109/CONIITI51147.2020.9240375.

[21] S. Furnell, J. Haney, M. Theofanos, Pandemic parallels: what can cybersecurity learn from COVID-19? Computer 54 (3) (2021) 68–72, https://doi.org/10.1109/mc.2020.3046888.

[22] R.O. Andrade, I. Ortiz-Garces, M. Cazares, Cybersecurity attacks on smart home during Covid-19 pandemic, in: Proceedings of the World Conference on Smart Trends in Systems, Security and Sustainability, WS4 2020, 2020, pp. 398–404, https://doi.org/10.1109/WorldS450073.2020.9210363.

[23] C. Stolojescu-Crisan, B.P. Butunoi, C. Crisan, IoT Based Intelligent Building Applications in the Context of Covid-19 Pandemic, 2020, https://doi.org/10.1109/ISETC50328.2020.9301124.

[24] L. Tawalbeh, F. Muheidat, M. Tawalbeh, M. Quwaider, G. Saldamli, Predicting and preventing cyber attacks during COVID-19 time using data analysis and proposed secure IoT layered model, in: 2020 4th International Conference on Multimedia Computing, Networking and Applications, MCNA 2020, 2020, pp. 113–118, https://doi.org/10.1109/MCNA50957.2020.9264301.

[25] G. Forni, et al., COVID-19 vaccines: where we stand and challenges ahead, Cell Death Differ. 28 (2) (2021) 626–639, https://doi.org/10.1038/s41418-020-00720-9. Springer Nature.

[26] M.C. Mills, D. Salisbury, The challenges of distributing COVID-19 vaccinations, EClinicalMedicine 31 (2021) 100674, https://doi.org/10.1016/j.eclinm.2020.100674. Lancet Publishing Group.

[27] A. Kumar, K. Sharma, Digital transformation and emerging technologies for COVID-19 pandemic: social, global, and industry perspectives, in: Artificial Intelligence and Machine Learning for COVID-19, 2021, pp. 73–96.

[28] A. Kumar, K. Sharma, H. Singh, P. Srikanth, R. Krishnamurthi, A. Nayyar, Drone-based social distancing, sanitization, inspection, monitoring, and control room for COVID-19, in: Artificial Intelligence and Machine Learning for COVID-19, 2021, pp. 153–173.

[29] S.S. Gill, A. Kumar, H. Singh, M. Singh, K. Kaur, M. Usman, R. Buyya, Quantum Computing: A Taxonomy, Systematic Review and Future Directions, arXiv preprint arXiv:2010.15559, 2020.

[30] A. Kumar, K. Sharma, H. Singh, S.G. Naugriya, S.S. Gill, R. Buyya, A drone-based networked system and methods for combating coronavirus disease (COVID-19) pandemic, Future Generat. Comput. Syst. 115 (2021) 1–19.

[31] A. Kumar, K. Rajalakshmi, S. Jain, A. Nayyar, M. Abouhawwash, A novel heuristic simulation-optimization method for critical infrastructure in smart transportation systems, Int. J. Commun. Syst. 33 (11) (2020) e4397.

[32] A. Kumar, S. Jain, Drone-based monitoring and redirecting system, in: Development and Future of Internet of Drones (IoD): Insights, Trends and Road Ahead, 2021, pp. 163–183.

[33] K. Sharma, H. Singh, D.K. Sharma, A. Kumar, A. Nayyar, R. Krishnamurthi, Dynamic models and control techniques for drone delivery of medications and other healthcare items in COVID-19 hotspots, in: Emerging Technologies for Battling Covid-19, vol. 324, 2021, p. 1.

[34] A. Kumar, D.K. Sharma, An optimized multilayer outlier detection for internet of things (IoT) network as industry 4.0 automation and data exchange, in: International Conference on Innovative Computing and Communications, Springer, Singapore, 2021, pp. 571–584.

[35] L. Atzori, A. Iera, G. Morabito, The internet of things: a survey, Comput. Network. 54 (15) (2010) 2787–2805.

[36] R.H. Weber, R. Weber, Internet of Things, vol. 12, Springer, Heidelberg, 2010.

[37] Y.I.N. Yuehong, Y. Zeng, X. Chen, Y. Fan, The internet of things in healthcare: an overview, J. Industr. Inform. Integr. 1 (2016) 3–13.

[38] A. Papa, M. Mital, P. Pisano, M. Del Giudice, E-health and wellbeing monitoring using smart healthcare devices: an empirical investigation, Technol. Forecast. Soc. Change 153 (2020) 119226.

[39] N. Menachemi, R.G. Brooks, Reviewing the benefits and costs of electronic health records and associated patient safety technologies, J. Med. Syst. 30 (3) (2006) 159–168.
[40] B. Farahani, F. Firouzi, V. Chang, M. Badaroglu, N. Constant, K. Mankodiya, Towards fog-driven IoT eHealth: promises and challenges of IoT in medicine and healthcare, Future Generat. Comput. Syst. 78 (2018) 659–676.
[41] A. Kasthuri, Challenges to healthcare in India-The five A's, Indian J. Commun. Med. 43 (3) (2018) 141.
[42] S. Nakamoto, A. Bitcoin, A Peer-To-Peer Electronic Cash System. Bitcoin, 2008, p. 4. URL: https://bitcoin.org/bitcoin.pdf.
[43] Z. Zheng, S. Xie, H. Dai, X. Chen, H. Wang, An overview of blockchain technology: architecture, consensus, and future trends, in: 2017 IEEE International Congress on Big Data (BigData Congress), IEEE, 2017, pp. 557–564.
[44] D. Mingxiao, M. Xiaofeng, Z. Zhe, W. Xiangwei, C. Qijun, A review on consensus algorithm of blockchain, in: 2017 IEEE International Conference on Systems, Man, and Cybernetics (SMC), IEEE, 2017, pp. 2567–2572.
[45] A. Meneghetti, M. Sala, D. Taufer, A survey on PoW-based consensus, Ann. Emerg. Technol. Comput. 4 (1) (2020) 1–11. Print ISSN, 2516-0281. p2.
[46] V. Gramoli, From blockchain consensus back to Byzantine consensus, Future Generat. Comput. Syst. 107 (2020) 760–769.
[47] S. Alla, L. Soltanisehat, U. Tatar, O. Keskin, Blockchain technology in electronic healthcare systems, in: Proceedings of the 2018 IISE Annual Conference, 2018, pp. 1–6.
[48] A.D. Dwivedi, G. Srivastava, S. Dhar, R. Singh, A decentralized privacy-preserving healthcare blockchain for IoT, Sensors 19 (2) (2019) 326.
[49] G. Rathee, A. Sharma, H. Saini, R. Kumar, R. Iqbal, A hybrid framework for multimedia data processing in IoT-healthcare using blockchain technology, Multimed. Tool. Appl. (2019) 1–23.
[50] D.W. Prak, S.H. Lee, Hyperledger blockchain design for sharing, spreading, and protecting national cybersecurity information, J. Inform. Commun. Converg. Eng. 18 (2) (2020) 94–99.
[51] M. Shah, M. Shaikh, V. Mishra, G. Tuscano, Decentralized cloud storage using blockchain, in: 2020 4th International Conference on Trends in Electronics and Informatics (ICOEI)(48184), IEEE, 2020, pp. 384–389.
[52] A. Yadav, J. Ahmed, Blockchain: An Assured Technology for Protecting Healthcare in Post COVID-19 Era, J. Eng. Sci. (2020).
[53] C.C. Agbo, Q.H. Mahmoud, J.M. Eklund, Blockchain technology in healthcare: a systematic review, Healthcare 7 (2) (2019) 56 (Multidisciplinary Digital Publishing Institute).
[54] L.A. Ajao, J. Agajo, E.A. Adedokun, L. Karngong, Crypto hash algorithm-based blockchain technology for managing decentralized ledger database in oil and gas industry, J. Multidiscipl. Sci. 2 (3) (2019) 300–325.
[55] S.M.H. Bamakan, A. Motavali, A.B. Bondarti, A survey of blockchain consensus algorithms performance evaluation criteria, Expert Syst. Appl. (2020) 113385.
[56] P. Sasidharan, T. Rajalakshmi, U. Snekhalatha, Wearable cardiorespiratory monitoring device for heart attack prediction, in: 2019 International Conference on Communication and Signal Processing (ICCSP), IEEE, 2019, pp. 0054–0057.
[57] L. Ismail, H. Materwala, S. Zeadally, Lightweight blockchain for healthcare, IEEE Access 7 (2019) 149935–149951.
[58] M. Walton, E. Murray, M.D. Christian, Mental health care for medical staff and affiliated healthcare workers during the COVID-19 pandemic, Eur. Heart J. 9 (3) (2020) 241–247.

[59] J. Gruber, M.J. Prinstein, L.A. Clark, J. Rottenberg, J.S. Abramowitz, A.M. Albano, A. Aldao, J.L. Borelli, T. Chung, J. Davila, E.E. Forbes, Mental health and clinical psychological science in the time of COVID-19: challenges, opportunities, and a call to action, Am. Psychol. 76 (4) (2020) 409–426. 32772538.
[60] S.B. Thapa, A. Mainali, S.E. Schwank, G. Acharya, Maternal Mental Health in the Time of the COVID-19 Pandemic, 2020.
[61] R. Antunes, R. Frontini, Physical activity and mental health in Covid-19 times: an editorial, Sleep Med. 77 (2021) 295.
[62] M. Soga, M.J. Evans, K. Tsuchiya, Y. Fukano, A room with a green view: the importance of nearby nature for mental health during the COVID-19 pandemic, Ecol. Appl. 31 (2) (2021) e2248.
[63] Y. Huang, N. Zhao, Mental health burden for the public affected by the COVID-19 outbreak in China: who will be the high-risk group? Psychol. Health Med. 26 (1) (2021) 23–34.
[64] Blockchain's potential role in the history-making plan to deliver the COVID-19 vaccine | World Economic Forum, 2021. https://www.weforum.org/agenda/2020/07/blockchain-role-in-distributing-covid-19-vaccine-could-make-history/. (Accessed 15 June 2021).
[65] India COVID-19 Vaccination Distribution Report, 2021. URL: tica_distribution_report_web_v1.pdf (idfcinstitute.org). (Accessed 16 June 2021).
[66] D. Roy, S. Tripathy, S.K. Kar, N. Sharma, S.K. Verma, V. Kaushal, Study of knowledge, attitude, anxiety & perceived mental healthcare need in Indian population during COVID-19 pandemic, Asian J. Psychiatr. 51 (2020) 102083.

CHAPTER FOURTEEN

A blockchain approach on security of health records for children suffering from dyslexia during pandemic COVID-19

Megha Jain[1], Dhiraj Pandey[1] and Kewal Krishna Sharma[2]
[1]JSS Academy of Technical Education, Noida, UP, India
[2]Sanskriti University, Mathura, UP, India

1. Introduction

In India, 10% of children in India have learning disabilities (LDs). Delayed identification leads to mental health problems. Therefore, due to the lack of current assessments, we propose an automated approach that is objective, fast, and cost-effective. To develop a machine learning model to detect dyslexia and design computerized cognition assessment tests to identify developmental disorders, which include all the environmental factors and other factors as they also affect his/her situation. Dyslexia, also known as reading disorder, is characterized by trouble with reading despite normal intelligence. It is a neurologically based neurodevelopmental condition in which children find it difficult to read despite having appropriate IQ, education, and socioeconomic background. Dyslexia affects areas of the brain that process language. The percentage of people with dyslexia is not exactly known, but it has been estimated to be as low as 5% and as high as 17% of the population [1].

According to research by Panicker and Chelliah (2016), a greater number of students with a specific LD reported severe stress (16%), severe anxiety (23%), and/or severe depression (14%). An increasing amount of data shows that children and adolescents with dyslexia are more likely to have mental health issues. Poor readers were found to be at moderate risk of experiencing anxiety and depression in a meta-analysis by Francis et al. (2019), and it was also discovered that students with dyslexia have worse depression symptoms than those with nonverbal LDs. Dyslexia not only causes major difficulties for students, but it also results in severe consequences for their parents

Artificial Intelligence, Machine Learning, and Mental Health in Pandemics
ISBN: 978-0-323-91196-2
https://doi.org/10.1016/B978-0-323-91196-2.00004-1

(mothers, in particular). Guardians of children having dyslexia are seen to have greater levels of stress and anxiety. Because of the enormous and widespread health threat posed by the coronavirus (COVID-19) pandemic, several governments throughout the world have imposed home-based quarantine as a means of limiting COVID-19's spread. Schools and universities all around the world were forced to close campuses and libraries, reduce face-to-face interactions, and transition to virtual instruction in a short period as a result of the epidemic. This sudden requirement to rely only on web-based instruction may be viewed as a significant shift in how we approach learning and teaching. Although new technologies for online learning existed, the bulk of face-to-face courses provided by different institutions and e-learning platforms were not very popular [2].

Many educational institutions performed online questionnaires to assess student satisfaction with remote learning, the efficacy of remote teaching, and how they were dealing with stress linked to the COVID-19 epidemic. The findings show that a solid Internet infrastructure and digital equipment, teaching staff support, computer abilities in using remote learning platforms and applications, living situations, as well as motivation, self-discipline, and self-initiative, all play key roles in effective remote studying. Although all children have been affected by abrupt and drastic changes in all aspects of their lives since the start of the COVID-19 epidemic, the group of kids with developmental learning difficulties and other impairments requires special attention. To our knowledge, no research has looked at learning difficulties of any type faced by higher education students with dyslexia who were enrolled in remote learning during the COVID-19 epidemic [3].

With the growing revolution and automation, i.e., the use of technology in every field of work, it is often observed that the actual load on humans depreciates drastically. Be it in the technical and corporate sector, or the production houses, the automobile industry, and many more, technology has spread its web across nearly every corner of them. One such area is the healthcare sector. Data involved in the medical healthcare sector, known as Electronic Health Records (EHR), consists of the details and records of the patients, their appointments, the diagnosis, the medicines, and prescription. For example, in the department of dentistry, the data stored is generally the history of the patients, their surgeries, and procedures that the patient has gone through such as cavity fillings tooth decay, etc. [4].

Medical Health Record (MHR) includes the various kinds of paper notes filled over time by the specialist of the health care, orders for the smooth management of the medicines and therapies, X-rays, test results, and many other things. MHRs have originally been organized and monitored by healthcare professionals. Today, the facility to store data online has helped the patients to keep a record of their health records (PHR) by themselves, and this can be easily facilitated by the presence of third-party organizations that give online storage at a very minimal cost. Scientifically, EHRs are the records and data of the patients that are stored virtually in a digitized format. These data may range from very basic allergies of the patients to their transaction records at various healthcare institutions to the medications and the treatments that a patient has received. Online storage providers are utilizing the data from the patient's EHRs to maintain various types of medical data, which in turn helps them to identify the ill patients. EHR systems are developed in such a manner to keep the patient's data secure and precise. EHR documents help to eliminate the risks of losing the patient's medical history. Besides, EHR also enhances accessibility and reduces the burden of data duplication, and it has a negligible chance of data losses [4].

The traditional patient records require a large number of human work hours. For instance, suppose a patient visits a clinic or a hospital, now his/her documents must be found and then transported to the required department, and then the actual examination of the patient can start. Besides, the high chances of mishandling of the patient record files also exist. Through blockchain, every record is protected with a unique blockchain id that not only protects the records but also makes them easily accessible to authorized personnel only. When the dentistry sector is considered, the doctors and their assistants get control over the details of the patients and can easily check their histories with the help of controlled blockchain architecture. The architecture establishes the functions and the powers of each entity involved in the system, and it is used to encapsulate the relationship between the entities. Thus, blockchain is used to implement both security and efficiency [5].

The basic needs of the healthcare system are the problems of authenticity, data transportation, interoperability, considerations of mobile health, and the transfer of health records. All these important parameters have been explained below to see more insight on this. Blockchain can be an influence to mark some of the medical care greatest difficulties. In the case of traditional EHR, if a user needs to get to his health records, he would need to follow the process to get access to them. Data is centralized to just a medical services association and its control are just given to the medical care area or associations. This problem makes it reasonable for a system that would be useful in changing the medical care area to be more transparent and reliable among all the users [6].

The article is structured as follows. Section 2 presents the related study in the healthcare sector, and Section 3 explains healthcare use cases. Section 4 and 5 discuss the proposed framework and technology used to implement the proposed framework. The details of implementation and results have been discussed in Section 6. Finally, Section 7 concludes the whole approach as suggested.

2. Related study

Most of the research done on LD detection includes primitive and simplistic methods such as pen and paper tests, a survey on parents. Very few of the research studies focus on doing it with machine learning models. Moreover, these already established methods may or may not be suitable from the perspective of Indian children. These past methods are mostly designed only for the detection of one of the LDs. To make the foundation frameworks straightforward, a systematic literature review has been done in many areas. A summary of a detailed review of major research works in direction of various approaches toward healthcare management is presented below.

2.1 Healthcare approach

Various approaches toward health care management have been suggested by researchers. Uddin et al. discuss that the increased usage of the IoT in the day-to-day life of human beings has also led to the concept of Remote Patient Monitoring, and a Patient-Centric Agent using the blockchain technology is commendable.

Agbo et al. [7] worked extensively on the research paper Blockchain Technology in Health Care: security because the data of health care of a patient not only contains the records of his or her health and treatments but also personal information such as contact address, contact number, and other sensitive information such as social security number.

Matthias Mettler and MA [8] studied the different areas and various fields where Blockchain can be used and how it can be used in other nonfinancial sectors. The major areas in which Blockchain can be implemented successfully are the areas of Smart Healthcare Systems, to fight the counterfeit drugs in pharmaceutical companies, for digitally signing of emails as well as contracts of legal purposes. The use of Blockchain helped the companies that were already existed in storing and transferring the data more quickly and securely without any third-party intervention.

Ramani et al. [9] discussed the field of healthcare records securing and efficient data accessibility by using blockchain technology. Blockchain as a decentralized and circulated innovation can assume a key function in giving such medical care administrations. Smart contracts and ethereum platforms maintain authenticity, security, and prevent data alteration.

Tanwar et al. [10] proposed that medical aid frameworks are described as being exceptionally remarkable technology. The utilization of blockchain in medical aid frameworks assumes a basic part of the current medical services market. They will try to show current difficulties looked at by the medical services industry; propose framework engineering and calculation for control access strategy for members to accomplish protection and security for tolerant data inside the EHR framework.

Vora et al. [11] proposed BHEEM: A Blockchain approach-based system for securing medical records in 2018. Blockchain innovation settles the plans dealing with the security of EHRs, which have brought about information being commonly unavailable to patients. They have proposed a Blockchain framework that gives secure and data access to health records by patients, doctors, and outsiders while securing the patient private data. The goal is how the proposed system satisfies the requirements of patients, doctors, and outsiders and to see how the system maintains the protection and security concerns in the EHR system.

2.2 Pandemic survey

Cherish et al. [12] analyzed the students' views regarding online education, which were collected through google forms and were analyzed using a mixed-method (both qualitative and quantitative) along with a machine learning approach. The results showed varying responses of the students with 66.55% being negative, 29.39% were neutral, and only a small percentage, i.e., 4.05%, had positive emotion regarding the online study.

Akash [13] gave an analysis to examine how the citizens of 12 different countries were trying to cope with COVID-19 by conducting sentiment analysis and text mining and on the tweets collected. The result showed that citizens of eight countries were more optimistic as compared to the remaining four countries where citizens were disheartened.

Richard et al. [14] gave an analysis by examining tweets of different users related to COVID-19. Around 50% of the tweets were demoralizing with a sense of fear. The results indicated that the demoralizing tweets filled with pessimistic emotions had a high impact on the occurrence of COVID-19 positive cases.

Simon et al. [15] proposed a deterministic forecasting algorithm, Monte-Carlo model (CMCM) coupled with GROOMS methodology, taking input as random samples of deterministic and nondeterministic data and the results obtained to predict the highest spans of upcoming possibilities about the outbreak.

V.S. [16] analyzed by taking input parameters as patient characteristics, patient age, patient gender, fatality and mortality rates, viral spread, epidemiological curve construction, and subgroup analysis, by extracting data from China's Infectious Disease Information System and concluded that COVID-19 speeded with a high speed within a month only.

Zhong et al. [17] proposed an SIR model, which analyzes available epidemiological data to obtain the reasonable estimation of the key parameter, i.e., infection rate, and the results are supposed to provide important information for the crisis management against the novel coronavirus.

Stephen et al. [18] proposed a study for analysis of mortality ratio among various age groups of Wuhang taking epidemiological information as input parameters, research is done based on statistical method, and the result achieved shows that mortality rate was higher for development of systemic complications.

2.3 Blockchain survey-based approach

Casino et al. [19] proposed that blockchain-based applications provide a logical writing survey over different areas, which commit to research on blockchain and its applications and become more developed; their applications are required to enter more areas.

Konstantinidis et al. [20] completed a survey on Blockchain innovation generally called the mechanical premise on which bitcoin is made. This innovation has made elevated standards, as exchanges of every sort are executed in an extremely decentralized manner, without the necessity of an outsider. Shen and Mora did a survey on Blockchain use cases and work may be preliminary to limit various gaps by utilizing the combination information from use cases by the monitoring on the network.

Ahmed et al. [21] survey Blockchain Technology and summarize that it can be a progressive innovation that has great possibilities in settling problems with the transaction, improving scalability, upgrade security, founded trust, and protection.

2.4 Additional research on children suffering from dyslexia

A study in terms of focusing on kids with reading issues, who may be affected differentially by the epidemic and distant learning due to the nature of their reading and writing difficulties. While the challenges manifested themselves in different ways, it was noticed that they were also encountered by those students at previous levels of study. Furthermore, persons with dyslexia may require additional family support and professional assistance throughout their school careers, as they struggle with more than just learning challenges. Secondary symptoms including excessive anxiety and low self-esteem are common in youngsters and can persist into adulthood.

According to the findings, university students diagnosed with dyslexia had greater anxiety levels and poorer self-esteem than those without learning challenges. Dyslexia is frequently accompanied by other diseases. They investigated how children with dyslexia dealt with the new environment and what their main obstacles were during a period of fast change in the teaching and learning process as a result of the COVID-19 epidemic in the current study [22].

Another research study was done by Manuel Soriano-Ferrer, Manuel Ramón Morte-Soriano, John Begeny, and Elisa Piedra-Martínez (2021), to examine the psychoeducational impact of the required COVID-19 quarantine in Spain among children with dyslexia and their families. The findings showed that children with dyslexia experienced higher levels of despair and anxiety symptoms during quarantine, and parents regarded their children to have greater emotional symptoms, hyperactivity inattention, and behavior issues. Children and adolescents with dyslexia demonstrated less reading activity and motivation during the quarantine period. In comparison to prequarantine settings, parents reported much more stress during quarantine. Some demographic and psychological factors, as well as parental stress, predicted children's state anxiety. Several significant conclusions emerged from the questionnaire on the effects of quarantine. For example, virtually all parents of dyslexic children said they had trouble creating study routines, that the quarantine had a detrimental impact on their child's studying, and that they did not get enough advice from teachers on how to support their child's learning. Furthermore, the clear majority of parents were concerned about their child's learning and school progress, as well as the child's motivation and interest in reading, peer relationships, and the teacher's professional qualities. The research also looked at the effects of quarantine and the emotional well-being of parents who have a dyslexic child. Mothers reported much more stress and unwanted interactions with their kids during quarantine compared to prequarantine conditions, according to the findings. These findings are novel and significant in the context of evaluating parents of dyslexic pupils, although the data appear to be consistent with what may be expected during a quarantine.

2.4.1 Observation from study

Observations indicated that the senior citizens were more prone to COVID-19 for which WHO even circulated guidelines, but recent research indicates that more young adults are suffering from acute COVID-19 symptoms (Shreshth et al. (2020)), making it a more complex problem, and a result rapid decline is noticed in the mobility rate of population (Micheal et al. (2020)) of countries affected by the novel virus. After following the guidelines of WHO and a decrease in mobility rate, the virus is transmitting at a very high rate within a short period (V.S et al. (2020)). The best way to protect one from the COVID-19 virus is to be well informed about the disease and its causes; it will also help slow down the transmission rate of the virus. At this point, the entire world is facing a difficult time as there is no vaccine or specialized treatment to cure the patients, and this results in a high mortality rate. Therefore, to justify the following objective, the subobjectives are stated as to collect COVID-19 information using secondary data collection techniques. To preprocess the COVID-19 information using text cleansing and vectorization in respect to converting the input text into tensors. To create a training and prediction model by splitting training and testing data and using various regression techniques. To verify and validate (V&V) the developed model. The study deals with the mortality rate in India using various machine learning techniques. The secondary data collection is done using various websites such as Kaggle. The dataset collected contains a lot of noise, which is preprocessed and the inputs are converted by using hot encoding. The pandemic flare-up is ending up being an unrivaled calamity, particularly in the most influenced nations including China, Italy, Iran, Russia, the United Kingdom, India, and the United States in all angles, particularly well-being and social. It is too soon to gauge any reasonable situation, yet it is anything but a solid effect around the world. The outcome demonstrates that Lasso Regression gives the best outcomes [18].

Mala R Naranjan, an educator trained to teach children with dyslexia, shared her story about how special educators at the Madras Dyslexia Association (MDA) jumped into action early to devise remedial sessions that leveraged technology while staying as close to the best ways to reach out to children with dyslexia as possible when the pandemic hit. She discussed the numerous inventive techniques that special educators used to deal with certain common difficulties, such as attention deficiencies and sitting tolerance that she encountered while educating a kid with dyslexia. She believes that for a youngster with dyslexia, the teaching-learning process is centered on the idea "Teach me the way I learn." This is best accomplished by adopting a multimodal strategy to make the process both profitable and enjoyable. They believed that an encouraging touch can reduce the frustration built inside the child rather than just a verbal form of appreciation. Occupational Therapy (OT) sessions were conducted online and were able to assist the child in coping with fine motor, gross motor, attention, and executive function challenges.

Students, instructors, and parents all had different perspectives and expectations of the online sessions at the outset of the epidemic, ranging from joy to skepticism. Technology, network difficulties, and the abrupt switch to a no-paper, no-text environment all created challenges. Instructors and students rapidly adjusted to the new standards, and teachers and parents were happy that remedial sessions could continue uninterrupted. However, COVID-induced worry in the parents rubbed off on their children in certain situations. Until the pandemic, educational technology (Edtech) was an obscure word; nevertheless, special educators have become willing users of different software, computers, web cameras, and other gadgets for successful instruction in the last few months. It is now extremely easy to include these into the lesson plan. When in-class instruction resumes, the majority of the instructors indicated a willingness to continue integrating Edtech into remedial education. Once in-class sessions restart, the institutions hope to carry forward the beneficial outcomes of the teaching-learning process from this pandemic and bridge the gaps [3].

The findings of the study underline the necessity of providing prompt assistance to children with dyslexia, as well as implementing prevention programmed to counteract any future harmful effects of COVID-19 on children with dyslexia and their parents. At a time when there is a critical dearth of research-based guidance, a swift and focused effort on prevention, intervention, and comprehensive evaluation of intervention success are critical. COVID-19 outbreak, we may expect hybrid/blended learning to become the standard in the academic environment. Due to the volume and timeframe of implementation, this shift from traditional teaching to a new e-learning strategy presents challenges to lecturers and students. As a result, we must identify potential benefits and drawbacks for teachers and students, particularly for those who are most vulnerable, students with LDs [23].

3. Healthcare use cases

Several use cases have been discussed in this section to highlight their several utilities toward efficient data transfer and the fast decision made for patient's treatment.

3.1 Sharing of information between traditional care and telemedicine

Scalable and secure information sharing is essential for EHR decision-making. Telemedicine allows a user to access a medical record in any remote area, it removes the barriers to efficient data transfer and the fast decision made for patient's treatment. Without losing time and waiting for a health specialist's office and on-demand patients get immediate treatment.

3.2 Patient-controlled cancer data sharing

Sharing the data is important in most cancer care in instances where generally cases are complex and healing procedures are rarely identical. However, it could additionally agglomerate intelligence collected to lessen unwanted repetitions in medical trials. It permits distributed medical trials to gain a significant result that accelerates the technology of extra powerful most cancer treatment.

3.3 Medical insurance claim adjudication

The medical insurance claim is to help individuals paying less from the large bills of major health issues, health emergencies, or in the treatment of a long and persistent sickness or to make certain medical care is supplied while needed. Patients might also get additional costs on the point of medical care; however, the extra closing charges are given as claims to the medical claim companies.

4. Proposed methodology

The implementation steps as depicted in Fig. 14.1 include data acquisition, preprocessing of the data, applying rule-based learning to label the data, and then using this marked data to train a suitable machine learning model

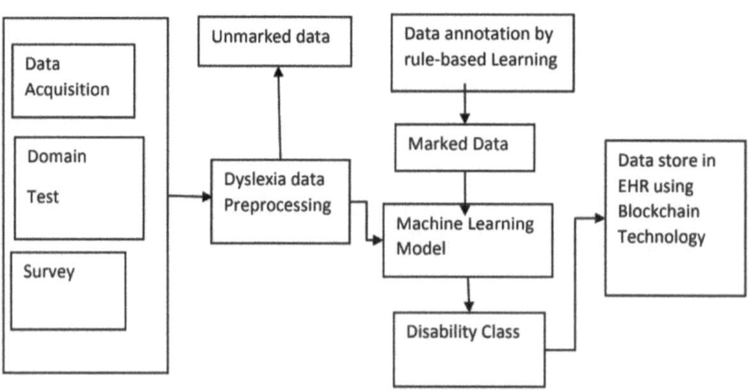

Figure 14.1 System design.

with cross-validation strategy. After the model is trained, predictions on unmarked data can be made. The data store in the EHR framework. The main idea behind developing a secure and transparent platform using blockchain is to mainly make the existing EHR system to be more precise, accurate, secure, and transparent. Objectives have been set to develop a secure, decentralized, and distributed platform for medical records using Blockchain [24].

5. Data acquisition

5.1 Sampling method

The sampling unit is children of age group 5–10 years and sampling are taken from Slum Swaraj Foundation students. Around 500 samples are taken for the machine learning model. In the classification model, 70% of samples out of total available are used for model training 30% and are used for model testing with cross-validation and hyperparameter tuning.

5.2 Methods of collecting data

A sampling of six-month data collected during pandemic through assessments tests and surveys.

5.2.1 Assessment tests

These are designed to test the ability of a child in the five different domains of dyslexia. These domains are—1. Language Vocabulary, 2. Memory, 3. Speed, 4. Visual Discrimination, and 5. Audio Discrimination. Each question is associated with one or more than one domain.

5.2.2 Surveys

A survey is taken from parents/guardians to obtain information about the environmental factors and development of a child.

5.3 Preprocessing of data – I

The scores obtained from each student in the five learning domains are combined with survey scores obtained from their parents/guardians. All obtained data is numerical. The five learning domains of dyslexia are—I. Language vocabulary, 2. Memory, 3. Speed, 4. Visual Discrimination, and 5. Audio Discrimination. When combined with survey scores, they make six columns in the dataset. The data is then preprocessed by dividing all the values by their corresponding ranges so the new range for every feature is between 0 and 1. Table 14.1 shows that the preprocessing is done before the labeling of data and is known as min-max normalization.

Table 14.1 Preprocessed data (min-max scaling).

Language vocab	Memory	Speed	Visual discrimination	Audio discrimination	Survey score
0.5	0.6	0.5	0.8	0.6	0.7
0.6	0.7	0.9	0.9	0.5	0.9
0.6	0.4	0.3	0.3	0.4	0.6
0.3	0.8	0.2	0.1	0.3	0.5
0.7	0.6	0.7	0.0	0.9	0.5
0.4	0.1	00	0.1	0.4	0.2
0.8	00	00	0.9	0.6	0.6
0.5	0.3	0.5	0.4	0.2	0.4
0.6	0.5	0.5	0.4	0.6	0.5
0.6	0.7	0.7	0.8	0.7	0.8

5.4 Fuzzy rule-based learning

In this step, we have to classify the dataset into three fuzzy subsets. The total number of fuzzy if—then rules generated by partitioning each attribute into K fuzzy subsets in an n-dimensional feature space is defined as K. In this problem, we use five features, which are generated from six features in the dataset. The first feature is calculated by the weighted sum of all the features, where weights are given to the features on basis of their priority. The priority order of features is—language vocabulary, memory, speed, visual discrimination, audio discrimination, and survey score. Output is converted 0—1 range by scaling. The second feature is calculated by taking an average of language vocabulary and memory. The third feature is Speed. The fourth is obtained by averaging over visual and audio discrimination, and the fifth feature is survey score. Thus, there are a total of 243 rules. The classification is done based on numerical values of these five features. The three fuzzy classes are 1. Dyslexia, 2. Probable Dyslexia, 3. No Dyslexia. The range of first-class is 0—0.4, second class is 0.3—0.7, and third is 0.6—1.0. We implement these rules with help of if—else statements in python language. After this step, a labeled dataset is obtained.

5.5 Classification techniques used in model

Two classification techniques are used in this paper. The first is Support Vector Machines. Support Vector Machines are used because they work well on small datasets and, with help of suitable kernel functions, can detect complex nonlinear relationships. They have less risk of overfitting and are not solved for local optima. The second technique used is Random Forests. Random Forest is considered one of the best methods for structured or tabular data. It can also handle unbalanced data and has low bias with moderate variance [25].

5.6 Preprocessing of data – II

Before the machine learning model is applied, preprocessing is performed again to balance the data. This is done by subtracting the mean from every feature of data and then dividing it by the corresponding standard deviation. Table 14.2 represents standardized scaling.

5.7 Secure data in HER using blockchain technology

The framework has two controllers: Administrator and User. The user is additionally separated into two classifications: doctor and patient. The system administrator has authorized access to two users (doctors and patients) of our framework. The main task would be that the administrator appoints jobs to incorporate the Name and Address of the user. Fig. 14.2 depicts user interaction with the administrator with DApp. Users of this framework have a patient's name and id for utilizing the framework [26].

The Blockchain-based medical service framework has three modules. These sections, when brought together, would keep our structure functioning.

5.7.1 User layer

The user can be Doctors, Users, staff, and so on. A user is a person who makes efficient use of the system and resources, user has many features and tasks on the system, such as interacting with the system and some simple

Table 14.2 Preprocessed data (standardized scaling).

Language vocab	Memory	Speed	Visual discrimination	Audio discrimination	Survey score
1.661885	1.484552	0.638225	1.1471165	1.121748	0.067094
−0.840954	−0.797034	0.188771	−0.282819	0.63647	−0.390367
0.160182	0.571918	0.188771	0.193842	0.129051	0.524556
2.162452	1.028235	1.537134	0.282819	0.625399	0.982018
−0.340386	−0.340717	0.188771	−0.759481	−0.367298	0.067094
0.660749	0.115600	1.537134	−0.282819	1.121748	0.982018
0.160182	−0.340717	−0.260684	−0.282819	0.863647	−0.847829
−0.340386	−0.340717	−0.260684	0.670504	0.863647	0.524556
−0.340386	−0.340717	0.188771	0.193842	0.863647	−0.390367
−0.840954	0.571918	0.638225	−0.759481	0.129051	0.067094

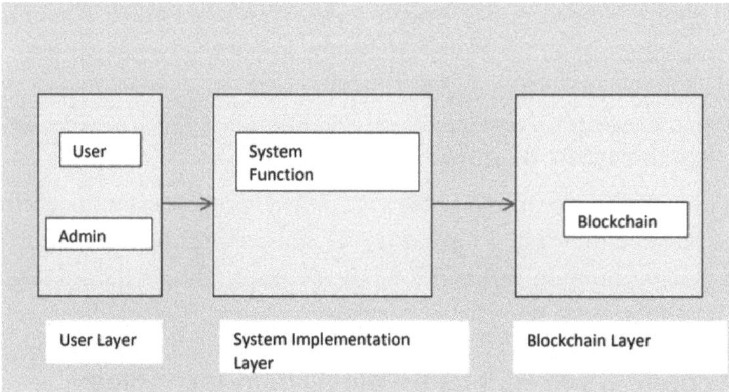

Figure 14.2 Admin and user interaction with DApp [24].

task operations such as create, read, delete, update, etc., which makes him identifiable on the system. Users can use system functions using GUI (Graphical User Interface), with the help of GUI users can communicate with the blockchain layer. By using this framework would get to the system functionality in specialized terms Distributed Application browser.

5.7.2 Blockchain layer

The following layer on the framework is the blockchain layer; this is the middle layer of the framework, which contains code for communication of the user with DApp functioning on the blockchain. This layer has three modules.

5.7.2.1 Blockchain assets

In 2005, Ethereum was launched, which is an open-source, blockchain-based, decentralized software platform. It uses transaction to be a piece of data that is transferred from one user to another so the only transaction can change the state of record. The transaction is handled as an asset by the blockchain as data that essentially stores it for utilizing later or the user can send this piece of information to another user [27].

5.7.2.2 Governance rules

In the Blockchain approach, it is observed that some rules for its transaction to be computed. There is a requirement of some agreement to keep the blockchain secure. The reason behind using the Proof of Work (PoW) agreement is for guaranteeing that governance of technology is kept up in a confident way, which is through all the nodes interconnected to the blockchain system [28].

5.7.2.3 Network

The basic idea is to create a decentralized distributed platform, which is achieved by a peer-to-peer network where every node is connected as peers so that every node has equal status. In a blockchain system, no node acting as the main node maintains all the basis of the organization. This Blockchain-based organization makes a decentralized system. Thus, utilizing an organization where every associated block has equivalent status and authority was the most ideal decision of this blockchain approach [29].

5.7.3 Implementation layer

By utilizing Ethereum, the framework is implemented. Smart contracts play a main role in the DApp. The health records agreement is made for implementing the usefulness of the system. It plays out the CRUD activities alongside defining the role to access these records. In other contracts, i.e., roles are a predefined agreement by the OpenZeppelin agreement libraries. These libraries contain most agreements that have been done in different functions that can be used for making your agreement [30].

6. Implementation

There has to be some algorithm used to keep the data analysis and for all its computations of data repository, dyslexic patterns, and a massive amount of data can be shared for further clinical research, statistical analysis, and quality assurance.

6.1 Model phase – I

Snapshot of Unlabeled data—The dataset used in this project is taken from samples of 500 students aged 5–10 years old shown in Table 14.3.

Correlation heatmap of data—This heatmap shows the correlation between the five domains (language vocabulary, memory, speed, visual discrimination, and audio discrimination) and survey score. The correlation coefficient is a value that lies between 0 and 1. A value closer to 1 signifies a high correlation between the variables. In this correlation matrix, all the values lie in between 0.53 and 0.63, which shows that the correlation present is not much significant. Fig. 14.3 show correlation heatmap of the unlabeled dataset.

Generating weights—These random weights are generated to calculate a weighted sum as shown in Fig. 14.4. This sum is used as the first new feature in the rule-based data labeling process. These weights are

Table 14.3 Unlabeled data.

Language vocab	Memory	Speed	Visual discrimination	Audio discrimination	Survey score
0.5	0.6	0.5	0.8	0.6	0.7
0.6	0.7	0.9	0.9	0.5	0.9
0.6	0.4	0.3	0.3	0.4	0.6
0.3	0.8	0.2	0.1	0.3	0.5
0.7	0.6	0.7	0.8	0.9	0.5
0.4	0.1	00	0.1	0.4	0.2
0.8	00	00	0.9	0.6	0.6
0.5	0.3	0.5	0.4	0.2	0.4
0.6	0.5	0.5	0.4	0.6	0.5
0.6	0.7	0.7	0.8	0.7	0.6

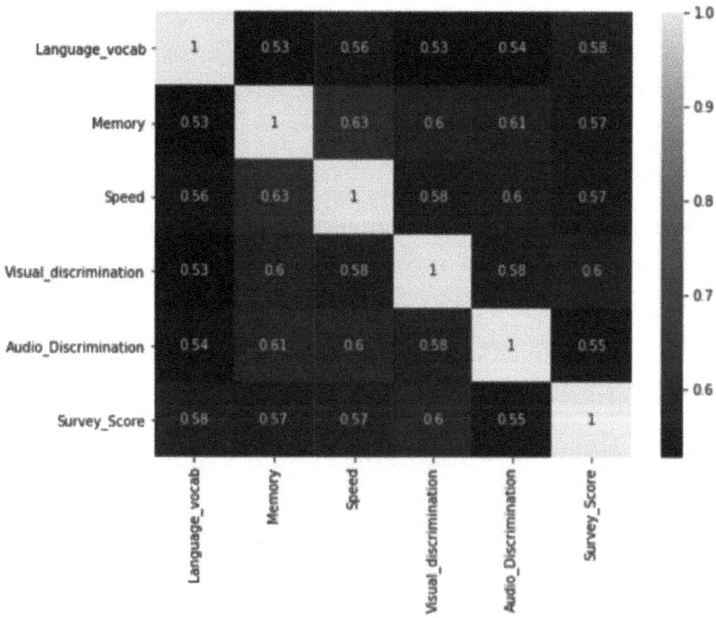

Figure 14.3 Correlation heatmap of the unlabeled dataset.

```
[3.7967676314200761,
2.679110831192357,
0.8519740822605654,
0.3636941502196O727,
0.2341400542487521 2]
```

Figure 14.4 Generated random weights.

assigned to these variables in a specific priority order, which is language vocabulary, memory, speed, visual discrimination, audio discrimination, and survey score. The weight assigned to visual discrimination and audio discrimination is the same.

Labeling of data into fuzzy subsets by generating rules—In this step, the unlabeled dataset is labeled using rule-based learning into three fuzzy subsets, which are dyslexia, probable dyslexia, and no dyslexia. This process is explained in detail in System Design and Methodology chapter.

6.2 Model phase – I

Snapshot of labeled data—The labeled data is split data into training and testing set with a 70:30 ratio as shown in Table 14.4.

Implementing SVM twice with linear and RBF kernel—Two machine learning models are trained on the dataset in this step. First is SVM with the linear kernel, which gives 0.905 precision, 0.935 recall, and 0 .91 9 F1 -score on the test set. The second is SVM with RBF kernel, and it gives 0.909 precision, 0.942 recall, and an F1 -score of 0.923.

Implementing Grid search with SVM to find best parameters—Grid search is a method where the best hyperparameters of a model are found through searching for them in a given search space and then comparing them. Here, a Grid search is used. SVM tries to find the best value of hyperparameter gamma and C where gamma can be 0.001 or 0.0001 and C can be m, 10, JOO, or 1000. It also tries to find the better-suited kernel between linear and RBF kernel. The best hyperparameters found in this case are 0.001 for gamma, 1000 for C, and RBF kernel.

Table 14.4 Labeled data.

Language vocab	Memory	Speed	Visual discrimination	Audio discrimination	Survey score	Label
0.5	0.6	0.5	0.8	0.6	0.7	1.0
0.6	0.7	0.9	0.9	0.5	0.9	2.0
0.6	0.4	0.3	0.3	0.4	0.6	1.0
0.3	0.8	0.2	0.1	0.3	0.5	0.0
0.7	0.6	0.7	0.8	0.9	0.5	2.0
0.4	0.1	00	0.1	0.4	0.2	0.0
0.8	00	00	0.9	0.6	0.6	1.0
0.5	0.3	0.5	0.4	0.2	0.4	1.0
0.6	0.5	0.5	0.4	0.6	0.5	1.0
0.6	0.7	0.7	0.8	0.7	0.6	2.0

When this model makes predictions on the test set, precision is found to be 0.9 I 9, recall is 0.949, and F I -score is 0.933.

Implementing Grid search with Random Forest Classifier to find best parameters—When Grid Search is used with Random Forest Classifier, it tries to search for the best value of hyperparameter n estimators, which denotes the number of a decision tree in a random forest. The possible values for n estimators are 10, 100, 500, and 1000.

Results obtained for five observations are shown in Table 14.5 with their actual output and predicted output by the SVM Grid search model.

There has to be some algorithm to keep the blockchain secure and for all its computations.

Transactions: Following transactions have been created to monitor the flow:

- **Add records** ()—to create user records containing ID, name, medical data.
- **Access grant** ()—to grant access to the database of a user to someone.
- **Update records** ()—to update the user records which is already stored.
- **View records** ()—to view the medical record of the user stored in the app.
- **Erase record** ()—to delete the record of a user.

Smart contracts: This includes user records and Task's contract. Through this contract, access is given in CRUD operations that are performed on the user record.

1. User Record contract— made for the only implementation of the functionality of the proposed framework. It defines tasks access as well as performs CRUD operations.
2. Task's contract—Tasks smart contracts belong to Asset's libraries, sublibraries of OpenZeppelin libraries. Various other smart contracts are defined in the asset library for defining the access tasks.

Table 14.5 Data of five students from the dataset.

Language vocab	Memory	Speed	Visual discrimination	Audio discrimination	Survey score
0.5	0.6	0.7	0.8	0.7	0.7
1.0	0.7	0.5	0.6	0.6	0.7
0.6	0.6	0.6	0.3	0.5	0.6
0.3	0.3	0.5	0.5	0.6	0.7
0.3	0.3	0.3	0.2	0.4	0.5

7. Conclusion

This paper provides a summarized study of the techniques that can be used for the detection of dyslexia. In this project fuzzy rule-based learning has been used to get the labeled data. This machine learning model takes care of almost all the domains, which are essential for detecting this LD. The experiment results and model accuracy show that this model is quite efficient in detecting the child suffering from dyslexia. It will help lots of people to get their child tested for dyslexia and if tested positive can get the proper medication for them so that they can also be a part of the mainstream society. We focused on improving the security aspects of health records data and in turn, it opens up new directions of other research to meet other security requirements. In future work, other security models that will be more generalized and cater to the need for health data security as well as identifying the untrusted hosts will be useful for critical application deployment for any medical purpose.

References

[1] J. Zawadka, A. Miękisz, I. Nowakowska, J. Plewko, M. Kochańska, E. Haman, Remote learning among students with and without reading difficulties during the initial stages of the COVID-19 pandemic, Educ. Inf. Technol. 0123456789 (2021), https://doi.org/10.1007/s10639-021-10559-3.

[2] M.S. Farooq, M. Khan, A. Abid, A framework to make charity collection transparent and auditable using blockchain technology, Comput. Electr. Eng. 83 (2020), https://doi.org/10.1016/j.compeleceng.2020.106588.

[3] M. Soriano-Ferrer, M.R. Morte-Soriano, J. Begeny, E. Piedra-Martínez, Psychoeducational challenges in Spanish children with dyslexia and their parents' stress during the COVID-19 pandemic, Front. Psychol. 12 (2021) 1–15, https://doi.org/10.3389/fpsyg.2021.648000.

[4] R. Guo, H. Shi, Q. Zhao, D. Zheng, Secure attribute-based signature scheme with multiple authorities for blockchain in electronic health records systems, IEEE Access 6 (2018) 11676–11686, https://doi.org/10.1109/ACCESS.2018.2801266.

[5] C. Latulipe, A. Gatto, H.T. Nguyen, D.P. Miller, S.A. Quandt, A.G. Bertoni, A. Smith, T.A. Arcury, ACM Press the 33rd Annual ACM Conference - Seoul, Republic of Korea (2015.04.18-2015.04.23) Proceedings of the 33rd Annual ACM Conference on Human Factors in Computing Systems - CHI '15 - Design Considerations for Patient Portal Adoption by Low-Income, Older Adults, 2015, pp. 3859–3868, https://doi.org/10.1145/2702123.2702392.

[6] W.J. Gordon, C. Catalini, Blockchain technology for healthcare: facilitating the transition to patient-driven interoperability, Comput. Struct. Biotechnol. J. 16 (2018) 224–230, https://doi.org/10.1016/j.csbj.2018.06.003. Elsevier B.V.

[7] C. Agbo, Q. Mahmoud, J. Eklund, Blockchain technology in healthcare: a systematic review, Healthcare 7 (2) (2019) 56, https://doi.org/10.3390/healthcare7020056.

[8] A. Al Omar, M.S. Rahman, A. Basu, S. Kiyomoto, " MediBchain, A blockchain-based privacy-preserving platform for healthcare data, in: Lecture Notes in Computer Science (Including Subseries Lecture Notes in Artificial Intelligence and Lecture Notes

in Bioinformatics), LNCS, vol. 10658, 2017, pp. 534–543, https://doi.org/10.1007/978-3-319-72395-2_49.
[9] T. Kumar, V. Ramani, I. Ahmad, A. Braeken, E. Harjula, M. Ylianttila, Blockchain utilization in healthcare: key requirements and challenges, in: 2018 IEEE 20th Int. Conf. e-Health Networking, Appl. Serv. Heal., vol. 2018, 2018, pp. 1–7, https://doi.org/10.1109/HealthCom.2018.8531136.
[10] S. Tanwar, K. Parekh, R. Evans, Blockchain-based electronic healthcare record system for healthcare 4.0 applications, J. Inf. Secure. Appl. 50 (2020) 102407, https://doi.org/10.1016/j.jisa.2019.102407.
[11] A. Gervais, G.O. Karame, K. Wüst, V. Glykantzis, H. Ritzdorf, S. Čapkun, On the security and performance of Proof of Work blockchains, in: Proceedings of the ACM Conference on Computer and Communications Security, Oct. 2016, vol. 24, 2016, pp. 3–16, https://doi.org/10.1145/2976749.2978341. 28-October.
[12] C.K. Pastor, Sentiment analysis of Filipinos and effects of extreme community quarantine due to coronavirus (COVID-19) pandemic, SSRN Electron. J. 3 (1) (2020) 1–6, https://doi.org/10.2139/ssrn.3574385.
[13] N. Nummela, E. Paavilainen-Mäntymäki, R. Harikkala-Laihinen, J. Raitis, When all doors close: implications of COVID-19 for cosmopolitan entrepreneurs, Int. Small Bus. J. Res. Entrep. 38 (8) (2020) 711–717, https://doi.org/10.1177/0266242620954127.
[14] R.J. Medford, S.N. Saleh, A. Sumarsono, T.M. Perl, C.U. Lehmann, An 'Infodemic': leveraging high-volume Twitter data to understand the early public sentiment for the Coronavirus disease 2019 outbreak, Open Forum Infect. Dis. 7 (7) (2020), https://doi.org/10.1093/ofid/ofaa258.
[15] S.J. Fong, G. Li, N. Dey, R.G. Crespo, E. Herrera-Viedma, Composite Monte Carlo decision making under high uncertainty of novel coronavirus epidemic using hybridized deep learning and fuzzy rule induction, Appl. Soft Comput. J. 93 (2020) 106282, https://doi.org/10.1016/j.asoc.2020.106282. December 2019.
[16] C. CDC, Analysis of epidemiological characteristics of novel coronavirus pneumonia, Chin. J. Epidemiol. 41 (2) (2020) 145–151 [Online]. Available: http://www.ncbi.nlm.nih.gov/pubmed/32064853.
[17] L. Zhong, L. Mu, J. Li, J. Wang, Z. Yin, D. Liu, Early prediction of the 2019 novel coronavirus outbreak in the mainland China based on simple mathematical model, IEEE Access 8 (2020) 51761–51769, https://doi.org/10.1109/ACCESS.2020.2979599.
[18] S.A. Lauer, et al., The incubation period of coronavirus disease 2019 (CoVID-19) from publicly reported confirmed cases: estimation and application, Ann. Intern. Med. 172 (9) (2020) 577–582, https://doi.org/10.7326/M20-0504.
[19] F. Casino, T.K. Dasaklis, C. Patsakis, A systematic literature review of blockchain-based applications: current status, classification, and open issues, Telematics Inf. 36 (2019) 55–81, https://doi.org/10.1016/j.tele.2018.11.006. May 2018.
[20] I. Konstantinidis, G. Siaminos, C. Timplalexis, P. Zervas, V. Peristeras, S. Decker, Blockchain for business applications: a systematic literature review, in: Lecture Notes in Business Information Processing vol. 320, 2018, pp. 384–399, https://doi.org/10.1007/978-3-319-93931-5_28.
[21] A. Kosiba, A. Miller, E. Shi, Z. Wen, C. Papamanthou, " Hawk, The blockchain model of cryptography and privacy-preserving smart contracts, in: Proceedings - 2016 IEEE Symposium on Security and Privacy, SP 2016, 2016, pp. 839–858, https://doi.org/10.1109/SP.2016.55.
[22] L.C. Wang, Effects of phonological training on the reading and reading-related abilities of Hong Kong children with dyslexia, Front. Psychol. 8 (2017) 1–13, https://doi.org/10.3389/fpsyg.2017.01904. OCT.

[23] M. Marlais, et al., COVID-19 in children treated with immunosuppressive medication for kidney diseases, Arch. Dis. Child. (2020), https://doi.org/10.1136/archdischild-2020-320616 archdischild-2020-320616.
[24] A. Shahnaz, U. Qamar, A. Khalid, Using blockchain for electronic health records, IEEE Access vol. 7 (2019) 147782–147795, https://doi.org/10.1109/ACCESS.2019.2946373.
[25] Ethereum: A Secure Decentralised Generalised Transaction Ledger.
[26] L. Chen, W.K. Lee, C.C. Chang, K.K.R. Choo, N. Zhang, Blockchain-based searchable encryption for electronic health record sharing, Future Generat. Comput. Syst. 95 (2019) 420–429, https://doi.org/10.1016/j.future.2019.01.018.
[27] D. Macrinici, C. Cartofeanu, S. Gao, Smart contract applications within blockchain technology: a systematic mapping study, Telematics Inf. 35 (8) (2018) 2337–2354, https://doi.org/10.1016/j.tele.2018.10.004. Elsevier Ltd.
[28] Q.V. Le, M. Rishi, Corruption and capital flight: an empirical assessment, Int. Econ. J. 20 (4) (2006) 523–540, https://doi.org/10.1080/10168730601027161.
[29] W. Wang, et al., A survey on consensus mechanisms and mining strategy management in blockchain networks, IEEE Access 7 (2019) 22328–22370, https://doi.org/10.1109/ACCESS.2019.2896108.
[30] A. Azaria, A. Ekblaw, T. Vieira, A. Lippman, MedRec: using blockchain for medical data access and permission management, in: Proceedings - 2016 2nd International Conference on Open and Big Data, OBD 2016, 2016, pp. 25–30, https://doi.org/10.1109/OBD.2016.11.

Index

'*Note*: Page numbers followed by "f" indicate figures, "t" indicate tables and "b" indicate boxes.'

D

E

F

G

H

I

N

X

Z

FSC
www.fsc.org
MIX
Papier | Fördert gute Waldnutzung
FSC® C083411

Kolibri 360 GmbH
Ferdinand-Jühlke-Straße 7
99095 Erfurt, Deutschland
produktsicherheit@kolibri360.de